MICROCOMPUTER
SOFTWARE
FOR
CIVIL ENGINEERS

MICROCOMPUTER
SOFTWARE
FOR
CIVIL ENGINEERS

Howard Falk

VNR VAN NOSTRAND REINHOLD COMPANY
_____ New York

Library of Congress Catalog Card Number: 86–5614
ISBN-13: 978-1-4684-6586-0   e-ISBN-13: 978-1-4684-6584-6
DOI: 10.1007/978-1-4684-6584-6

Published by Van Nostrand Reinhold Company Inc.
115 Fifth Avenue
New York, New York   10003

Van Nostrand Reinhold Company Limited
Molly Millars Lane
Wokingham, Berkshire, RG11 2PY, England

Van Nostrand Reinhold
480 Latrobe Street
Melbourne, Victoria 3000, Australia

Macmillan of Canada
Division of Gage Publishing Limited
164 Commander Boulevard
Agincourt, Ontario MIS 3C7, Canada

15   14   13   12   11   10   9   8   7   6   5   4   3   2   1

Library of Congress Cataloging-in-Publication Data

Falk, Howard, 1927–
   Microcomputer software for civil engineers.

   Includes index.
   1. Civil engineering—Data processing.   2. Microcomputers.   I. Title.
TA345.F35   1986   624′.028′553   86–5614
ISBN-13: 978-1-4684-6586-0

Preface

This is a book about software packages for use by civil engineers. It is written for engineers who need software that can do the job without requiring that they become computer experts or programmers.

The purpose of this book is to present a broad picture of the personal computer packages now available for use by civil engineers. Each chapter is devoted to an area, such as structures, surveying, hydrology, drafting, or equation-solving, in which a number of software packages are presently offered for use with personal computers. The chapter introductions explain what kinds of design or analysis or other tasks these packages perform, outlining the available choices, and comparing the capabilities of the various packages.

Detailed reviews of individual packages follow. The emphasis here is on what the user must know and do to employ the capabilities of the package. Going beyond general description, these reviews also explain what the packages actually will and will not do. Although many packages are covered, there is no attempt here at completeness. In every category covered in the book, many more packages exist than those that have been reviewed. In the fast-moving field of engineering software, many new packages are currently being written and marketed.

A new style of computing

Personal computers have become widely, perhaps universally, accepted as everyday tools for business applications. An essential prerequisite for this acceptance has been the availability of software packages designed for easy use by business people who have little or no background in computing. It is ironic that although engineers were using computers long before most business people dared approach a keyboard, personal computer software packages for engineering applications have been slow to develop.

When minicomputers and large, mainframe computers are used to solve engineering problems, the assumption has generally been that the user must know and use a computer language, such as FORTRAN or BASIC. And it has been assumed that operation of the computer system must be arranged for maximum effective use of computer resources, rather than for the convenience of engineering users.

The basic premises of personal computing are quite different. Users have exclusive access to their own computers, so the way they employ computing resources is shaped entirely by their own needs and whims. Although personal computer software can be created by the user, the software is usually purchased in the form of a package, shaped to perform the tasks the user wants the computer to do.

In this world of personal computing, the extent to which computers can be useful for performing engineering tasks depends largely on what kinds of engineering software packages are available. If there is a package for the structural design or surveying calculation or drafting task that needs to be done, then the personal computer can be used. If no such package exists, the engineer will probably turn to other means of doing the work.

A critical approach

The approach throughout this book is a critical one. Each application area and each software package is examined from the point of view of engineering users, specifically those users who may run a computer only occasionally, when particular problems have to be solved.

Toward the use of formal computer languages, the approach in this book is a skeptical one. It is useful for engineers to know how to program, if for no other reason than to gain a feeling of mastery over computers. But civil engineers are not, and probably should not be, programmers. Except for those few who decide to take up programming as their vocation, engineers use computers as they use any other tools—to help them carry out engineering tasks.

Some engineers spend much of their time at computer keyboards, doing analyses, design, planning, and similar tasks. For these users, learning a special computer language, such as COGO, or the special-purpose languages used by some finite element analysis, statistical, drafting, and other packages, can bring advantages both in speed and flexibility of problem solving.

For the most part, what engineers need are software packages that will allow them to continue to think in strictly engineering terms while getting the benefit of computing power. Writing programs that can offer this kind of capability is not an easy task, but it is what the field of programming for engineering applications is all about. It is the task that the vendors of engineering packages for personal computers have taken on. This book includes many examples of excellent packages that meet these requirements. Where packages fall short, they have been commented on in a critical manner.

HOWARD FALK

Contents

MICROCOMPUTER SOFTWARE FOR CIVIL ENGINEERS

Chapter 1
HVAC Design Packages

Calculation of building energy loads is the main task taken on by many personal computer HVAC packages. Although the computers used are small, the buildings that are modeled by these packages may be substantial in size. For example, the C-HVAC package can handle commercial buildings with up to 1000 rooms and as many as 100 heating-cooling systems. The R-HVAC residential package will also handle up to 1000 rooms. However some other packages are limited to only a few zones and rooms, so prospective users should take care to check the capacity of these packages as well as the types of answers they can provide.

California builders have the problem of demonstrating compliance with that state's Residential Building Energy Standards. These standards are strict compared with those of other states, but are indicative of a national trend toward designs that minimize energy use in all buildings, including single-family residences. Compliance of a building design with such standards can be demonstrated by using an approved calculation method such as that provided by the Micropas package.

Other HVAC packages, like REENERGY, are strictly preliminary design tools, intended for assessing the magnitude of estimated energy consumed for specific building components and for stimulating energy-efficient design concepts, rather than demonstrating energy code compliance.

Some HVAC packages, like DUCT 1-2-3, calculate size, velocity, pressure, and other design parameters for ducts used in air conditioning, ventilation, and exhaust systems.

Item and full-screen input editing

With HVAC packages, the overwhelming task facing the user is to get the required information into the computer. The number of different factors entering into a calculation of energy loads for a building can run into the hundreds. The practical usefulness of these packages must therefore be judged by the extent to which they can aid users in carrying through their input tasks.

These packages generally take advantage of the interactive, back-and-forth dialogue between user and display that personal computers typically use. Thus with the C-HVAC package, input from the keyboard is on an item-by-item question-and-answer basis. For the roof data, the package asks for the ASHRAE roof number, the user fills that in, then is asked for a U-factor, and so the dialog proceeds. In this package, the allowed answers are fixed in format. To indicate how many characters or digits are allowed, the package displays a string of dots above the answer space. When entries are to be changed, the previous value used for that item is displayed within the question that calls for a new value.

Full-screen editing offers an alternative and usually a more powerful, method of interactive data entry. For example, in the R-HVAC package, positions for many input items are provided on a single display. The user moves from one item to another on the screen, entering new data or revising existing entries. When finished, the user can visually review what has been entered, making corrections as needed before the entire screen is stored and committed as input for calculations.

In the DUCT 1-2-3 package, the user is completely free to move the display cursor to any location on the screen and edit the material displayed there. This is an ideal procedure when a few changes are necessary on an otherwise-acceptable screenful of information.

Working from existing data

One of the best ways to speed up the laborious input process is to work from existing, similar sets of data, replacing only those items that are unique to the current design problem. Thus the SYRSOL package retains input data in disk-stored files. When the data for a current analysis are similar to those of a previous one, the user can call up the previously entered input data file and make changes in selected items only. Most HVAC packages provide some sort of similar replacement feature.

Some packages come with typical or sample values already set, and the user then accepts or alters those values. For example, the HEATCOOL package comes with input parameters set for an office building in Sacramento, California. The parameters are displayed in three tables, each of which can be accepted as is or changed. When the user reviews a table and calls for changes, the items in that table are presented for revision one at a time, and the user can call for a printout of that table when the changes are completed.

The degree of freedom in editing existing data offered by different packages varies considerably. With the Micropas package, although arrays of screen-displayed data can be edited, the package does not provide full-screen editing in the sense that a cursor can be moved to a displayed item to guide changes. Instead the user must enter the number of changes to be made, then the column and row numbers of the items to be changed. The actual changes are then made as if isolated individual items were being altered.

The C-HVAC package allows users to skip from one input prompting question to another by pressing the Return key. At many of the questions the option of bypassing or "zapping" the remainder of the input process can be exercised simply by pressing the Z key.

Data replication is another technique that can be of great assistance in getting the needed data into the computer. In this regard C-HVAC allows up to 100 heating-cooling systems to be described. As these will probably not be individually unique, the package includes the ability to repeat the same description parameters for any desired number of air systems. Since zone data may likewise be similar or identical for many zones, the package also allows data from one zone to be copied into a new one. The user then has only to revise those items that differ between the two zones.

Design flexibility

In HVAC design, as in many other areas of engineering work, it is desirable to compare different design alternatives. With their ability to rapidly find answers that might otherwise take a long time to hand calculate, computers offer the ability to explore more and varied alternatives.

For example, "what if" analyses are not an accustomed part of residential design calculations, but a package like Micropas allows residential building designers to change their inputs and then repeat their simulation runs quite easily.

The C-HVAC package makes it easy for the user to "turn on" or "turn off" any of the air systems in a commercial building being simulated by that package. This feature is very useful when variations in number of building zones and associated air systems are being considered.

The HEATCOOL package provides for room-by-room trial and variation. Input data are entered separately for each room in the building. As the data for a given room are completed, the package calculates energy load totals for that room and displays the results. At this point the user can review these results and return to the input for that room to make any desired changes.

Although they give only approximate answers, packages like SEA are well equipped to aid in exploring design alternatives. With its relatively simple calculation methods, SEA can be used to quickly and effectively compare energy consumption with changes in design parameters. Once a building model has been set up, changes due to alternative parameters can be rapidly examined. Users must, however, keep in mind that those using a package in this way must have a sound background and experience in building energy calculations in order to have assurance that their results will be meaningful.

To give an idea of how long it might take to enter the data and solve an approximate-answer design problem, the vendor of the REENERGY package claims that, after two or three preliminary uses, it should take no more than 10 minutes to obtain a complete energy estimate for a simple building.

Controlling errors

With large amounts of data keyboarded by users, there is plenty of room for error; and, if the mistakes in the input data are not caught and corrected, the computed results cannot be expected to be correct. As the old computer adage goes, "Garbage in, garbage out."

Fortunately, most HVAC packages are designed with this need for input accuracy in mind. The SYRSOL package is particularly well equipped in this respect. When it comes to entering an item of numerical data, the user is first asked if entry of a new value for the item is desired. If so, the package will display acceptable upper and lower limits for the value, and the user then enters a number between these limits. If the typed value is outside the limits, the package will ask for another value. If the user finds the limits unacceptable, that feature can be turned off and the package will then accept a value outside the limits.

In addition to limits, SYRSOL also displays such useful items as the units in which values are expressed, commonly used values, and such other helpful hints as surface orientation sign conventions. The package also provides for deliberate user approval of all keyboard entries before they are actually accepted by the package.

The C-HVAC package provides several error-correction procedures to prevent improper design results. For example, if a leaving coil condition does not work psychrometrically with the calculated zone loads, the package will try out a number of alternative leaving coil conditions in an attempt to find one that is acceptable.

Users are not the only ones who make errors. From time to time HVAC packages may be used in ways their authors never considered; in such circumstances, weaknesses or bugs in the software may show up. If such a program error should occur, the package should display an error message containing a code that indicates the nature of the error. Unfortunately, these messages are usually incomprehensible to all but programmers familiar with the details of the software. At this point, all the user can do is to call the vendor, report what has happened, and hope for the best.

Computation speed

The notion is frequently put forward, particularly by those who have some attachment to large computers, that personal computers are too small to handle substantial engineering design problems. This may be the case for some special problems, but for most engineering calculations, the differences in speed and capacity between large and personal computers have little practical significance.

One instance where this comparison arises in HVAC computations is when weather conditions are to be accounted for hour by hour over a period of an entire year. On a large computer, the necessary data can be fed from a weather tape, and the great speed of large computer processing circuits minimizes the needed computing time. If these computations were to be exactly duplicated on a personal computer, it would have to be equipped with tape drives (unusual but available), and the runs would probably take about ten times as long as those on the large computers.

Vendors of personal computer HVAC packages use approaches designed to bypass the need for these lengthy calculations. For example, the Micropas package uses "compressed" weather data consisting of representative samples of hour-by-hour data. When the vendor compared Micropas results with those obtained from the mainframe program CALPAS1, the two were found to predict "essentially the same energy performance." The vendor cites Micropas run time for a "typical building," using an IBM/PC, as 9 minutes. For Apple II-type computers with CP/M, the time for the same problem is cited as 28 minutes. Our own reviewer ran a demonstration file provided by the vendor and found it took 17 minutes on an IBM/PC.

For HVAC packages where extended weather condition calculations are not involved, the differences in running time between large and personal computers seem truly trivial. For example, the vendor of the SYRSOL package (which is available in versions that run on both kinds of computers) measured the run time for a typical input data file on an IBM 4341 at 40 seconds. The same problem took just 1 minute, 56 seconds on an IBM/AT, 3 minutes, 33 seconds on an IBM/PC with a math chip, and 17 minutes, 14 seconds on an IBM/PC with no math chip.

As was pointed out earlier, the main effort, in using HVAC packages, is to get the information in, not to calculate answers. After all, while the computer is running by itself, all the user has to do is wait, or turn to other tasks, until the answers appear.

Primitive HELP features

One of measures of the extent to which a personal computer package takes the user's needs into account has come to be the presence of HELP messages that can be called onto the screen when the user is in doubt as to how to proceed. Only a few of the HVAC packages covered in this chapter provide such HELP messages, and they tend to be inadequately presented.

HELP in the C-HVAC package is provided to users in the form of messages that are on display at various points during input procedures. If users identify themselves as beginners, in answer to one of the general project information questions, all these help messages will appear. But if users say they are experts, all the messages will be suppressed. There does not seem to be any way to select display for specific messages.

The SYRSOL package handles HELP information in a different way. All the HELP messages are stored in four special files. These can be invoked with just a couple of keystrokes, but the user then has to search through the file, much as one would search through a user manual, to find the needed information. There is a nice feature here: in addition to the HELP file provided with the package, users can store their own HELP messages. These can be composed with a word-processing package and can be useful for training assistants and novice users of the package.

Few output options

Like many HVAC packages, C-HVAC produces voluminous output, including summaries for the entire building and individual sheets for the zones. To more easily handle this output, which may run to hundreds of pages for a large building, the package provides for printing four partial segments of the output. The user can further restrict the printed output by specifying which zones will be included in the zonal output, whether hourly loads or only peak loads will be shown.

Although some of the other packages provide similar partial selection of printed output, most of them have only a fixed printout format that must be accepted as is.

As for graphics, few of the packages offer any graphics output at all. That is a shame, because charts and graphs could be very helpful in interpreting the mass of data produced by these packages, and in locating critical parameters.

The Micropas package is one that offers some graphical output. Here graphics are used to present hourly data with separate graphs for mass and zone temperatures.

Analysis of cost and financing

Financial analysis is a concern that computers are able to address easily, so it is surprising that not many HVAC packages provide cost and financial analysis. The SEA package is one that meets this concern. It provides a financial analysis that covers time periods of up to 40 years. Factors considered include salvage value, fuel, and labor costs, yearly varying fuel escalation, maintenance escalation, and fixed costs. Among the financing methods that can be accounted for are bank loans, equity financing, and end-of-period payment. Output information includes a tabulation of yearly cash flow, fuel costs, interest charges, fixed charges, present worth, equivalent annual payments, and capitalized costs.

SYRSOL is another package that addresses cost considerations. Its output report includes an annual summary of simulated power bills and energy performance, and a breakdown of monthly energy use in kilowatt-hours and in dollars.

C-HVAC: COMMERCIAL HVAC LOADS

This package calculates heating and cooling loads for buildings with up to 100 air systems and 1000 rooms.

The package runs on IBM/PC and compatible computers and also on computers that use CP/M system software. The price of the package varies with the number of zones it can handle. A 2-zone version sells for $295, while one with full capacity sells for $1495. The vendor is Elite Software, P.O. Drawer 1194, Bryan, TX 77806. [(409) 846-2340].

The analysis procedures used by this package follow those outlined in the 1981 ASHRAE Handbook of Fundamentals. The package comes with stored tables of values for cooling load differences, maximum solar heat gain factors, and glass cooling factors, taken from this handbook.

Menu-based operation

The package operates from a series of menu displays, starting with a main "Master" menu. The second choice on this menu produces the "Master Data Input" menu through which parameters for the overall building are entered.

Master Data Input menu choices divide up the task of entering or revising these overall parameters into 13 areas, such as roof, wall, glass, and lighting. There is also a General Project Information area where other information, such as the project name, safety factors, and a number of other parameters, is entered.

When a Master Data Input menu choice is made, input from the keyboard for items is on a question-and-answer basis. Thus for the roof data, the package asks for the ASHRAE roof number, a U-factor, and whether the ceiling is suspended or not. Completion of these and other item entries returns the user to the Master Data Input menu, where another area can be chosen for input.

The allowed answers are fixed in format, only a limited number of characters are allowed for text (such as project name), and numeric answers are restricted to a certain number of digits. To indicate how many characters or digits are allowed, the package displays a string of dots above the answer space. When entries are to be changed, the previous value is displayed in the question.

When all the necessary parameters have been entered, the user makes a menu choice to display or print everything that has been entered for review. If satisfied, the user makes another menu choice to return to the Master menu.

Included in the Master Data Input are descriptions of the air systems to be used in the building. The package allows up to 100 such systems to be described. As these probably will not be individually unique, the package includes the ability to repeat the same description parameters for any desired number of air systems.

The package makes it possible for the user to easily "turn on" or "turn off" any of these air systems, a feature that is convenient when variations in number of building zones and associated air systems are being considered.

Entering zone data

But completion of the Master Data Input menu items does not finish the job of data entry. The next main menu choice will probably be the Project Zone Data menu. Here information on roof, walls, floor, glass, partitions, and other items are entered for each of the zones of the building. The data entry takes place for one zone at a time, and the user selects which zone is to be dealt with.

Since zone data may be similar or identical for many zones, the package allows data from one zone to be copied into a new one. The user then has only to revise those items that differ between the two zones.

It is left to the user to keep track of which zones have been specified and revised. The vendor provides a set of suggested input data forms on which the data can be manually entered. In a building with many zones, this may take a substantial amount of record keeping. If the package provided an overall displayed list of zones, showing entry and revision dates, this record keeping could be eased.

Segmented output report

The C-HVAC package produces voluminous output which includes summaries for the entire building and individual sheets for the zones. To more easily handle this output, which may run to hundreds of pages for a large building, users can call for printing segments of the output.

The first segment includes a printout repeat of all the Master Data Input. The second is a summary of all the loads in the overall building. The third is a summary of the loads under each air system in the building. And the final segment contains the zone load calculations.

The user can further restrict the printed output by specifying which zones will be included in the zonal output, whether hourly loads or only peak loads will be shown. Other options include a tabular summary of sensible hour-by-hour loads for each zone and indication of instances where the the heating supply CFM exceeds the cooling CFM supply for any zone.

Beginners and experts

Help is provided to users in the form of messages that are displayed at various points during input procedures. If users identify themselves as beginners, in answer to one of the general project information questions, all these help messages will appear. But if users say they are experts, all the messages will be suppressed. There does not seem to be any way to select display for specific messages.

The package provides several error correction procedures to prevent improper design results. For example, if a leaving coil condition does not work psychrometrically with the calculated zone loads, the package will try out a number of alternative leaving coil conditions in an attempt to find one that is acceptable.

If a program error should occur, the package should display an error message containing a code that indicates the nature of the error. Unfortunately, these messages will be incomprehensible to all but programmers familiar with the details of this package. At this point, all the user can do is to call the vendor, report what has happened, and hope for the best.

DUCT 1-2-3: DUCT DESIGN PACKAGE

This package calculates size, velocity, pressure, and other design parameters for ducts used in air-conditioning, ventilation, and exhaust systems.

DUCT 1-2-3 runs on IBM/PCs equipped with Lotus 1-2-3 software. The package sells for $40 from E. Jessup and Associates, 4977 Canoga Ave., Woodland Hills, CA 91364 [(213) 883-9021].

This package is for those who have or wish to purchase the popular Lotus 1-2-3 software package. DUCT 1-2-3 is what is called a template package. It takes advantage of the Lotus software, using spreadsheet and other capabilities of that software. DUCT 1-2-3 is inexpensive, but the Lotus package costs about ten times as much.

DUCT 1-2-3 works from screen displays already filled in with example data. The user types over this data with data of the design problem at hand, and the package finds a solution.

When the package is started, the user is confronted with a seven-choice menu. Three of these choices bring up displays on which all the input data are entered. The first two include a project description, and altitude, temperature, duct material, and velocity data.

The third, the main "Design" display, provides for listing each section and fitting of the desired duct system. This display shows duct length, fitting loss coefficients, CFM, and other system parameters in tabular form. The user enters design data into this table by moving the display cursor around to each table entry position, then keyboarding the new entry. When this display worksheet is completed, it can be printed or stored on keyboard command.

To perform the duct design calculations the user selects a menu choice called Construct. Design formulas are then brought in from memory and the calculations carried out. The Print menu choice will then produce a printout that repeats the input data, with computed results shown added to the table of duct sections and fittings.

HEATCOOL: WITH ROOM-BY-ROOM CALCULATION

This package is used to find BTUH and CFM requirements for heating and cooling buildings. The user can enter data and calculate results for one room at a time, for several rooms, or for the entire building.

HEATCOOL runs on IBM/PC and compatible computers and on TRS-80 Mod I,III,and 4 computers. It sells for $99.76 (PC) or $84.76 (TRS-80) from James J. Jordan, 5236 Overbrook Way, Sacramento, CA 95841. [(916) 332-6610].

The package comes with input parameters set for an office building in Sacramento, California. The user can accept these parameters, or review and change them to reflect conditions in another building. The parameters are displayed in three tables, each of which can be accepted as is or changed. When the user reviews a table and calls for changes, the items in that table are presented for revision one at a time, and the user can call for a printout of that table when the changes are completed.

There are some peculiarities. For example, where minus numbers are used for factors like temperatures, the numeral 2 is entered in place of the minus sign. Use of the minus sign is reserved for changes in any parameter that are made after initial design calculations have been made. Window, wall, ceiling, and door dimensions must be entered in decimal rather than in feet and inch format, but areas are immediately and automatically calculated and displayed. Areas that are not rectangular are attained by having the user add or subtract small rectangles until satisfied.

The package does not calculate attic temperatures, requiring the user to supply the figures through "experience or educated guess." Calculations for infiltration of air through outside windows and doors are based on the areas of these openings rather than on crack areas.

Room-by-room calculations

Input data are entered separately for each room in the building. As the data for a given room are completed, the package calculates totals for that room and displays the results. At this point the user can review these results and return to the input for that room to make any desired changes in parameters.

The package keeps running totals as calculations for one room after another are completed. Users may view these totals or break off the calculation process and resume it later on, once current data have been safely recorded for disk storage.

In addition to the room-by-room data there are also some overall parameters the user sets up for the building. These parameters can be changed as desired, but is a complication arises here. Some of these overall parameters are used in the individual room calculations, so if the overall parameters are changed, any existing room calculations have to be changed. Fortunately, the package does these room recalculations automatically.

Printout flexibility

The package produces a formatted output report showing design totals for the building as a whole and for each room. However, the user is given the option of printing only selected portions of this report, in almost any desired combination. The technique for setting up these selections is unfortunately quite complicated and confusing but, with patience, it can be done.

MICROPAS: FOR BUILDING ENERGY ANALYSIS

Reviewer: Victor E. Wright, PE, Louisville KY

Micropas is a well-written package useful for designers of residential and small commercial buildings. The package and it's manual assume that users have previous knowledge of building design, energy analysis by simulation, and heating-and cooling-system design. The package is a sound investment for designers or builders operating in states like California, that have performance energy codes. It's use with a single building, in those states, can result in savings that repay the user for the cost of the software.

Micropas runs on IBM/PCs and compatible machines. It also runs on most micro/personal computers that use CP/M system software. Required equipment includes a printer, two floppy disk drives (each with at least 125 KByte storage capacity). A CP/M version sells for $795; an IBM/PC and compatibles version for $895. Weather files sell for $125 per region, or $25 to $40 per location. The package is available from Enercomp, 757 Russell Blvd. #A3, Davis, CA 95616 [(916) 753-3400].

Micropas differs from some other energy analysis packages in that it does simulations for homes rather than for commercial, institutional, or industrial buildings. Yet it is a more sophisticated modeling tool than is normally used for residential building design. The reason for this is that the package is designed to help California builders demonstrate compliance with the state's Residential Building Energy Standards. These standards are strict, compared with those of other states, but are indicative of a national trend toward designs that minimize energy use in all buildings, including single-family residences.

California builders can demonstrate compliance with the standards by incorporating passive solar heating, or extensive insulation, or less-extensive insulation along with a solar water-heating system. Alternatively, the builder may comply by demonstrating, using an approved calculation method, that the building will meet the energy use standard. Micropas simulation runs provide the necessary calculation methods.

Three-zone modeling

Micropas allows the user to define up to 20 opaque and 20 glazed surfaces, up to 3 zones, and 5 thermal mass surfaces. The simulation can also include hourly internal heat-gain schedules, a heating and a cooling system for each zone, ventilation systems, thermostats for these systems, and air-to-air heat exchangers.

The package simulates weather from data files. The review copy of Micropas included a variety of these files, prepared from U.S. Department of Commerce Climatic Center weather tapes. Such files are available from Enercomp, the Micropas vendor, for about 150 locations in the United States.

Although use of a tool like Micropas is not required for residential building outside California, several other states are now considering energy performance codes. With the ablity to handle up to three zones, and it's calculation of annual energy consumption, the package can be used for system sizing and life-cycle analysis of small commercial buildings.

The package uses screen-displayed menus, starting with a main menu and then leading the user to more specific menus.

Input data may be keyed in as the user responds to prompts on the screen. Or the user can edit an existing input file to create the desired input data. For those HVAC designers who cannot, or do not wish to, use a computer keyboard (a skill that this reviewer believes every designer and engineer should have), the package prints out a set of blank input forms. The designer can write on these forms, then turn them over to a typist to key in the data.

Although arrays of screen-displayed data can be edited, the package does not provide full-screen editing in the sense that a cursor can be moved to a displayed item to guide changes. Instead the user must enter the number of changes to be made, then the column and row numbers of the items to be changed. The actual changes are then made as if isolated individual items were being altered.

Provides "what-if" analysis

Summary output reports provide abbreviated data adequate for demonstration of code compliance. Tabular output is also available with details on ambient conditions, zone loads and heat flows, mass, temperature, and peak conditions, all given in seasonal, daily, and hourly terms. This is the kind of information building designers can use to evaluate the effectiveness of their designs. By iterating the simulation runs, "what-if" analysis can be used, and that is certainly an unusual feature for a residential design method. Graphic output is also available, presenting hourly data with separate graphs for mass and zone temperatures. This is helpful in interpreting the computer data results.

The Micropas manual provides enough information to guide even the infrequent user through the package operations. The appendix on installation explains how to get started and make up working disks. After reading the manual once, this reviewer was able to go ahead and run the package with only minor difficulties. Users are invited to call the package vendor for technical consultation, a service included in the purchase price, and this reviewer found the service prompt and courteous.

A word of caution. Buyers of Micropas should be sure to order the version designed for the specific kind of computer on which it is to be run. The reviewer's attempts to run an IBM/PC version on a Zenith Z-100 system were unsuccessful, despite the fact that the Zenith, with its MS-DOS software, can run many IBM/PC packages.

The vendor cites the Micropas run time for a "typical building," using an IBM/PC, as 9 minutes. For Apple II-type computers with CP/M, the time for the same problem is cited as 28 minutes. This reviewer ran the demonstration file "Sunspace" provided by the vendor and found it took 17 minutes on an IBM/PC.

At one point the package was forced to stop because the reviewer had neglected to provide it with a weather file. The shutdown was orderly and no data were lost. During the long runs, Micropas provides a display of status to keep the user informed.

REENERGY: PRELIMINARY ENERGY ESTIMATES

This package is intended to be a preliminary design tool, for analyzing the magnitude of estimated energy consumed for specific building components and ideas for energy-efficient design concepts. It is not intended for use in determining energy code compliance.

REENERGY runs on IBM/PC and compatible computers. It sells for $150 from Reed Associates, P.O. Box 9863, College Station, TX 77840 [(713) 693-8793].

The user starts by making a pencil and paper sketch of the building that is to be analyzed. The vendor provides a blank data sheet with spaces for the needed design parameters. These include the areas of roof, floor, walls and glass, perimeters of glass and slab edge, net volume, winter and summer temperatures, weekday occupancy, watts per square foot for lighting and equipment, equipment heat, type of heating system, boiler efficiency, air-conditioner COP, R numbers for building spaces and materials, and similar items.

These items of information are entered one by one through the keyboard, in response to displayed prompts from the package. For example, one of the first such prompts is WHAT IS THE BUILDING FLOOR AREA IN SQ. FT?

Along the way, the user is given the choice of calculating infiltration by the crack or the air-change method.

Since the list of input prompts is a long one, the package divides them up into six groups. At the end of the input for each group, the user is asked if there are any revisions to make for that group. If so the prompts for that group are repeated. If not, the package proceeds to the next steps.

When the last group of inputs is completed, the package calculates the results, displays them, and, if desired, prints them out. Calculated results include electric and fossil fuel requirements for heating, cooling, lighting, equipment motors, and hot water. Also, estimated total fossil and electrical fuel consumptions, site, and source energy estimates.

The vendor claims that, after two or three preliminary uses, it should take no more than 10 minutes to obtain a complete energy estimate for a simple building.

R-HVAC: RESIDENTIAL HVAC LOADS

Reviewed by John W. Sheffield, University of Missouri-Rolla

This package is designed to calculate heating and cooling loads for residential and modestly small commercial buildings. The package uses the analysis procedure of the Air Conditioning Contractors of America's Manual J, titled "Load Calculation for Residential Winter and Summer Air Conditioning."

Residential HVAC Loads is available in versions to run on micro/personal computers using CP/M MS-DOS or PC-DOS operating systems. It sells for $295 from Elite Software, P.O. Drawer 1194, Bryan, TX 77806 [(409) 775-1782].

The package does accurate calculation of the peak heating and cooling loads for residential buildings. Each room in the structure may have as many as 10 walls, 10 windows, 5 ceilings, and 5 floors. The package is designed to handle up to 1000 rooms per project and determines optimal room CFM quantities. All input data are stored so they may be reviewed at almost any time.

Full-screen input

Input and editing are done with full-screen displays. That is, many input items are entered on a single screenful of data. The user moves from one item to another on the screen, entering new data or revising existing entries. When finished, the user can visually review what has been entered, making corrections as needed before the entire screen is stored and committed as input for calculations. This use of input data screens makes for easy organization of data input. The user's manual includes sample worksheets showing the input data needed to process an example project. As they are entered, the input data are subjected to some automatic error checking.

One screen is used to enter overall project data. Then there are four screens for each room: one for general room data, another for ceiling and floor data, the third for wall and door data, and the last for window and glass data.

Input project data include the following: date, user name, floor plan, client name, address, outside and inside dry-bulb temperature for winter and summer, temperature range, choice of temperature swing, humidity, ventilation CFM, BTUH per person, BTUH equipment, latitude degrees, and air changes per hour.

Input data for room parameters include the following: room name, active status, perimeter of exposed room walls; ceiling height, width, depth; BTUH appliances; number of people per room, BTUH per person; duct gain and heat loss multipliers; ceiling and floor construction type, materials, depth, and width; wall and door construction type, material, height, width, direction, and reference to wall; window and glass construction type, material, height, width, number of panes, shade type; overhang and offset.

The user's manual gives special attention to setting up the system disks and proper installation of the package, in terms a personal computer novice can understand.

There are HELP screens that can be called up. Assistance on many package procedures is available by keying in a question mark, a useful feature. However, several text errors were found in the HELP instructions, and a few of the HELP files were not available in early releases of the package.

Package-provided output reports are fixed in their structure. There are four of these reports. Together, they give an excellent summary of the project, including calculations, room loads, and a room-by-room analysis that includes the details of all heating and cooling loads for each room.

The reviewer did not find any problems in the way the package handles user errors or hardware failures. Several test cases were analyzed for errors. A strong recommendation to the vendor is to add a graphics option for both screen display and printed output.

SEA: SIMPLIFIED ENERGY ANALYSIS

Reviewer: John W. Sheffield, University of Missouri-Rolla

This package provides for simplified energy analysis of commercial buildings with greater than 20,000 square feet of conditioned space. It uses a modified bin weather method.

SEA can be used to quickly and effectively compare energy consumption with changes in design parameters. Once a building model has been set up, changes due to alternative parameters can be examined in a reasonable amount of time. This package effectively reduces the time and cost that might otherwise be encountered in using a large computer to perform relatively simple energy calculations. However, those using the package must have background and experience in building energy calculations in order to obtain meaningful results.

SEA runs on IBM/PC, TRS-80, and CP/M computers. It sells for $995 from Ferriera and Kalasinksy Associates, 13 Welby Rd, P.O. Box L6, New Bedford, MA 02745 [(617) 996-4499].

Based on the ASHRAE Technical Committee 4.7 proposed calculation procedure for energy analysis, SEA uses a modified bin method. It allows the designer to perform "trade studies," comparing and evaluating energy consumption for various building characteristics and different HVAC systems.

Models and results

The package includes sections on building models, bin weather data, peak and diversified load analysis, air side system simulation, heating and cooling plant simulation, financial analysis, and tabular and graphic output.

Supplied in the package are 13 disk-stored weather files. These are organized in 5-degree bins from -50 to 115 degrees, tallied in three equal periods. Added data can be obtained from Air Force Manual 88-29 titled "Engineering Weather Data."

Calculations of peak and diversified loads are made for all building zones, considering summer, winter, and setback temperatures, along with plenum, orientation, heat factors, and multiwalls per zone. The calculations allow for user-assigned occupied time periods.

System simulation is for unitary or central plant systems, with constant or variable volume air, and water, and power boxes. The simulation can take both double ducts and water loop heat pumps into consideration. Simulation control options include economizers, humidification, discriminator, VAV fan control, return air fans, resets, thermostats, and VAV box minimums. A major feature of the package, relating to the air side system simulation, is the use of multiple secondary systems per the primary plant.

The package provides heating and cooling plant simulation for sizing. It also allows direct input of data for equipment items such as plant chillers and pumps, as well as selection of fuel and caloric value. Auxiliaries can be employed on a multiple basis.

The financial analysis covers time periods of up to 40 years. Factors considered include salvage value fuel, and labor costs, yearly varying fuel escalation, maintenance escalation, and fixed costs. Among the financing methods that can be accounted for are bank loans, equity financing, and end-of-period payment. Output information includes a tabulation of yearly cash flow, fuel costs, interest charges, fixed charges, present worth, equivalent annual payments, and capitalized costs.

Possible improvements

SEA is accompanied by a user manual with detailed instructions and examples of how the package can be used. There is also a worked out test problem to illustrate the building model.

Needed is a reminder that, to obtain meaningful and accurate results, good engineering judgment and experience are essential. The user should be cautioned to verify the accuracy of the answers the package produces by experimental variation of the input data.

The reviewer found no fault with the package related to hardware failure of handling of user errors. However, it would be useful to have tutorial material added to the package. In future versions it would also be helpful to add a graphics feature to better display the financial analysis results and the bin weather data.

SYRSOL: BUILDING ENERGY ANALYSIS

This package is for energy simulation and design of commercial, institutional, industrial, and residential buidings. It will handle up to 60 zones and a total of 1200 surfaces.

SYRSOL runs on IBM/PC/XT/AT and compatible computers. It sells for $799 from SYRSOL, 734 Westcott St., Syracuse, NY 13210 [(315) 479-7820].

SYRSOL was originally developed to run on mainframe computers like the IBM 370 and 4341. This package is a personal computer version of the mainframe program. The vendor states that nothing has been lost in adapting the software for personal computer use. On the contrary, the PC version is actually more powerful than previous mainframe versions. What is more, it has been written with greater care for ease of use.

As for differences in running time, the vendor measured the run time for a typical input data file on an IBM 4341 at 40 seconds. The same problem took just 1 minute, 56 seconds on an IBM/AT, 3 minutes, 33 seconds on an IBM/PC with a math chip, and 17 minutes, 14 seconds on an IBM/PC with no math chip.

Preparing the input

As with many HVAC packages, most of the user effort that goes into a SYRSOL run is taken up with entering data. There are about 125 different items of input information that this package can take account of in its computations.

To avoid the need to reenter data that has been keyboarded in previous runs, the package retains input data in disk-stored files. When the data for a current analysis are similar to those of a previous one, the user can call up the previously entered input data file and make changes in selected items only.

When it comes to entering an item of numerical data, the user is first asked if entry of a new value for the item is desired. If so, the package will display acceptable upper and lower limits for the value, and the user then enters a number between these limits. If the typed value is outside the limits, the package will ask for another value. If the user finds the limits unacceptable, that feature can be turned off and the package will then accept a value outside the limits.

In addition to limits, the package also displays such useful items as the units in which values are expressed, commonly used values, and such other helpful hints as surface orientation sign conventions. The American engineering system of units (Btu, ft., F) is used for all input items, except weather data which are in SI units. There is no provision for converting from other units to those used in the package, so users must do all such conversions on their own.

The package provides input control features including user approval of all keyboard entries before they are actually accepted by the package and automatic questioning of unreasonable and unlikely entries. And these controls can be invoked or turned off by the user.

Users can skip from one input prompting question to another by pressing the Return key. At many of the questions the option of bypassing or "zapping" the remainder of the input process can be exercized simply by pressing the Z key. When data input is completed, the user can call for a printout of the input file, useful for a final check on correctness.

Input oautiono

The input process is designed to give the user a lot of assistance, but it is not foolproof, and there are some danger points.

Beware of accidentally touching the F6 function key. Users who do so will terminate the input process.

Beware of starting work with a disk that has insufficient room to store the data that are to be input. This is a sneaky problem, since everything that is keyboarded will be stored nicely in the computer memory until the input process is completed. At that point the package will attempt to store the input on the disk. If there is not enough disk space to hold the data, the run will be terminated, destroying all the input work that has been done. A similar problem exists for storing the results of a comutation run, and users are cautioned to check the available disk space before initiating such a run.

Modeling capabilities

The package includes capabilities to do hour-by-hour and zone-by-zone simulation. Both centralized and decentralized heating and cooling systems can be modeled, with simultaneous heating and cooling in different zones. The package has five active solar models, including flat plate and tracking systems, as well as a passive solar heating model. There are three heat pump models, three domestic hot water models with heat pumps and two with heat exchangers.

The output report includes an annual summary of simulated power bills and energy performance, a list of simulated thermal loads, a breakdown of monthly energy use in kilowatt-hours hand in dollars, daily total insolation intensities, and design loads for each building zone.

Changeable HELP instructions

The SYRSOL package handles HELP information in a unique way. As with many other packages, HELP can be invoked with just a couple of keystrokes. But in addition to the HELP file provided with the package, users can store their own HELP messages in auxiliary HELP files. These messages can be composed with a word-processing package and can be useful for training assistants and novice users of the package.

HELP files can grow very large. For example, they contain a weather database covering over 200 cities, with reference numbers used to denote city locations used in the analyses. To help in maneuvering around in the HELP files, the package has a browse feature that will display every *n*th line. Nevertheless, the organization of HELP files is a problem that does not seem to have been satisfactorily solved in this package.

Thought has been given to providing information in a form that can be easily used by other packages. All input and output files, as well as the HELP files, are in standard (ASCII) format, so they can be handled readily by word-processing and graphics packages.

TRACE: HVAC FOR PC PLUS TELEPHONE

This package allows the user to perform various analyses on a personal computer and also to access a larger computer via telephone, to solve larger problems. The stand-alone analyses include equal friction duct sizing, coil selection and optimization, fan and air handler sizing, load calculations for a 150-zone building, and static regain duct sizing for VAV systems.

TRACE runs on IBM/PC and compatible computers and on CP/M computers. It is available for $975 from The Trane Co., 3600 Pammel Creek Rd., LaCrosse, WI 54601 [(608) 787-3936].

The stand-alone capabilities of the TRACE package calculate loads for up to 150 zones. Trane's large computer capabilities can also be tapped, via telephone, using the TRACE package. The personal computer is used to compile the necessary input data and check them for errors. Then using communications software that is part of the TRACE package, and appropriate modem equipment, users log onto the Trane computer. Displays that originate in that computer instruct the user on how to make the large computer run and retrieve results.

Batch-style data entry

Data entry for this package is heavily influenced by the large computer programs from which it was developed. Information is keyboarded by users with each piece of data separated by a slash in the kind of tabular order that punched card operators are trained to handle. Users have to remember that the numbers they are entering represent floor area, wall area, and so forth, all in a prescribed order and format. For occasional users of this package, the procedure is likely to be difficult to remember, and a new learning process may be necessary at each use.

If users wish, the data can be keyed into a separate input file; then that file can be used to run the analyses. An editing program called VEDIT is included in the TRACE package, to handle this kind of input. It allows the use of full screen editing of multiple lines of input data. This kind of laborious input, like the line-by-line TRACE input, can be given over to non-engineering personnel, if they are available.

The TRACE package does include some automatic input data checking, for detecting values that are out of range or in incorrect format. However, there is no provision for letting the user know of these errors at the time of input. Instead, batch processing style again, when the input is used, an error listing will be produced that can be read to make input corrections.

According to one reviewer, preparing TRACE input for a building with 20 or 30 zones, and for one or two alternative designs, would take an experienced designer less than a day. If the data are sent in to the remote large computer, results can generally be obtained after about 4 hours.

ASHRAE methods

Like several other packages, TRACE calculations are based on the design methods in the ASHRAE Handbook of Fundamentals. The large computer version of the package has had more than 10 years of regular use, so it is well tested and relatively free of bugs. It has been used to design over 800 buildings.

TRACE calculates peak and hourly loads by zone to create an hourly load schedule. The package then calculates heating and cooling loads and air quantities and performs an economic analysis. The output accounts for such items as fuel rates, interest rates, maintenance costs, and economic life.

Chapter 2
Concrete Structure Design

Many concrete structure design packages are simply computer implementations of manual design procedures. In addition to rapid calculation, these packages provide the user with planned, organized solution procedures, and they compel the user to follow those procedures.

For example, based on the entered data, the DiscoTech footing design package will calculate the minimum dimensions needed for the footing. With this information displayed, the user is then asked to enter the desired width if the footing is to be continuous, or the length and width for a rectangular footing.

Some of the packages allow users to iterate the calculations by cycling back and entering new design data. Typically it will take several design iterations to achieve a satisfactory result. This kind of user-initiated iteration can be supplemented by largely automatic design optimization procedures. For example, to provide for vertical reinforcement, the ECOM column design package automatically runs successive trials for each load case, adding reinforcement as needed. It also checks the need for reinforcement for shear, in the case of tied columns. If all goes well, the governing load case is identified, and the required reinforcing is described, along with required spiral size and pitch and moment magnification factors. However, if any case is encountered that cannot be satisfied by using 8-percent vertical steel, that fact is displayed and the procedure ends.

Interacting with the ongoing design process, user and computer package can cooperate to produce the desired results. Thus the ECOM concrete column design package does an internal check of the column slenderness ratio (kl/r), based in the input data. If the ratio is less than 22 in both directions, the column is considered short and the computation proceeds. If the ratio is larger than 100, the procedure ends, since the computation method being used is not applicable. For slenderness ratios between 22 and 100, the user is asked for added data.

In many cases these packages offer use of alternative design methods.

Thus, in the ECOM reinforced concrete column package, users can choose to run either a complete design or a "flexural section" design, used when shear design is not required. They can also choose whether the ultimate strength or the working stress design method is to be used.

Finite element packages

A quite different approach to analysis and design is offered by packages that use finite element methods. These depart from manual design methods and use solution techniques more uniquely appropriate to computers.

The main task of finite element packages is to solve a large system of equations that will yield the key answers. These packages are discussed in detail in the chapter on finite element design. Those that are particularly appropriate to concrete structure design will be discussed here as well.

Easing data input

The extent to which the packages described in this chapter manage to reach the goals of easy learning and use varies. Most of the packages use interactive dialog between the computer display and the user to shape the way information is entered and package capabilities are employed. However, some of the packages continue to use the "batch" entry procedures familiar to users of computer programs that run on larger computers. For these, the user must prepare the necessary input items in correct format, then enter them into the computer as a group. For example, in the DiscoTech Footing design package, data are entered a screenful at a time. When the last item on a screen has been entered, the package display will ask if the user wishes to change any of the entries for that screen. If the answer is yes, the user can review each item on the screen, one at a time, to make desired changes.

This is a marked improvement over the input method used in DiscoTech's Retwall package. Here, the only way to deal with incorrect items, once they have been entered, is to start the package all over again. If almost all the needed data on a screen have been correctly entered and the user makes an error in just one final item, then all that has been previously done is lost. None of us is perfect, but this package does not seem to want to acknowledge that fact. The consequences can be infuriating.

The Softek plane frame analysis package uses a novel spreadsheet tabular format to input data. There are tables to be filled out with data on members, joints, member properties, connectivity, and loading. The user can maneuver within a displayed table, making entries and corrections as desired before entering the entire table for processing.

From sketch to solution

One notion promoted by some package vendors is that the user can come to the computer keyboard with just a rough sketch of the structure that is to be analyzed. However, the user also has to be prepared with the same kind of data on dimensions, properties, and loading needed for any analysis and design procedures.

Thus, in the Icon 2D package, the user works from a sketch of the structure to be analyzed, entering data for one member at a time. If all the members are of the same type, have the same moment of inertia and elastic modulus, and the same shear form factor, then the user will have to enter this information only once and automatically it will be applied to all. Otherwise, it will be necessary to enter separate data for each member. For each load case, the user provides the locations of the loads, with orientation angle and magnitude of moments.

Many packages require the user to make calculations outside the package. For example, in the DiscoTech Pier and Grade Beam (PGB) package, pier bearing is always calculated as a function of skin friction. If the pier design is actually based on end bearing pressure, this must be converted by the user into an equivalent skin friction which is then entered into the computer. The necessary conversion formula is given in printed form in the PGB package user manual, but it is not incorporated into the package itself.

Built-in computer files can ease the input burden on the user by collecting and storing frequently used input information. The storage capability is often referred to as a library or database. In the Icon 2D package, for example, sets of input data can be stored in files and called upon when a problem is to be run. Once retrieved, this information can be edited, using the display screen and keyboard, to modify the input data as desired. This minimizes input effort when the same structure is to be analyzed numerous times with only minor changes from one run to another.

Keeping track of units

The units of input and result quantities are an important concern. For correct results, units of input parameters must be not only correct but consistent with one another. Some packages cue the user on the units of input data that are to be entered. Thus, in the ECOM concrete column design package, the first prompt asks the user to choose whether to employ U.S. Customary units or MKS or SI metric units. When U.S. units are chosen, stored data for standard spiral sizes come with the package. If metric units are chosen, the user is prompted to input data (which will then be stored for future use) to describe the desired spiral system. But other packages, such as those that use finite element analysis, usually rely entirely upon the user to monitor correctness and consistency of units.

Internal program checks

Another way that computers can ease the laborious process of entering data is by providing internal controls or checks on the accuracy of the input. Both logical and typographical errors can be checked in this way. For instance, the ECOM reinforced concrete beam design package checks to see if the data the user inputs are inconsistent with the basic design specifications (spacings too small or too large, reinforcement too light). The package will detect these faults and notify the user so these can be corrected and the calculations can proceed.

Check the package assumptions

Virtually every engineering analysis and design package includes some built-in assumptions needed for the particular design method being used. Users should not make the mistake of ignoring these assumptions simply because they are not evident on the computer display screen.

ECOM slab analysis calculations, for example, assume that there is no shearhead reinforcement. It is also assumed that the critical section is located within the drop panel area for solid slabs, or within the solid panel for waffle slabs. Another assumption implicit in the design procedure is that the slab is centered over the columns, so that the critical shear is governed by Section 11.11.1.2 of the ACI Code. It is up to the user to verify whether or not assumptions like these are correct for each individual design case.

BEAM DESIGN PACKAGES

PGB: PIER AND GRADE BEAM DESIGN

ElFan: ANALYSIS OF GRADE BEAM ON ELASTIC FOUNDATION

The PGB package aids users in the design of pier and grade foundation spans. These are designed one at a time. When the design of one span is complete, the user can go on to the next span. Up to 99 spans can be handled, each with its own specific load development. The package offers a choice of three design procedures; all use the ultimate strength method.

The ElFan package allows the user to predict how a grade beam will perform. Up to 99 point loads can be applied, and the package will calculate deflection, slope, bending moment, shear, and soil pressure for each load point, and up to 99 analysis locations as well. The computation follows formulas developed by M. Hetenyi in his book Beams on Elastic Foundation *(Univ. of Michigan Press, 1979).*

Both packages are for use with the IBM/PC and compatible computers and with micro/personal computers that use CP/M system software. PGB sells for $150, Elfan for $220. They are available from DiscoTech, Morton Technologies, 600 B Street, P.O. Box 1659, Santa Rosa, CA 95402 [(707) 523-1600].

EASI: CONCRETE BEAM DESIGN

Concrete beams are designed to meet ACI codes. Steel requirements and geometric dimensions are calculated for given loadings and boundary conditions. This package runs on IBM/PC, TRS-80, and CP/M micro/personal computers. It sells for $100 and is available from EASI Software, Inc., 2891 Livonia Center Rd., Lima, NY 14485 [(716) 346-2022].

CD-1: REINFORCED CONCRETE BEAM DESIGN

This package is used to design reinforced continuous concrete beams. Two methods are offered, ultimate strength and working stress—both are in accordance with ACI 318-77. The package generates reinforcement requirements for rectangular, T-beam, and ledger (inverted T) cross sections. It also generates vertical stirrup requirements based on the user's choice of size and spacings. Calculations can be for cantilevers or spans. End sections and midsections can be different sizes. The user can choose a bar size and the package will calculate appropriate cutoff locations. Each individual span or cantilever can have as many as nine changes of slope or steps in its shear diagram.

The package is available in versions that run on a variety of micro/personal computers. Versions for the IBM/PC, Apple II+, DEC Rainbow, TRS-80, Wang PC, and HP-150 sell for $600. Versions for the Wang PC, HP-9845, and HP-9816 sell for $850. Versions for the HP-85, HP-86, and HP-87XM sell for $575. Available from ECOM Associates, Inc., 8634 West Brown Deer Rd., Milwaukee WI, 53224 [(414) 354-0243].

SD-3 COMPOSITE STEEL BEAM ANALYSIS AND DESIGN

This package is used to check or design simple span beams of composite steel and concrete construction. The package finds the reactions, the maximum moment, and its location. Bending stresses, web shear stresses, and midspan deflections are also calculated. The required number of shear connectors can be determined for a given connector load.

SD-3 runs on IBM/PC and compatible computers, HP 9816, 9845, 85, 86, and 87 computers, and CP/M computers. It sells for $550 from ECOM Associates, 8634 West Brown Deer Rd., Milwaukee, WI 53224 [(414) 354-0243].

To operate the package and enter data, users keyboard replies to displayed queries. There are quite a lot of data to be entered for this package. The queries are made a few at a time. Then the user is asked if there have been any errors. If so, the package returns to the beginning of that short sequence and reenters the data.

This is an improvement on those packages that require the user to finish the program sequence, then restart at the beginning of the entire program whenever a keyboarding error is included in entered material. However, the method used in this package, and in the other packages from this vendor, is still inconvenient when compared to full-screen entry, pull-down, windows and other entry techniques now widely used with personal computer packages.

The input load pattern is limited to nine steps or slope-changes in the shear diagram, between the supports.

ST16M: CONCRETE BEAM DESIGN

ST16M uses the ultimate strength design method from ACI 318-77. Rectangular and T-section beams can be handled. Either English or SI metric units can be used. The user inputs load conditions, material properties, cross-section dimensions, span and stirrup size. The package calculates the area of reinforcing steel and bar cutoff data. Cutoff locations are calculated for all the bar sizes selected by the user. Other outputs include stirrup spacings, design moments, and inflection points.

The package comes in formats that can be run on IBM/PC, TRS-80, Apple, Hewlett-Packard, DEC, and other micro/personal computers. It *sells for $395 and is available from MC2 Engineering Software, 8107 S.W. 72nd Ave., P.O. Box 430980, Miami, FL 33143 [(305) 665-0100].*

RAND BEAM ANALYSIS

This continuous beam analysis procedure can include columns above and below the beam, as well as cantilevers. The procedure is for use with distributed, partially distributed, concentrated, and pattern loads. It calculates deflection at mid-span and maximum positive and negative moments.

A separate concrete beam capacity check procedure handles rectangular, T and joist cross sections, with both compression steel and multiple-layer tension steel. It computes the ultimate bending capacity, conforming to ACI 318-83.

These procedures are among several included in the Rand Structural Utilities package. The package runs on IBM/PCs and other micro/personal computers. It sells for $450 and is available from The Rand Group, 17430 Campbell Rd. #114, Dallas, TX 75252 [(214) 661-0124].

COLUMN DESIGN PACKAGES

EASI: CONCRETE COLUMN DESIGN

This package is used to design spiral, square tied, and rectangular columns in accordance with ACI codes. Eccentric loads are allowed. Calculation results include geometric dimensions and steel requirements. It runs on IBM/PC, TRS-80, and CP/M micro/personal computers, sells for $100, and is available from EASI Software, Inc., 2891 Livonia Center Rd., Lima, NY 14485 [(716) 346-2022].

CD-2: REINFORCED CONCRETE COLUMN DESIGN

This package is for design and capacity checking of reinforced concrete columns. The computations are in accordance with ACI 318-77. One of the two main procedures in the package is a design routine that finds the re-

quired reinforcement needed for a given set of design loads and moments. Reinforcement is always assumed to be symmetrically placed. The second main procedure calculates the allowable axial load for given eccentricities.

Bending may be in either or both directions. Slenderness effects are handled by the moment magnification method (Section 10.11 of the ACI Code) with slenderness ratio limited to 100. Column cross sections may be rectangular (tied), round (tied or spiral), or square with circular bar (spiral or tied). Loads are applied to the column ends, and there is no provision for lateral loads between the ends.

The package is available in versions that run on a variety of micro/personal computers. Versions for the IBM/PC, Apple II+, DEC Rainbow, TRS-80, Wang PC, and HP-150 sell for $575. Versions for the Wang PC, HP-9845, and HP-9816 sell for $800. Versions for the HP-85, HP-86, and HP-87XM sell for $550. From ECOM Associates, Inc., 8634 West Brown Deer Rd., Milwaukee, WI 53224 [(414) 354-0243].

ST18M: STRUCTURAL CONCRETE COLUMN DESIGN

Near-optimum reinforced concrete columns can be designed with the help of this package. The columns can be round-spiral, square tied, or rectangular tied. The basic design method used is that of Gaylord and Gaylord, which is extended to deal with eccentric axial loads and rectangular columns. The concrete is assumed to be in compression, with no bending other than eccentricity. The results conform to ACI 1972 Concrete Design Code requirements.

The user inputs data on dead and live axial loads, ultimate strength and weight of the concrete, yield strength of the longitudinal rebar, eccentricity, longest laterally unsupported length, total column length, and column-end fixity factor. Either English or SI metric units can be used. Calculated information supplied by the package includes needed spiral reinforcing, size, and axial spacing of the longitudinal rebar. A number of combinations of reinforcing and rebar choices are given, and the best choice is identified.

Versions of the package can run on TRS-80 computers and other micro/personal computers that use CP/M system software. ST18M sells for $295 and is available from MC2 Engineering Software, 8107 S.W. 72nd Ave., P.O. Box 430980, Miami, FL 33143 [(305) 665-0100].

RAND CONCRETE COLUMN ANALYSIS

Interaction diagrams for reinforced concrete columns, round or rectangular, are produced by this procedure, which can analyze bar patterns, using actual rebar locations. The columns can be subject to a combination of axial loads and bending moments. The ACI 318-83 code is used.

This procedure is one of several included in the Rand Structural Utilities package. The package runs on IBM/PCs and other micro/personal computers. It sells for $450 and is available from The Rand Group, 17430 Campbell Rd. #114, Dallas, TX 75252 [(214) 661-0124].

SLAB AND WALL DESIGN PACKAGES

RETWALL: RETAINING WALL DESIGN

TILTWALL: CONCRETE TILT-UP WALL DESIGN

Using either poured concrete or concrete block, stemwalls up to 30 feet high can be designed and analyzed with the help of this package. Calculations are based on the ACI 318-77 standard and on the Reinforced Masonry Handbook *by Amrhein.*

Tiltwall provides a method of designing concrete walls with thickness less than what would normally be prescribed by height-thickness ratios. The designs are said to meet Uniform Building Code Section 2610 and ACI requirements.

Both packages are for use with the IBM/PC and compatible computers and with micro/personal computers that use CP/M system software. Retwall sells for $250, Tiltwall for $125. They are available from Disco-Tech, Morton Technologies, 600 B Street, P.O. Box 1659, Santa Rosa, CA 95402 [(707) 523-1600].

EASI: ONE- AND TWO-WAY SLAB DESIGN

Either one-way or two-way slabs can be designed in multiple bay patterns. Slab thickness and steel requirements are calculated to meet AISC Code *requirements. This package runs on IBM/PC, TRS-80, and CP/M micro/ personal computers. It sells for $100 and is available from EASI Software, Inc., 2891 Livonia Center Rd., Lima, NY 14485 [(716) 346-2022].*

CD-3: FLAT SLAB ANALYSIS AND DESIGN

Flat slab and waffle slab floors are analyzed and designed to conform with ACI 318-77. Either the ultimate strength or the working stress design method may be used. A strip of floor one bay wide and up to 10 spans long can be handled, with cantilevers at the ends.

The package is available in versions that run on a variety of micro/personal computers. Versions for the IBM/PC, Apple II+, DEC Rainbow, TRS-80, Wang PC, and HP-150 sell for $700. Versions for the Wang PC, HP-9845, and HP-9816 sell for $1150. Versions for the HP-85, HP-86, and HP-87XM sell for $825. From ECOM Associates, Inc., 8634 West Brown Deer Rd., Milwaukee, WI 53221 [(414) 354 0243].

RETWALLS: FOR RETAINING WALL DESIGN

This package does calculations for poured concrete or concrete block retaining walls. It sizes the concrete elements and determines the needed steel reinforcement. The output includes a graphic representation of the wall design with data included.

Retwalls runs on an IBM/PC with 64K main memory; it sells for just $78.44, from J.J.Jordan, Architect-Engineer, 5236 Overbrook Way, Sacramento, CA 95841 [(916) 332-6610].

ST19M: ONE-WAY, TWO-WAY CONCRETE SLAB DESIGN

One-way and two-way slabs under uniform applied loads can be designed. The ACI 318-77 direct design method and procedures of Winter and Nilson are used. Either English or SI metric units can be employed. Users input the span, minimum desired thickness, live and dead loads, reinforcing steel yield strength, concrete density, and compressive strength. For the two- way design column dimensions, interior and exterior beam dimensions must also be given. The package calculates the minimum slab thickness required by the codes, flexural steel bar sizes, design moments, and actual and allowable shear stresses.

The package comes in formats that can be run on IBM/PC, TRS-80, Apple, Hewlett-Packard, DEC, and other micro/personal computers. It sells for $395 and is available from MC2 Engineering Software, 8107 S.W. 72nd Ave., P.O. Box 430980, Miami, FL 33143 [(305) 665-0100].

RAND: SLAB AND WALL ANALYSIS

The Rand concrete slab-punching shear check procedure can take account of uni-axial and bi-axial moments and accommodates interior, edge, or corner columns. It not only calculates the punching shear for a concrete flat plate but also the required sizes and limits on drop panels, if those are used. And it conforms to ACI 318-83.

For design of cantilever retaining walls, a procedure calculates the necessary stem heights and thicknesses, heel and toe length and thickness, and all required reinforcing. The procedure will accommodate various patterns of stem-load distribution and handle tapered stem design. It also checks overturning moment, bearing pressure, and factor of safety against sliding. ACI 318-83 is used.

These procedures are among several included in the Rand Structural Utilities package. The package runs on IBM/PCs and other micro/personal computers. It sells for $450 and is available from The Rand Group, 17430 Campbell Rd. #114, Dallas, TX 75252 [(214) 661-0124].

DESIGN OF PRESTRESSED ELEMENTS

PD-1: PRESTRESSED CONCRETE BEAM ANALYSIS AND DESIGN

This package is used to analyze or design prestressed concrete beams that may have cantilevers at each end. The calculations conform to ACI Code 318-83. The beams must have constant cross section but may be of composite construction. Prestressing strands may be sleeved or "slipped" for a portion of their length, and the design will account for this. Calculated results include flexural and shear stresses, moment capacity, web reinforcement, and deflection.

The package is available in versions that run on Hewlett-Packard and Wang micro/personal computers. Versions for the Wang PC, HP-9845 and HP-9816 sell for $1200. Versions for the HP-85, HP-86, and HP-87XM sell for $800. Available from ECOM Associates, Inc., 8634 West Brown Deer Rd., Milwaukee, WI 53224 [(414) 354- 0243].

SPAN: PRESTRESSED BRIDGE GIRDER ANALYSIS AND DESIGN

Span allows users to design major types of bridge girders according to 1983 AASHTO specifications. It performs 10th point analysis, automatically generates loads, and carries out automatic stand pattern and sheilding calculations. The package is intended for use by consultants, contractors, and precast producers.

Span runs on the IBM/PC and compatible computers. It sells for $2500 and is available from LEAP Associates, P.O. Box 16007, Tampa, FL 33687 [(813) 988-6870].

FINITE ELEMENT PACKAGES

ICON 2D: FOR PLANE STRUCTURES WITH A VARIETY OF MEMBERS

The Icon 2D package provides for the use of prismatic, tapered, and curved beams as members, as well as for beams with rigid offset joints and shear beams. Smaller structures are analyzed by rapid processing within the computer main memory, but very large structures can also be handled. The processing takes longer, since it transfers chunks of the problem from disk to main memory for solution.

Icon 2D runs on IBM/PC/XT computers and on HP 86, 87 computers. The package sells for $695. An added graphics program, used to view deformed shapes and other output, sells for $195. An added input program that replicates data and geometries also sells for $195. The package is available from Advanced Structural Technology Inc., P.O. Box 16659, Clayton, MO 63105 [(314) 725-8282].

P-FRAME: FOR DESIGNING PLANE FRAMES

P-Frame analyzes two-dimensional structural systems like trusses, frames, beams, arches, or rings. Up to 99 load combinations and 99 load cases can be handled. Structures with up to 960 members, 480 joints, 100 springs (elastic restraints), and 50 sections can be analyzed. The package is said to be able to process a frame with 250 members and three load cases in under three minutes.

P-Frame runs on IBM/PC and XT computers with a minimum of 92,000 bytes of main memory (64,000 bytes is needed to take advantage of the maximum analysis parameters mentioned above). A color-graphics adapter is also needed. P-Frame sells for $1395, and there is an annual fee of $140 for maintenance and updating services. It is produced by Softek Services in Vancouver, Canada, and is available in the United States from ECOM Associates, 8634 West Brown Deer Rd., Milwaukee, WI 53224 [(414) 354-0243].

OTHER DESIGN PACKAGES

FOOTING: DESIGN OF ISOLATED FOOTINGS

The Footing package aids in designs of concrete footings, with or without steel reinforcement. Six different types of footings can be designed using ultimate-strength techniques.

Footing is for use with the IBM/PC and compatible computers and with micro/personal computers that use CP/M system software. The package sells for $110 and is available from DiscoTech, Morton Technologies, 600 B Street, PO Box 1659, Santa Rosa, CA 95402 [(707) 523-1600].

EASI: PRECAST CONCRETE VAULT

This package computes design moments and steel requirements for top, bottom, and side sections of precast vaults. This package runs on IBM/PC, TRS-80, and CP/M micro/personal computers. It sells for $100 and is *available from EASI Software, Inc., 2891 Livonia Center Rd., Lima, NY 14485 [(716) 346-2022].*

RAND: STRUCTURAL UTILITIES PACKAGE

Ten structural analysis and design procedures are included in this package. Most of them conform to ACI 318-83. The procedures for analysis of beams, columns, slabs, and walls have already been described. Others include:

A pile cap design procedure takes both axial loads and bi- axial moments into consideration. It accommodates virtually any pile configuration, including misplaced and compression-only piles. The procedure determines cap thickness, required rebar quantities, and sizes. It also checks punching shear and conforms to ACI 318-83.

For spread footings, a procedure analyzes axial loads and uni-axial and bi-axial moments. It provides required footing dimensions, rebar quantities, and sizes, gives the bearing pressure distribution of the footing, and checks punching shear, using ACI 318-83.

Capacity of drilled piers and caissons is checked by a procedure that takes friction load transfer and end bearing capacity into account. It allows for skin friction variation with depth and conforms to ACI 318-83.

Steel bearing capacity, the required dimensions of steel base plates bearing on concrete, is calculated by a steel column base plate procedure. It can also be used to determine the number of anchor bolts needed and their placement. The designs are based on axial load as well as uni-axial moments.

A steel section properties procedure calculates the properties and detailing dimensions of built-up wide flange shapes constructed of rolled steel plate. The procedure calculates the area, moments of inertia, and tortional and other constants needed for design of columns, girders, and beams according to the AISC Code.

The Rand Structural Utilities package runs on IBM/PCs and other micro/personal computers. The package sells for $450 and is available from The Rand Group, 17430 Campbell Rd. #114, Dallas, TX 75252 [(214) 661-0124].

ACI-214: ANALYSIS

This package works together with the widely used Lotus 1.2.3 software. It follows the ACI guideline 214, to prepare graphs and reports on the breaking strength of concrete samples.

The package runs on an IBM/PC with 192K main memory. It sells for $495 (plus the cost of the Lotus 1.2.3 package) from Systemics, 3050 Spring St., West Bloomfield, MI 48033 [(313) 851- 2504].

Chapter 3
Structural Design and Analysis

Packages discussed in this chapter include those that allow users to calculate the characteristics of wood, steel, and other beams and to select appropriate beams to meet design needs. There are also two packages that provide similar capabilities for columns and several packages for analysis and design of truss and frame structures.

This is not the only chapter in this book in which structural design packages are discussed. There is a chapter on structural design using members made of concrete as well as one on general finite element packages. Some truss and frame packages use the same basic stiffness-matrix computation method as do finite element packages, but they concentrate on these specific types of structures rather than providing the more diverse elements that the more general packages have.

One of the packages, STRESSPAC, is a potpourri of seven different programs, concerned with such diverse matters as stresses in cylinders. It is included here because more of its programs seem concerned with beams than with any other single subject covered in this book.

There is little, in the packages discussed in this chapter, that touches specifically on the important problem of dynamic analysis. However, the TRUS-ILPC package calculates influence lines for the member forces in a plane truss, and these are useful for calculating maximum member forces that can be produced by moving loads.

Help with data entry

Calculations that involve a single beam usually require only a few items of input information. If methods used for data entry are difficult, the pain for the user will be short-lived. However, entering the data for frame and truss structures can involve keyboarding geometry, material properties, and other items for many members. If the data input methods provided by a package are not convenient, users may find themselves spending many extra hours at the keyboard.

Compared to most of the other packages, STRESSPAC is a model of input design. Data entry for the programs in this package is done on full-screen displays. By pressing cursor-positioning arrows, and other keys, users write data onto the display, erasing and changing the information as needed. Any screen of data can be stored in a disk file and retrieved for use.

Many of the other packages suffer from inappropriate input techniques. In the SD-1 package, keyboard data input is in response to a string of 25 or 30 screen-displayed queries. Then the package goes right ahead with calculations. Those users who make entry mistakes have to start all over again from the beginning. The SD-2A package from the same vendor is a bit more forgiving. After a short sequence of queries and replies, the package asks the user if there have been any errors. If so, it will return to the beginning of the sequence for reentry of the data.

Little mainframes

Some of the packages seem to be designed in the belief that personal computers are just little mainframe computers that should really be getting their input from punched cards. Their input is in rather rigid line-by-line formats.

With FATPACK, for example, numeric values are entered a line at a time. If there are errors, the user retypes the whole line. But once a group of data has been entered, it has to be edited in file format. Over 30 pages of the manual for this package are devoted to spelling out the formats for input files. To check BEAMDS data the user has to understand the symbolic notation and format this package uses for 12 different arrays of input data.

Other packages handle data using computer programming methods. Thus FASTRAN has a special command language to set up structure geometry and specify loads and other conditions. The SET command is used to enter point coordinates; L/D defines linear displacements; L/A defines angle-distance location. Each of these and other commands have their own rules, which the user must learn to operate the package. The USA-STRESS package has commands that call up input data queries. For example, the MEI command calls up queries on data for a member. If the structure has 48 members, the MEI command must be given 48 times.

Keyboard commands are sometimes used to increase the flexibility with which users can manipulate a package. In BEAM-1, a set of 10 keyboard commands allow users to move the display cursor, delete or insert characters, and maneuver during data entry.

Entering multiple members

In frame and truss structures containing many identical members, it can be very handy simply to duplicate already entered input data. To help with identical joints, joint restraints, members, and loads, the FA-3 package allows users to indicate how many of these items they want; then it adds them automatically. Along the same lines, the Frame80 package has a "same as" feature that allows data for the current member to be copied from those for a previously entered member.

Pre-stored data

Input to design and analysis packages can be greatly simplified whenever it is possible to provide stored data with the package, from which needed input information can be transferred. In the BEAM ANALYSIS AND DESIGN package most of the input data come from such stored tables. Included are data on U.S. standard structural steel sections (AISC WF, S, and M shapes), timber beams (including single, double, triple, and a few quadruple sections), and on 256 concrete reinforcing bar combinations.

The SD-1 package comes with built-in files containing data on W6 through W36 sections normally used as beams, and also on C and S shapes. And the SD-2A package comes with stored data on pipe sections 1-inch and larger in diameter, and on all square and rectangular tubes three inches or larger listed in the AISC Manual of Construction.

Beam design alternatives

Design of a single beam is a fairly simple procedure that can be handled with a calculator. One advantage that beam design packages like those discussed in this chapter can offer is to give the user a look at different design alternatives. For example, the BEAMJOIS package will search through it's stored data to find the cheapest grade of lumber that will meet the specified conditions. If one is not found, the package increases the depth of the beam by two inches and goes through the calculations and table search once again. Two more automatic searches follow—one for a deeper beam of a cheaper grade; and for a wider but shallower beam.

The BEAM ANALYSIS AND DESIGN package will choose the lightest steel section whose properties meet those specified. Three alternate choices, with different depths, are presented. In a similar manner the package will choose the smallest, most efficient timber section and present three alternative choices.

Tracking units

BEAM ANALYSIS AND DESIGN can operate in metric and S.I. units. A UNITS command allows a choice of units (kips,ft; lbs,ft; kg,m; or kN,m) in which data will be entered and answers will appear. The package then prompts for the correct units for input data and displays results with the correct units.

Most frame and truss packages are neutral with respect to units. They calculate with numbers-only and leave it up to the user to enter numbers that correspond to consistent units and to interpret the units for the computation results. An exception is the FA-3 package. At the beginning of data entry, the user is asked to enter the type of units being used. Quantities are entered as numbers, but the package questions whether member properties and frame dimension units are consistent with the indicated type.

Variety in elements and loads

In truss and frame structures containing rod, truss, or beam-type elements, cross-section properties may be significant. Usually the packages are designed to handle elements with constant cross sections. The common practice is to represent tapered elements by setting up a series of constant cross-section elements, each larger than the next. Some packages allow the user to call for elements with nonconstant cross section included. For example, beams analyzed with the BEAMDS package may have variable or fixed cross section with variable material properties across each cross section.

Types of loading available with packages may include concentrated loads or moments at the nodes and concentrated or distributed loads on the members. With the Frame80 package, up to 99 cases can be entered; and these can then be assembled into up to 99 combinations of load cases, with factors applied to the constituent load cases. Thus, if one load case represents a wind load and another a dead load, the two can be combined so the total is, say, 0.8 wind + 1.2 dead.

What users have to know

The ideal structural design package would probably require that the user be knowledgeable about engineering but not necessarily know very much about using computers. However, most packages require some minimal computer knowledge on the part of the user. For example, the S/SAM package assumes that users can load and run programs, and that they are able to copy and transfer files from one disk to another to facilitate package operation.

In almost every case it is either expected or advisable for the user to make a sketch of the structure involved before trying to use the computer to analyze or design it. USA-STRESS package users are specifically advised to start by making a hand sketch of their structure, and to use it to determine the coordinates of the joints, to number the members, and to set up loading arrangements. Frame80 advises that a hand sketch be used to count the number of joints, members, and supports. These numbers are required initial inputs to the package. In fact, assignment of such numbers is an important item for many frame and truss analysis packages, since the way these numbers are assigned can affect the speed and efficiency with which the package will reach a solution.

One final point that applies to virtually any engineering design package is that users must continue to exercise prudent engineering judgment, even though they are using a computer package that readily churns out answers. For example, the shear and bending analysis performed by the BEAM ANALYSIS AND DESIGN package assumes that there is adequate bracing to assure lateral stability. If not, the analysis is not valid. It is the user's responsibility to see that this and other limitations of the packages are taken into account when interpreting the computed results.

BEAM ANALYSIS AND DESIGN

This is a well-designed package that evidences some concern for ease of learning and use. It can be used to analyze and select steel, concrete, and wood beams.

This beam analysis package runs on IBM/PC/XT/AT computers. It sells for $500 from C2 B2 Software Design, 763 27th Ave., San Francisco, CA 94121 [(415) 751-1337].

The designer of this beam analysis package evidently loves little boxes. The screen display for the package is divided up into six of them. At the lower left is a box in which menu displays appear: first a main menu, then submenus, each with several one-word choices available. A tiny box at the top reminds the user of the name of the package. The other four boxes are for describing the beam, setting out load and material specifications, and displaying computation results.

This arrangement is convenient, since the boxes that require data input from the user can be quickly filled by use of menu choices. Most of the data come from stored tables that are part of the package. Other data items are keyboarded by the user as the display cursor appears in the proper location. Users can skip from one menu choice to another by pressing the space bar, or they can invoke menu items by keyboarding the first letter of the desired item.

Some of the procedures can only be characterized as cute. For instance, the choice of type of beam support is made by selecting from tiny diagrams that show the four available arrangements.

There are a few things new users need to learn to operate this arrangement, mainly to understand the meaning of the various windows and the needed keyboard actions. But all this can be absorbed in an hour or two.

Defaults plus

This package comes with built-in data on U.S. standard structural steel sections (AISC WF, S, and M shapes) timber beams (including single, double, triple, and a few quadruple sections), and on 256 concrete reinforcing bar combinations. The vendor also provides a custom version of the package that allows users to choose beams from data on aluminum extrusions whose properties the user can specify.

Material properties required by the package include such items as the modulus of elasticity, allowable bending and shear stresses, and deflection. The package will pull standard "default" values for these properties from stored data for the material chosen by the user. These can be accepted, or users can change individual property values as desired.

Immediate recalculation

Point, uniform, or moment loads can be specified. Loads are entered one at a time. Users choose which of the three they want and the package prompts for information on that particular load. There are good editing facilities. Particular loads, identified by number, can be changed as needed. New loads can be added. Existing loads can be deleted.

The package does immediate recalculation of analysis results. As changed load information is entered, this calculation proceeds, so the user can call for and see new analysis results immediately.

Beam files

Once created, descriptions of beams can be stored for future use. Each disk-stored file created by the package can contain up to 50 such descriptions, and ten such files will fit on one disk. So hundreds of beam descriptions can be kept ready for use in designs. The package includes, on its

SYSTEMS menu, commands to list, save, retrieve, and delete beam descriptions and files.

Calculations are done in single precision with seven significant figures, then rounded to display results containing four significant figures. The package can operate in metric and S.I. units. The design itself is based on U.S. codes of practice. A UNITS command allows a choice of units (kips,ft; lbs,ft; kg,m; or kN,m) in which data will be entered and answers will appear. The package then prompts for the correct units for input data and displays results with the correct units.

Users are warned that they must exercise prudent engineering judgment with this package. For example, the shear and bending analysis performed by the package assumes that there is adequate bracing to assure lateral stability. If not, the analysis is not valid. It is the user's responsibility to see that this and other limitations of the package are taken into account when interpreting the computed results.

The package will display shear, moment, slope, and deflection diagrams on systems equipped with color displays and plug-in graphics boards. It will also find the shear, moment, slope, and deflection at any designated point along the beam.

Design routines

In addition to beam analysis the package performs design procedures. For steel beams it will choose the lightest steel section whose properties meet those specified. Three alternate choices, with different depths, are presented. In a similar manner the package will choose the smallest, most efficient timber section and present three alternative choices.

For concrete beam design, the package will calculate a preliminary beam size. The user can accept this or change the specified proportions. The package then selects steel reinforcing, usually at three points along the beam, using the smallest number of bars that satisfy area of steel requirements.

Help for the user

The user manual for this package is comprehensive. It gives explanations of each of the possible menu choices the user can make. A tutorial section goes step by step through analyses and design of one steel and one concrete beam.

The manual also gives references and briefly discusses the analysis and design techniques used. Some of the possible pitfalls of the analyses are mentioned. This discussion could be enlarged, and similar information on design methods would be most helpful to users. A list of references is given to which users can refer for this kind of information.

The manual also has printed versions of the beam section data built into the package, useful for those who want to see the alternatives from which the package makes its design choices. The manual we saw had a place for an index, but none was provided.

BEAM DESIGN

Reviewed by: Mendel Nock, Houston, TX

This package computes the required rectangular section for a beam to resist a specified force or deformation loading, for any of four end conditions. Data for steel and copper- and aluminum-alloy beams come as part of the package.

Beam Design runs on IBM/PC computers. It sells for $115 from Don Willis Assoc., 12562 Loraleen St., Garden Grove, CA 92641 [(714) 539-4498.]

Design of single-bay beams is a fairly simple procedure. But it can become tedious when performed repeatedly. Engineers have usually tackled this problem with a programmable calculator. More recently, personal computer spreadsheet packages have been pressed into service. Special-purpose packages like Beam Design are a third alternative. The choice between the three will depend on the availability of a suitable computer, software already purchased, and the engineer's personal attitude.

Beam Design operates through displayed menus for making choices of material, end conditions, and load type. Data are entered in response to screen-displayed queries.

The initial menu allows 14 responses, which define the end conditions and load type. Permitted end conditions are: simply supported at both ends; fixed at both ends; cantilevered; and fixed at one end but simply supported at the other. Permitted load types are: concentrated at any point along the beam; uniform over the beam length; and graduated, varying from zero at one end to a maximum at the other. Only one load can be applied during any given run.

A material selection menu comes next. The standard materials are carbon steel, stainless steel, aluminum alloy, and copper alloy. Alternatively, users may define their own material. Data associated with a material are its name, tensile elastic modulus, and specific weight. Allowable stresses are defined later and are not associated with any particular material. User-defined material can exist for the current run but is not stored for future runs.

As in any stress analysis, force and deflection are mated variables. This package queries as to which one to use as the solution variable. Next, there are queries for beam width, length, allowable stress, and load. The package then calculates the solution and displays the input data, and the resulting section, along with such data as the shear stress, moment of inertia, section modulus, and beam weight. Users can change the input, one parameter at a time, and rerun to optimize the design.

Handling of user errors is adequate. The range of menu choices is protected by automatic checks. However, data ranges are not automatically checked. An inappropriate zero or negative number will result in a system error. To recover, the user has to restart the package.

No knowledge of programming or special computer expertise is needed to use this package. All of the system commands needed to set it up and run it are described in the user manual. No special equipment is needed. The user manual describes program use and provides examples. In some respects the manual is overdone. It is a rare engineer who needs to be told what a simply supported beam is.

Improvements to the package should include the ability to combine several of the linearly superposable load primitives into a single loading condition for a design. It would be convenient to be able to store user-specified materials permanently in a library, and to associate an allowable stress to each material as a default. Expansion of the design capability to include simple H shapes would also be desirable.

BEAMDS: BEAM DEFLECTION AND STRESS

Beams analyzed with this package may have variable or fixed cross section with variable material properties across each cross section. There can be up to ten point loads and one variable running load.

BEAMDS runs on IBM/PC Apple II, TRS-80, and most other personal computers. It sells for $39.95 from Dynacomp, 1064 Gravel Rd., Webster, NY 14580 [(716) 671-6160].

BEAMDS comes with a separate program for creating and editing input data files. This program steps through a series of screen-displayed queries to which the user replies by keyboarding appropriate data.

However, to check the data, or to review an existing file of input data that are to be modified, the user has to understand the symbolic notation and format this package uses for input data. It is fairly complex, since there are 12 different arrays of numbers to handle.

The vendor warns that the calculation process can be slow, and that no claims are made for the accuracy of the package in producing deflection and stress figures.

BEAMJOIS

This package is designed to select Douglas Fir wood beams for simple and cantilevered spans with distributed or concentrated load.

BEAMJOIS runs on IBM/PC, Apple IIe,IIc, and TRS-80 computers. It sells for $96.96 from James J. Jordan Sr., 5236 Overbrook Way, Sacramento, CA 95841 [(916) 332-6610].

The manual, which is a bit difficult to read since it is made up from dot-matrix printer output, gives a detailed, step-by-step explanation of how to use the package. Like this explanation, the package operates through a step-by-step sequence of queries and other displays which call for keyboard responses from the user.

After some preliminary queries, there is a display of data depicting a simple single beam with normal wood moisture content. The user can change items by pressing an item number, then making new choices or entering new values. Users can opt to specify member width and depth or allow the package to choose these. Types of loads can be chosen and specified.

Based on such choices and options, selected by the user during this dialog, the package then makes its calculations. While these are running, the package displays a rough symbolic diagram of the beam with its loads. Results include required moment, shear, and moment of inertia.

The procedures include many options and these are only explained in narrative form. About the only way to discover what choices there are is to go through the entry, calculation, and output procedures with an actual problem and explore the possibilities.

Stored lumber tables

The package comes with stored tables of allowable stress for various sizes of lumber. These are searched to calculate the moments, reactions, and stresses, taking the weight of the beam into account. The package then searches for the cheapest grade of lumber that will meet the specified conditions. If one is not found, it then increases the depth of the beam by 2 inches and goes through the calculations and table search once again. Two more automatic searches follow—one for a deeper beam of a cheaper grade and for a wider but shallower beam. In this way, the package comes up with three possible choices of beams.

Printed results seem to be compact, perhaps a bit crowded, but clearly presented.

BEAM-1

This package is for the analysis and design of beams made of wood and other homogeneous materials. Uniform and point loads may be applied. The package computes reactions, maximum shears, bending moments, and deflections.

BEAM-1 runs on IBM/PC and compatible computers and on CP/M computers. It sells for $145 from DiscoTech, 600 B Street, PO Box 1659, Santa Rosa, CA 95402 [(707) 523-1600].

BEAM-1 operates from a main menu with 12 choices for data entry, calculation, and output functions. A set of 10 keyboard commands allows users to move the display cursor, delete or insert characters, and maneuver during data entry. Most of the entries for this package are responses in a space provided at the end of a displayed query. Some, like the data for point loads, are entered in tabular format.

For data entry, the package displays a group of items to be filled in. Starting with the top item, the user keyboards appropriate letters of numbers, then presses the Enter key to move to the next item. Point loads are entered in a tabular format through which the user moves in a similar fashion.

Enter and calculate

The package will calculate shear and moment at any points along the beam that the user specifies. This procedure operates through a tabular display. The user enters a position for the first desired point in the first row of the table; then the computer displays the shear and moment for that point on the same line. Subsequent point positions are entered, one to a line, and the shears and moments for each are displayed in the same way.

Users enter material properties: elastic modulus, allowable bending stress, horizontal shear, and overstress. The package then provides a method for calculating required section properties for wood beams. For nonwood beams (the shapes must lend themselves to calculation of a unit shear), users are required to enter a section modulus and area for shear, and for nonrectangular beams, a moment of inertia.

BEAM-1 then calculates the maximum deflection for the beam and a deflection factor. If that factor is too small, the user can obtain a minimum beam depth for wood beams or a maximum moment of inertia for other beams. Section property calculations and entries can than be repeated to increase the beam depth.

The line-by-line procedure for calculating deflections at desired points is similar to that described for calculating shear and moment.

The package can produce a beam geometry diagram that shows point and uniform loads. Various results and input data items can be printed, and users can select which items will appear in the printout.

CONTINUOUS BEAM ANALYSIS

This package analyzes up to 20 spans with as many as 40 concentrated loads and a uniform load on the beam. Beams may be prismatic or have variable cross-sections. Ends may be fixed, free, or cantilevered. Outputs include end shears and moments.

Continuous Beam Analysis runs on IBM/PC computers and sells for $127 from Systek, P.O. Drawer JJ, Mississippi State, MS 39762 [(601) 323-6905].

Data input to the package is through answers to a sequence of screen-displayed queries. To get ready for these, the user is expected to make a hand sketch of the beam and its loading. The entries are formatted, with formats varying from one item to another. Thus spans are entered on one line with spaces between the length figures. Loads are each entered on a separate line with entries for load type, magnitude, distance from left support, and the span number where the load is applied.

The entry line for properties of prismatic beams is quite simple. Not so for beams of variable cross section, where users must learn to respond properly to some mysterious-looking prompt symbols.

The format for the calculated results from this package is cryptic. Columns of data are headed by abbreviated titles such as DL for left end distribution factor, and FEML for left end fixed moments.

FASTRAN

This package is designed to analyze structures under static loads. Loads can be uniformly distributed on members or concentrated on members or joints. Temperature deformations can be handled.

FASTRAN runs on IBM/PC computers and sells for $127 from Systek, P.O. Drawer JJ, Mississippi State, MS 39762 [(601) 323- 6905].

FASTRAN uses a special command language to set up structure geometry and specify loads and other conditions. Data can be entered from the keyboard, or an input file can be set up using a separate editor or word processor package. Input files are in ASCII format.

Input by command

Data input of structure geometry begins with node definitions. The SET command specifies the coordinates of a single point. The L/D command defines linear displacements from a point; the L/A command locates a point at a given angle and distance from another. The DIV command allows lines to be divided by equally spaced nodes. The DUM command produces a listing of point coordinates. Each of these commands has its own rules, which the user must learn to operate the package.

Member data are entered in a somewhat different manner. The package displays four prompts. After each one, the user enters a formatted line of data.

For support and member end-release data, and for differential temperature data, there is another set of commands and formats for the user to remember. And still another set of commands is used to enter the load data.

To check the correctness of the data, the user has to be quite familiar with the various commands and formats and be able to refer to a carefully drawn and labeled sketch of the structure. The package itself offers no assistance in this data-checking process.

Fixed printout

When these data have all been satisfactorily entered, the user starts the actual computation with an EXE command. The package then produces a fixed output that includes a table of displacements and rotations for the joints, a table of moments, axial forces, and shears for the members, and a table of reactions and moments for the joints that are constrained.

Smaller structures are handled by fast solutions in the computer main memory, and the package will automatically switch over to slower, disk-based solutions for larger problems.

User manual explanations of how to operate the package are disjointed and confusing. The reader has to hop about from one page to another to reconstruct what this package is all about.

FA-3: PLANE FRAME AND TRUSS ANALYSIS

This package calculates critical moments shears and axial loads for all members of 2D frame structures. It also calculates displacements at the joints and reactions and displays deformed and undeformed structures.

FA-3 runs on IBM/PC and compatible computers ($1150) on HP 9816 9845 ($1150) HP 85 ($750) HP 86 and 87 ($850) computers and on CP/M computers ($600). The vendor is ECOM Associates 8634 West Brown Deer Rd., Milwaukee, WI 53224 [(414) 354-0243].

Members may have uniform or variable cross sections. They may have initial axial displacements, thus allowing settlement, shrinkage, or temperature change to be accounted for. Loads on members can be concentrated or uniformly distributed.

Frames to be analyzed can include up to 120 members and 80 joints. As many as 78 different types of members can be used; members must have the same orientation, loading, and cross-section properties and must be within one percent of each other in length in order to be considered as the same type.

Data entry follows a query-answer routine in which joints are described by coordinates and numbers, and members are defined by type and the joint numbers at their ends. After these data have been entered, the user can get a graphical display of the structure that has been entered.

If some error has been made in entering these joint or member data, the user can go to revision procedures.

At the beginning of data entry, the user is asked to enter the type of units being used. Quantities are entered as numbers, but the package questions whether member properties and frame dimension units are consistent with the indicated type.

Cross-section data are entered, and users can then define a table of numbered sections with an area and moment of inertia for each. These section numbers can then be applied to the members of the structure to define their properties.

The input procedures for loading first ask for uniform loads, then for concentrated loads. These can be defined for horizontal, vertical, or inclined members. Hinged ends are specified by the user. Four combinations of dead and live load factors can be defined. So can initial axial displacements and joint loadings. The procedures seem a bit complicated.

To help with inputting joints, joint restraints, members, and loads where many identical items appear one after another in a structure, the package allows users to indicate how many of these items they want; then it adds them automatically.

The package calculates critical moments, shears, axial loads, and displacements for all the joints in the structure. Users can see graphical displays of the deformed and undeformed structures.

FATPAK

This package includes four modules for 2D and for 3D analysis of truss and of frame structures.

FATPAK runs on IBM/PC and compatible computers and sells for $249 from Structural Software Systems, 4440 Gateway Dr., Monroeville, PA 15146 [(412) 325-4117].

Input data can be entered from the keyboard in response to displayed prompts. Numeric values are entered a line at a time, in the exact order requested by the prompt, and with the values separated by commas. If there are errors in a line, the user retypes the whole line. However, once a group of data (such as joint coordinates) has been entered, the only way to correct items is to store the input in a file and edit the file with other software.

Alternatively, input data files can be set up with the help of the user's word processor or editing software. Over 30 pages of the manual for this package are devoted to spelling out the formats for these input files. They are similar, for all four modules, but there are some variations and differences. The formats do not seem difficult to handle. However, these input procedures are not designed for the kind of user convenience that the typical personal computer business package provides.

For computers equipped to display graphics, the package allows users to view a display of the frame or truss geometry they have entered.

Careful numbering needed

To allow the package to store and calculate efficiently, users have to number joints carefully, since the package does no automatic renumbering for this purpose. Users also have to keep track of the coordinate system assumed by the package, so they can enter the correct signs for force, translation, rotation, and moment components.

For both 2D and 3D truss analysis, the forces must be concentrated at the joints. Forces for 2D frames can be concentrated at joints (where moments can also be applied) or on members, and linearly distributed member forces are also permitted. For the 3D frames, the forces and moments must be concentrated at the joints only.

The members are assumed to be slender prismatic beam elements. Users specify the cross-section properties as part of their input to each computation run.

It is up to the user to keep the units for input quantities consistent. The package itself simply takes numerical data and assumes that the use of units is consistent.

Multi-minute calculations

The computation method used in this package is to develop and solve a set of linear stiffness equations. The vendor states that when a 2D building frame structure with 126 joints and 220 members was analyzed, the solution was obtained in 55 minutes.

Although the package uses single precision arithmetic, the vendor found that the results for maximum moments in a member at the base of this structure varied only 0.01 percent from those calculated with the help of mainframe computer software.

The computed results for each of the modules include joint translations, axial forces, and support reactions. For the frame modules, additional output includes joint rotations, shear force, and bending moment at the end of each member. The 3D frame module also calculates twisting moments.

There is some error trapping built into the package, so some user errors can be corrected on the spot and the program resumes operation from that point. However, some errors, including errors made while inputting data from the keyboard, result in abrupt termination of package operation. When this happens, the user must start the program all over again.

Users are invited to contact the package vendor by mail or telephone for help in handling any problems or errors that continue to puzzle them.

FRAME80

This package is for analysis of plane frame structures with joints, members, and supports. Up to 99 load cases and 99 combinations of those cases can be applied.

Frame80 runs on IBM/PC and compatible computers and on CP/M computers. It sells for $1200 from DiscoTech, 600 B Street, P.O. Box 1659, Santa Rosa, CA 95402 [(707) 523-1600].

Users are advised to make a hand sketch of the structure before using the computer. From this sketch, the number of joints, members, and supports, should be counted, since these are required initial inputs to the package. Users must number the joints, and the way these numbers are assigned can affect the speed and efficiency with which the package will reach a solution.

Data are entered from the keyboard in response to screen-displayed queries. The package asks for each joint by number, and it is specified by keying in x- and y-coordinates, separated by commas. The package also has a feature that will automatically generate these data for a sequence of joints, provided they are in a straight line and equidistant from one another.

Member data are entered in a similar way, but there are more items to enter for each member. The user must give the numbers of the joints at each end of the member, the cross-section area, moment of inertia, and a code (users must memorize the four alternative codes) that indicates which ends are rigid or pinned. As with joints, members can be automatically generated; for this they have to be identical and sequentially numbered.

To aid further in entering member data, there is a "same as" feature that allows data for the current member to be copied from those for a previously entered member. The package automatically calculates member lengths from the node coordinates.

Data for supports are entered, one support at a time, indicating whether they are free to move in the x- and y-directions and to rotate.

Error checks and correction

As the data for each item are entered, the package will check for such conditions as use of valid numbers for member end joints and non-zero member length. If erroneous data are found, the package will not go on to the next node or member but will wait for the user to reenter correct data for the current item.

There seems to be no means to correct data items until all are entered. Then joint, member, and support data can be viewed and printed to locate any errors. An editing mode allows users to call for items by number and change them one by one.

Load cases and combinations

When the structure description data are complete, the user goes on to enter load data. The procedure is similar to those already described. Member loads (uniformly distributed, point, and moment) are entered for the first load case, then nodal loads. This process is repeated for each load case. The completed load data can be viewed and printed for correction; then an editing mode can be used, as with joint, member, and support data.

Up to 99 cases can be entered; and these can then be assembled into up to 99 combinations of load cases, with factors applied to the constituent load cases. Thus, if one load case represents a wind load and another a dead load, the two can be combined so the total, is say, 0.8 wind + 1.2 dead.

Fixed output

An analysis can be run for a structure with any desired load combination. Results can be displayed or printed, giving member forces and support reactions. A load summation is also given, checking applied loads against calculated reactions. Large differences here indicate calculation accuracy problems.

ICON 2D

The Icon 2D package provides for the use of prismatic, tapered, and curved beams as members, as well as for beams with rigid offset joints and shear beams.

Smaller structures are analyzed by rapid processing within the computer main memory, but very large structures can also be handled. The processing takes longer, since it transfers chunks of the problem from disk to main memory for solution.

Icon 2D runs on IBM/PC/XT computers and on HP 86 and 87 computers. The package sells for $695. A 3D version is available for $895. An added graphics program, used to view deformed shapes and other output, sells for $195. An added input program that replicates data and geometries also sells for $195.

The package is available from Advanced Structural Technology Inc., P.O. Box 16659, Clayton, MO 63105 [(314) 725-8282].

The user works from a sketch of the structure to be analyzed, entering data for each member and its end nodes, one member at a time. If all the members are of the same type, have the same moment of inertia and elastic modulus, and the same shear form factor, then the user will have only to enter this information once and it will automatically be applied to all. Otherwise, it will be necessary to enter separate data for each member. For curved members, the user must supply a radius of curvature. Nodes with rigid reactions, inclined supports, translational or rotational freedom, elastic support (with spring stiffness specified), must all be identified by the user in response to screen displayed questions.

For each load case the user provides the locations of the loads, with orientation angle and magnitude of the moment for point loads at the nodes. For loads on the members, orientation and magnitude must be given for running loads, and location and magnitude for point loads.

An added-cost input program allows the user automatically to replicate input data and generate data for repetitive geometries. There is also an input option that allows files in the format used by the mainframe finite element program STRUDL to be used as input to Icon 2D.

To verify the accuracy of the input, a graphical display of the geometry can be viewed. Graphical display of the output, deformed geometry can also be viewed, along with graphs of applied loadings, global moment and shear, with the help of an added program.

Sets of input data can be stored in files and called upon when a problem is to be run. Once retrieved, this information can be edited, using the display screen and keyboard, to modify the input data as desired. This minimizes input effort when the same structure is to be analyzed numerous times with only minor changes from one run to another.

The output provides data on nodal displacements, member end forces, and support or spring reactions. A post processing routine will locate maximum and minimum values of bending moment and shear for each member. These will be shown as overall values and also at 11 equally spaced points along the member.

The output can be produced without units or with the user's selection from six different choices of unit types. There are no automatic checks in the package for consistency of use of the units; the choice affects only the labels on the output. The extent to which they truly represent the quantities shown is the user's responsibility.

MSAP4

The MSAP4 package is designed for analyzing static equilibrium problems for structures consisting of beam and truss elements. For those who want to get into finite element analysis with a low-priced package, MSAP4 may have some attraction. It is bare bones in that no interactive input capability exists, no graphics are provided, and the available element types are limited.

MSAP4 sells for $295. It runs on the IBM/PC and compatible computers. Required equipment includes 256K main memory, a printer, and at least two floppy disks. Use of a hard disk is recommended. The package is available from Syscon Computers, 1609 Bridge Ave., Northport, AL 35476 [(205) 339-8241].

MSAP4 is derived from the SAP IV program which was developed at the University of California, Berkeley, by Edward Wilson. SAP IV is in the public domain (not copyrighted) and has been a very popular piece of software. It was turned over to a user group that added preprocessor and postprocessor capabilities and now markets it for use with mainframes and minicomputers.

MSAP4 solves static problems. It is strictly for small deformation linear elastic analysis. The continuum elements of SAP IV have been removed and there is no dynamics capability.

The package uses a disk-based solution process in which the size of the problems that can be solved is limited by the amount of disk storage available. Single-precision arithmetic is used, and the practical limit on nodes is 400–500. Roundoff errors limit the size of problems that can be solved, producing answers that are increasingly inaccurate for larger problems.

Elements available with the package are a 3D beam and a truss element.

Flexible loading capability

The assumption in the package is the usual one, that the loading applied to the members of a structure will always be in the principal planes of inertia. To identify a beam, the user has to suitably specify the principal planes of inertia.

Loads may be at the nodes or upon the elements. There can be concentrated loads, couples, distributed loads, and linearly varying (ramp) loads. The package has a provision for general transverse in-span loading involving combinations of couples and concentrated forces.

Output parameters include nodal displacements and member end forces. At the end of each member are two transverse loads, an axial load, and two bending moments.

There is no interactive input. The user prepares a batch data file, which can be in column format. And a considerable amount of input may be involved. For example, it is a 3D package, so users have to provide the orientation of the principal axes of the beam elements (not needed in a 2D program).

MSAP4 does have a node generation capability. Successive nodes can be generated along a line. And it provides storage for input material. The user can specify and store material property sets. To specify any given element later, one of those stored sets can be identified with it.

The package has no graphics capability, and there is no built-in checking of the input data. Since the package is derived from SAP IV, transfers to and from larger machines can be done relatively easily.

According to the vendor, a user who had been exposed to similar software would have little difficulty in learning to use the package. A bright person should be able to start solving problems within a few days.

Inquiries about user problems are responded to on the telephone, but it is preferred that printed input and results be sent through the mail for troubleshooting.

P-FRAME

P-Frame analyzes two-dimensional structural systems like trusses, frames, beams, arches, or rings. Up to 99 load combinations and 99 load cases can be handled. Stiffness matrix finite lement analysis is the computational technique used by the package. Structures with up to 960 members, 480 joints, 100 springs (elastic restraints), and 50 sections can be analyzed. The package is said to be able to process a frame with 250 members and three load cases in under 3 minutes.

The package runs on IBM/PC and XT computers with a minimum of 192,000 bytes of main memory (640 thousand bytes is needed to take advantage of the maximum analysis parameters mentioned above). A color-graphics adapter is also needed.

P-Frame sells for $1395, and there is an annual fee of $140 for maintenance and updating services. It is produced by Softek Services In Vancouver, Canada, and is available in the United States from ECOM Associates, 8634 West Brown Deer Rd., Milwaukee, WI 53224 [(414) 354-0243].

As with most finite element analysis packages, the major task the user faces with P-Frame is to input the needed data. To get started, the user is asked to enter some initializing data. In order to get these data, the user must first sketch out, on paper, the details of the structure that is to be analyzed. From this sketch the number of members, nodes, sections, and elastic support "springs" are counted and the totals are entered. The user must also enter the number of load cases to be analyzed, the Young's and the shear modulus of elasticity to be used, and indicate whether metric or imperial units are to be used.

A spreadsheet (row and column) format is used to input most of the data needed to describe a structure that is intended for analysis. What this amounts to is that the data are entered into screen-displayed tables. There are tables to be filled out with data on members, joints, member properties, connectivity, and loading. Several single-key commands are used to make this process easier, including replication and generation commands that allow the user to quickly insert repetitive or sequential data. The user can maneuver within a displayed table, making entries and corrections as desired before entering the entire table for processing.

Truss structure geometries and distributed loads can be automatically generated. The user inputs just a few parameters, and the rest comes from a stored library of patterns that is part of the package.

In the member property table, users must enter cross-sectional areas and moment of inertia of the members. If calculation of shear deflection is desired, shear area must also be entered. All members and joints are numbered; the connectivity data indicate the way they are connected to one another. Curved and tapered members are represented by breaking them down into small segments connected by "fictitious" joints.

The input process is aided by a number of internal logical checks including those on the number of members and joints used and data missing or improperly entered. Deformed and undeformed graphical displays can be shown to provide visual checks of loading effects and of correct data input. The deformed shape can be magnified if the user wishes, and there are zoom and windowing capabilities, but members are ordinarily displayed to scale. Axial forces, shear forces, and bending moments can also be displayed graphically.

When all the needed inputs have been entered, the package proceeds to analyze the structure. Since this may take several minutes, screen displayed messages inform the user of the progress of these calculations. The output data include displacements and rotations at each joint for each load case, deflections and internal forces at each end of each member for each load case, and the reactions at each support joint for each load case.

PolEm: POLE EMBEDMENT DESIGN

This package calculates embedment depths up to 12 feet, for laterally loaded poles.

PolEm runs on IBM/PC and compatible computers, and on CP/M computers. It sells for $80 from DiscoTech, 600 B Street, P.O. Box 1659, Santa Rosa, CA 95402 [(707) 523-1600].

Like other packages from this vendor, entry of data into this package is facilitated by 10 keyboard commands that allow the user to position the display cursor, add, and delete characters, and maneuver around the display screen.

PolEm presents the user with a display with eight items that are to be filled in to describe the pole that is being used. When these are entered, the package calculates an embedment depth.

The calculation formulas are taken from the 1979 Uniform Building Code. An iterative solution is used for unconstrained poles. Since depths greater than 12 feet are not compatible with the UBC formulas, the package will display a warning message when the calculated result exceeds 12 feet.

SD-1: STEEL BEAM DESIGN

This package designs and checks steel W, S, and Channel sections. Traverse loads and end moments can be applied. It determines maximum moments, reactions, stress ratios, and the ratio of actual working load maximum shear stress to AISC-allowable shear stress.

SD-1 runs on IBM/PC and compatible computers, HP 9816, 9845, 85, 86, and 87 computers, and CP/M computers. It sells for $325 from ECOM Associates, 8634 West Brown Deer Rd., Milwaukee, WI 53224 [(414) 354-0243].

Users can choose, at the beginning of each run, to do design. In that case the package will choose the lightest section for a user-specified depth. Or users can choose to use the package for checking. In that case, it will verify a specified section for its adequacy.

The package comes with built-in files containing data on W6 through W36 sections normally used as beams, and also on C and S shapes.

Data can be input from the keyboard or taken from the results of the vendor's FA-3 Plane Frame and Truss Analysis package. A special data transfer package (DF-3, $300) is used for this purpose.

Keyboard data input is in response to screen-displayed queries. In all, depending on the kind of run and user options, there may be as many as 25 or 30 such queries and replies. There is little room for error in these entries once the user presses the Return key. The package will simply proceed to do its calculations when the last required entry has been made. If there have been mistakes in the entries, the answer will be wrong and the user can begin all over again.

The package designs one span at a time, with up to eight lateral braced points for a span. Loads can be applied up to a maximum that causes nine steps or slope changes in the shear diagram. Cantilever sections are not designed by this package, but cantilever loads can be included at either end of a span.

SD-2: STEEL COLUMN AND BASE PLATE DESIGN

This package designs and checks W-shape steel sections subjected to axial loads. Bending moment about the x- and y-axes can also be applied. The lightest W-shape for any desired depth section is selected.

There is also a calculation to design "pin-ended" base plates. Users can specify either the desired length or width of these base plates.

SD-2 runs on IBM/PC and compatible computers, HP 9816, 9845, 85, 86, and 87 computers, and CP/M computers. It sells for $425 from ECOM Associates, 8634 West Brown Deer Rd., Milwaukee, WI 53224 [(414) 354-0243].

This package comes with stored data on the W6 through W36 sections normally used as columns. Like some other packages from the same vendor, this one operates through a long sequence of screen-displayed queries to which users respond. This package does have two error correction pauses in the column design sequence. After four keyboard data entry queries, the user is asked if there are any errors. If the answer is yes, the program goes back to the first data query. There is a similar correction pause seven queries later, just before the package begins calculating its results.

Column data can be input from the keyboard, or taken from the results of the vendor's FA-3 Plane Frame and Truss Analysis package. A special data transfer package (DF-3, $300) is used for this purpose.

The base plate design procedure is not so flexible. Here the user must go through the entire sequence of about a dozen steps; the package then does its calculations. If any inputting mistakes have been made, the user has to start over again from the beginning.

The column design portion of the package selects the lightest section that satisfies equations 1.6-1A, 1.6-1B, or 1.6-2 of the AISC Specification for Design, Fabrication and Erection of Structural Steel for Buildings (Nov. 1978).

SD-2A: STEEL TUBE AND PIPE COLUMN DESIGN

This package can be used to design or check steel tube and pipe sections subjected to axial loads and bending moments. It will select the lightest tube or pipe for a desired tube dimension or pipe diameter.

SD-2A runs on IBM/PC and compatible computers, HP 85, 86, and 87 computers, and CP/M computers. It sells for $375 from ECOM Associates, 8634 West Brown Deer Rd., Milwaukee, WI 53224 [(414) 354-0243].

Like some other packages from this vendor, the operation of this one proceeds through a sequence of screen displayed queries to which the user responds by keyboard actions.

Data can be input from the keyboard or taken from the results of the vendor's FA-3 Plane Frame and Truss Analysis package. A special data transfer package (DF-3, $300) is used for this purpose.

Keyboard data input follows short sequences of queries and replies; then the package asks the user if there have been any errors. If so, it will return to the beginning of the sequence for reentry of the data.

When the needed data have been entered, the user can choose to have the package calculate a design for a specific tube or pipe depth, or for the lightest useable section, or to go on to the base plate design portion of the package where it selects base plates large enough to accommodate anchor bolts.

The package comes with stored data on pipe sections 1-inch and larger in diameter, and on all square and rectangular tubes three-inches or larger listed in the AISC Manual of Construction (Eighth Edition).

S/SAM

This package analyzes 2D and 3D truss and frame structures. Loads may be concentrated forces and moments at the nodes, temperature variations between members, or displacements and rotations of nodes. Results consist of node translations and rotations, member forces, moments, and stresses.

S/SAM runs on Apple II+,IIe, IBM/PC/XT, and compatible computers. It sells for $385 from Kern International, 433 Washington St., P.O. Box 1029, Duxbury, MA 02331.

Users of this package are expected to be minimally familiar with the operation of their computers. The package actually consists of 8 separate programs. To use any one of these, and they must be used one after another to do structural analyses, users have to load that program, then run it.

Users also have to access several files in the course of running a typical problem. Thus there will be a file for the model of the structure, and another for each load case. There is also a file for properties of up to 10 materials (five sets of material properties come with the package), and for beam cross-section dimensions. And results are stored in their own file. Users are expected to be able to copy and tranfer files from one disk to another to facilitate package operation.

Entering node and member data

Program functions are accessed through menu displays. For example, the MODEL program, used to set up a data file describing a structure, has menu choices for adding and removing nodes and members, defining member properties, applying restraints, and filing and printing the data.

Users must assign numbers to each node and member. These are used to select nodes for removal. To keep track, users will want to work from a hand-drawn sketch of the structure. A copy option is provided to easily apply the same properties or restraints to several members or nodes.

Loads are defined for each node and member where they exist. Uniform loads must be approximated by applying equivalent loads at joints. Although force-moment, displacement, and thermal loads can all be applied, only one type can be used for any single solution run. To get combined effects of different types of loads, the results of two or three runs are summed, using the PRINT program.

Rotated plots

The VIEW program is used to display models. Three-dimensional plots of deflected or undeflected structures can be rotated for better viewing, and both can be displayed together.

The package uses the stiffness method. It solves problems with up to 180 active degrees of freedom. For example, it can handle a truss structure with up to 90 unrestrained nodes (two degrees of freedom per node), or a 3D frame with 30 nodes (six degrees of freedom per node). Memory limitations restrict structures to 150 members and 151 nodes with 128K computer main memory.

The solution process is a relatively slow one, and larger problems can take hours to solve. If the package is compiled by the user and put into machine language form, it can be expected to run faster and even accommodate larger structures. Outputs include node displacements (translations and rotations), member forces, and moments.

To do a stress analysis, the STRS program must be run. One of the inputs to this program is member cross sections. The package allows use of just five cross-section shapes, and users can set up 50 cross-section descriptions involving different dimensions for these shapes. The STRS program calculates section properties from these descriptions.

Clear manual

The user manual for this package is a model of clarity. It is well organized and very well written. However, it does lack specific operating instructions for using the various menu options, and there is no index.

STRESSPAC

There are seven different programs in this package. BEAM1 finds deflections and stresses in beams with step changes in cross section. CONTACT finds the contact stress and factor of safety for contact between spheres, sockets, cylinders, grooves, and planes. CURBEAM calculates bending, axial stress, and factor of safety for beams with various cross-section shapes. PORTFORM finds stresses and displacements for portal frames. RPLATE calculates deflections and stresses in thin rectangular plates. SST calculates principal stresses given strains (or vice-versa) for isotropic materials. THICKWL calculates stresses in pressurized cylinders

STRESSPAC runs on IBM/PC and compatible computers. It sells for $250 from Engineering Software Company, 3 Northpark E. #901, 8800 N. Central Expressway, Dallas, TX 75231 [(817) 261-2263].

Data entry for the programs in this package is done on full-screen displays. Using cursor-positioning arrows and other keys, users write data onto the display, erasing and changing it as needed.

Any screen of data can be stored in a disk file and retrieved for use as needed. The main menu for this package is displayed across the bottom of each such display screen. It offers users the option of accessing the files, calculating results, printing the display, erasing it, or quitting the package.

The package seems quite simple and convenient to operate. In each case the calculations seem to be rapid, and the output is conveniently displayed.

The user manual consists mainly of an example of each of the seven programs. The vendor has relied on these and on the package displays to be self-explanatory. They are not, and users will wish that the manual also included specific explanation of the procedures to be used with each program. The manual also lacks explanations of the calculation methods used and of the analysis limitations users need to be aware of when running these calculations.

TRUSILPC

This package calculates influence lines for the member forces in a plane truss. These are useful for calculating maximum member forces that can be produced by moving loads.

TRUSILPC runs on IBM/PC and compatible computers. It sells for $149 from Structural Software Systems, 4440 Gateway Dr., Monroeville, PA 15146 [(412) 325-4117].

The input to this package is handled in much the same way as that for the FATPAK package from the same vendor. Data can be keyboarded in response to screen inquiries or can be fed in from previously created files. Comments on the limitations of this type of input made in the description of FATPAK apply here as well.

On computers equipped with graphics capabilities, users can view the geometry of the trusses they input as well as a plot of each influence line that is generated.

Like FATPAK, this package performs all calculations in single-precision arithmetic. It uses the stiffness method to find its results, and computations can be be lengthy, running many minutes for larger structures with several hundred members and joints.

TRUSILPC comes with a sample data file that can be used to check out the operation of the package.

Once influence lines have been calculated for a given structure, the users can calculate alternative load cases with greatly reduced computation time.

USA-STRESS

This package is designed to analyze statically loaded trusses, continuous beams, and plane frames. Outputs include calculated forces, moments, and displacements.

USA-STRESS runs on IBM/PC, CP/M, and TRS-80 computers. It sells for $500 from Universal Software Applications, 13001 Cannes, St. Louis, MO 63141 [(314) 878-1277].

Users are advised to start by making a hand sketch of the structure they wish to analyze, and to use this sketch to determine the coordinates of the joints, to number the members, and to set up loading arrangements.

When the package is started up, a main menu is displayed that gives the user a choice of creating/editing an input file, of running calculations, or of ending the session.

Data entry by your command

From that point on the user is prompted to enter commands, and these control the data entry process. For example, the JOC command calls up a series of six queries to elicit data for a joint; the MEI command calls up a series of 8 queries on data for a member. If the structure has 48 members, the MEI command must be given 48 times.

The package accumulates these commands, and the data entered with them, in a program-statement list. To delete a joint or member or load from this list, the user steps or scrolls through it. When the proper item is reached, it can be deleted by keyboard action. Additions are made in a similar manner.

There is a prescribed order for the items in this list: general structural data first, then joint data starting with joint #1, then member data and load data. The way to tell if everything is in order is to scroll through the list observing whether the correct commands appear in the right order.

Formatted output

Data files can be stored and retrieved for use as needed. Once such a file is ready, the package will use it for computation when the user makes the main menu choice to run the material.

The package uses the stiffness method to calculate its results. Inputs and results are in the form of numbers without units. It is up to the users to see to it that the units for quantities in the input data are consistent, and to figure out the units that should be applied to output quantities. The output appears in a fixed format display or printout .

All this is explained in the user's manual, which restricts itself to rather minimal exposition of how to use the package but provides no insight on the calculation methods used and their limitations. There is no advice on the best ways to number joints and members. There are no explanations of error messages nor is there an index.

Chapter 4
Hydrology Design Packages

The software packages discussed in this chapter are designed to deal with problems related to flow and drainage. Some are specifically for the analysis of flow through pipes and channels. Others are focused on analysis of drainage and runoff in storm sewers and drainage basins. A number of the packages are specifically concerned with the calculation and routing of hydrographs. Finally, there are a few packages that deal with flood prediction and analysis.

Flow through pipes and channels

The HYDRAL package is for design and evaluation of open channels. It can be used for design of storm drains, sanitary sewers, canals, flood channels, and spillways. Like many hydrology packages, this one comes with multiple capabilities, allowing the user to analyze floodplains, bridge hydraulics, tailwater, flow over roadways or dam crests, and to make discharge computations from high water marks.

HYDROPAK is another multiple-use package that includes five different hydrology modules. One of these, called CHANNEL, performs a normal depth analysis on a variety of different channel shapes.

The WATERFLO/PLUS package calculates water surface profiles for flow through a natural channel such as a river or stream. The calculations are valid only for tranquil (subcritical) flow. However, the package is designed to take account of the effects of bridges and culverts, and there is an encroachment feature to assess the effects of levees and fill areas.

Two of the four modules in the Hydraulics Package are concerned with channel flow. The HYDROL module includes procedures for routing through pipes and streets, natural mountains and valleys, and designated channels. PBACK uses the standard step method to analyze backwater curves in circular conduits flowing partially full. The TBACK module uses the same method to develop backwater curves for trapezoidal, triangular, or rectangular open channels.

Flow in both full and partially full pipes can be analyzed with the help of the SDNET package, and minor losses and headwater effects can be included.

Analysis of drainage and runoff

The Hydraulics Package has already been mentioned. The HYDRAU module in this package performs loss analysis at junctions in a storm drain system as well as pipe hydraulics analyses for the various reaches of the system.

The USA-STORM package is also concerned with analysis of sewer systems. This package calculates hydraulic properties for pipe culverts, box culverts, and open ditches for systems with up to 100 separate reaches.

The HYDRO PLUS III package analyzes drainage systems and produces storm water detention reports.

Calculation and Routing of Hydrographs

Several of the packages discussed in this chapter can generate and route hydrographs. One of the most capable seems to be HYDROSIM, a package designed to model drainage basins. It can calculate and use up to 145 hydrographs with combinations of subareas, channels, diversions, reservoirs, and inflows.

Two of the five modules included in the HYDROPAK package have related applications. The HYDROGRAPH module calculates basin and unit hydrographs, and the RESERVOIR ROUTING module takes a hydrograph and routes it through a reservoir.

Flood prediction and analysis

Two of the remaining HYDROPAK modules are specifically concerned with floods. The USGS REGRESSION EQUATIONS module is used to calculate flood flows for basins in different states and areas. And the STREAMFLOW GAGE ANALYSIS module analyzes yearly peak flood data to determine the flood peak for any interval greater than a year.

A statistical analysis technique is used by the FFAN package to calculate flood frequency. The method is taken from a 1981 U.S. Water Resources Council Report.

Designed for use by state and local government units that need to predict

the effects of bridges and culverts on the flood profile within their jurisdictions, the HOBCW package calculates the backwater effects of culverts
and bridges.

Exemplary data entry

Although the packages discussed in this chapter seem to be competent as
far as their calculation capabilities are concerned, most of them are poorly
designed when it comes to easing the tasks of potential package users.

Almost invariably, the main user task is to enter the often extensive
amounts of data that are needed for the calculations these packages perform. One package that handles this task in an exemplary fashion is
SDNET.

Data entry into SDNET is made on full-screen display forms. As the user
completes each entry on the form, the cursor moves on to the next entry
position. When the entries on a screen are complete, the user can review
them and make changes before entering the entire screen.

Working from a hand sketch of a pipe network, the SDNET user consecutively numbers each pipe and node, then keys in the total number of
pipes. A data entry screen is then displayed for the first pipe in the system,
and the user enters upper and lower node numbers, length, diameter, flow,
and Manning number for that pipe. Similar screens are then filled out for
each of the other pipes in the system. Node data are entered on a similar
set of screens. This system allows not only for orderly entry of large amounts
of data but for easy checking as well.

Other input methods

Other packages fall short in data entry procedures, using a variety of
unsatisfactory methods. For example, the HOBCW package is an adaptation of a large computer program, and it accepts input as if it were punched
on computer cards. As in most situations where this kind of input is used,
a rigidly defined and demanding format has to be followed.

The Hydraulics Package divides up the input into sections, each consisting of a series of displayed comments, prompts, and user entries. At the
end of a section, the user can indicate that material from that section was
incorrectly entered and can recycle through the section. However, if a user
should make an incorrect entry and pass the section check point, there seems
to be no way to correct the data, so the entire program must be restarted
from the beginning. This approach is fine for those who make few mistakes
in their data entry, but not many of us are so gifted.

With the USA-STORM package, instructions for data entry are followed by the entries themselves, all packed onto adjacent lines of displayed text in capital letters. The screen display is difficult to read and seems to have been set up with little thought for ease of entry or for checking the accuracy of the entries.

The main task for the user of the WATERFLO package is to enter data describing the cross sections of a channel. This input is done from the keyboard in response to sequences of screen-displayed queries. Unfortunately, the instructions in the manual for this package tend to get a bit vague. Thus, the user is told to enter data pairs for all the points in a natural cross section, but is not told what spacing or punctuation to use during this keyboard entry process. And the explanation for entering Manning's n values and corresponding ground points seems to be completely incomprehensible.

Built-in data

With the disk storage capacity offered by personal computers, it is feasible to provide users with direct access to the kind of data found in manuals and handbooks. Most of the packages discussed in this chapter do not seem to have taken advantage of this capability. One exception is the HYDRO-PAK package. SCS standard storm data for 6- and for 24-hour storms come as part of this package.

Calculation aids

Well-designed software generally offers users some shortcut procedures that take advantage of the computer's capabilities. For example, HYDRO PLUS III facilitates repeat calculations with revised parameters. It allows users to quickly revise the basin area, curve number, 24-hour precipitation, or basin lag and then get a recalculated hydrograph.

In some cases, the packages offer users a choice of several different computation methods. Thus for the subarea component of the model, the HYDROSIM package allows use of either the SCS Dimensionless Unit Hydrograph, a user-supplied hydrograph, or a kinematic wave computation. Unfortunately, the manual provides no hints on the relative merits of these choices.

For friction slope calculations, the WATERFLO user is given a choice of four different methods. In this case, the manual provides a reference that discusses the merits of each of these methods. This package even allows different calculation methods to be applied to different cross sections.

Output formats

Even the most perfect calculations must often be presented in a form that can be understood at a later time and by persons other than the one who ran the computer. The printed reports produced by the packages discussed here seem largely to ignore this need for clear communication. Most of the printed results seem designed to conserve paper but make it difficult to interpret the results they present, unless the reader is thoroughly familiar with the formats and abbreviations that are used.

Documentation

User manuals for these packages are, for the most part, neither well written nor thoughtfully designed. In the case of such packages as FFAN, users must rely almost entirely on screen-displayed instructions and formats. The vendor has apparently decided to eliminate most of the work and expense involved in putting together detailed user instructions in printed form.

DRAINCALC

This package generates hydrographs using the Soil Conservation Service method. It will also route hydrographs through circular pipes and trapezoidal or rectangular channels. The package can handle up to 30 reaches, generating outflow hydrographs and calculating velocities and storage values for various depths of flow in each reach.

DRAINCALC also does detention pond routing using the Storage-Indication method. For outflow control devices, the user has a choice of V-notched or rectangular weirs, circular or rectangular submerged orifices, or circular or rectangular culverts. The package can handle up to 10 detention ponds.

The package can do hydrograph addition so that subcatchments, reaches, and detention ponds can be added to one another. It will also plot hydrographs.

Draincalc runs on Apple, IBM/PC, TRS-80, and CP/M computers. It sells for $1500 from Hydro Systems, 48 Robin Hood Rd., Arlington, MA 02174. [(617) 683-2662.]

FFAN: FLOOD FREQUENCY ANALYSIS

FFAN uses a statistical analysis technique to calculate flood frequency. The method is taken from a 1981 U.S. Water Resources Council Report.

The package runs on IBM/PC/XT/AT and compatible computers. It sells for $225,or $275 for a version with graphics display of results. The vendor is Hydrasoft, P.O. Box 194, American Fork, UT 84003. [(801) 756-8313.]

The user of this package must rely almost entirely on screen-displayed instructions and formats in order to enter the necessary data and to obtain desired results. The vendor has decided to eliminate most of the work and expense involved in putting together detailed user instructions in printed form. Instead, the manual presents a brief description and commentary on the formulas used for calculation. It also provides a list of error and cautionary messages with a brief explanation for each. And sample printouts of results are given without explanation.

When it comes to running the package, the user is told that input will be done on "page" displays, and that there are seven keyboard commands that can be used to move from page to page or mode to mode. Beyond that, users are pretty much on their own.

HOBCW: HYDRAULICS OF BRIDGE AND CULVERT WATERWAYS

HOBCW calculates the backwater effects of culverts and bridges. It is designed for use by state and local government units that need to predict the effects of bridges and culverts on the flood profile within their jurisdictions.

HOBCW runs on IBM/PC/XT/AT, Compaq, and Corona computers. It sells for $200 from Galileo Software, 226 Buell St., Madison, WI 53704 [(608) 244-6062.]

This package is an adaptation of a large computer program, and it accepts input as if it were punched on computer cards. Data entry is first set up, with the help of the user's own word processing package, in an input file. This file can then be read into HOBCW and run to produce answers.

As in most situations where this kind of input is used, a rigidly defined format has to be followed. Data must appear in eight-character units, starting on columns 9, 17, 25, and so forth. If any of the data units happen to be shorter than eight characters, they have to be filled out with spaces. Users have to be careful with their punctuation, since stray commas and misplaced decimal points will cause incorrect output.

Most of the user's manual is taken up with detailed instructions on how to set up this input. The vendor advises that "HOBCW is unfortunately not the easiest progam to use" and backs up this candor with a phone number which users can call for any advice they may need.

The calculation method is based on a U.S. Department of Commerce Bureau of Public Roads publication, "Hydraulics of Bridge Waterways," by Joseph N. Bradley (1973), and the U.S. Department of Transportation, Federal Highway Administration publication, "Hydraulic Charts for the Selection of Highway Culverts" (1961).

HYDRAL · OPEN CHANNEL HYDRAULICS

HYDRAL is for design and evaluation of open channels and can be used for design of storm drains, sanitary sewers, canals, flood channels, and spillways, for analysis of floodplains, bridge hydraulics, tailwater, flow over roadways or dam crests, and to make discharge computations from high water marks.

The package runs on IBM/PC/XT/AT computers. It sells for $145 from HYDRASOFT, PO Box 194, American Fork, UT 84003 [(801) 756-8313.]

Two equations are used for the calculations. Manning's equation is used for uniform flow conditions, and there is also an equation for critical flow conditions. These calculations do not meet all conditions, so the limitations of the package must be kept in mind by users. There are some assumptions in the design method that must be kept in mind. Areas in channels that are below the water surface, but do not actually carry flow, must be deleted from the user's input cross-section description, and some user ingenuity must be exercised to describe complex channel cross sections.

As with other packages from this vendor, the user manual is very brief and sketchy, giving mainly the error and caution messages and some sample output. Users are advised to rely on the package itself to explain, through its screen displays, how it is to be used.

HYDRAULICS PACKAGE

This package includes four separate programs. HYDRAU is for design of storm drain systems. HYDROL calculates storm runoffs. TBACK develops backwater curves for open channels. PBACK calculates similar curves for circular conduits flowing partially full.

The Hydraulics Package sells for $395 from First Principles Software, 1110 Holly Ave., Rohnert Park, CA 94928 [(707) 584-0321].

The programs in this package operate in a serial mode that runs from the beginning through displayed comments and prompts to printout of the results. Along the way, at section intervals, the user can indicate that material from that section was incorrectly entered and can recycle through the section. If a user should make an incorrect entry and pass the section check point, there seems to be no way to correct the data and the entire program must be restarted from the beginning. This approach is fine for those who make few mistakes in their data entry, but sloppy typists beware. You may find yourself doing the same lengthy input procedure over and over again.

Storm drain system analysis

HYDRAU performs loss analysis at junctions in a storm drain system as well as pipe hydraulics analyses for the various reaches of the system. Either one or two flow rates can be calculated in a single analysis. Thus the effects of a 10-year and 100-year storm frequency can be calculated in the same analysis.

The package does some immediate calculation during the data entry process. Thus after the user enters the pipe diameter and length and flow rate, calculated values for velocity, velocity head, and friction slope will be displayed. When the user enters the energy grade line, and the exit, entrance, and junction loss figures, the package will calculate the friction loss and velocity head and new energy and hydraulic grade lines.

At the end of the program input run, the results that have been displayed along the way are repeated in printed form.

Channel flow analysis

HYDROL uses formulas for channel flow developed by M. Hudis and Associates. It includes procedures for routing through pipes and streets, natural mountains and valleys, and designated channels. Up to three storms can be analyzed in a single run; the storms are described by two user-supplied constants in an intensity vs. time equation.

When the input process is completed, the package displays all the input data along with computed times, intensities, flow rates, velocities, and, where appropriate, depths of flows.

Flow in conduits and channels

PBACK performs an iterative calculation using the standard step method for backwater curves in circular conduits flowing partially full. Slopes can be mild, steep, or adverse.

The program solves for normal and critical depths and advises the user of the slope condition. Velocities at each section and percent change in velocity between sections are also calculated. If the change exceeds 20 percent, a warning message is displayed. If the water level in a pipe exceeds 0.8`of the diameter, another warning message will be displayed, and full-pipe analysis is recommended.

TBACK uses the standard step method to develop backwater curves for trapezoidal, triangular, or rectangular open channels. It solves for normal and critical depths and notifies the user whether the slope condition is mild, steep, or critical. Velocities at each section and percent change in velocity between sections are also calculated. In addition, pressure plus momentum is calculated at each reach to help the user locate hydraulic jumps.

HYDROPAK

This package includes five different modules. USGS REGRESSION EQUATIONS are used to calculate flood flows for basins in different states and areas. HYDROGRAPH calculates basin and unit hydrographs. RESERVOIR ROUTING takes a hydrograph and routes it through a reservoir. STREAMFLOW GAGE ANALYSIS analyzes yearly peak flood data to determine the flood peak for any interval greater than a year. CHANNEL performs a normal depth analysis on a variety of different channel shapes.

The package runs on IBM/PC/XT/AT and compatible computers. It sells for $150 for the first module, plus $100 for each additional module. The vendor is Galileo Software, 226 Buell St., Madison, WI 53704 [(607) 244-6062].

Data are entered into these programs in response to series of screen-displayed queries. There are some points to watch; for example, use of commas in entered text such as titles can cause computation problems.

Results computed by these modules can be viewed on the screen, printed, and saved in disk storage. And graphs of the results can be displayed. Reruns with altered input data are simplified by a procedure that allows the user to edit what has been previously entered or stored.

USGS REGRESSION EQUATIONS follow methods established in USGS publications discussing estimation of floods in various states. These use regression equations developed for watersheds based on records at gaging sites within each state.

To use this module, the user selects the state of interest, and may also be asked to specify a targeted geographical area, within that state. The vendor apparently does not supply equations for every state and area, so prospective users should verify that the geography they desire is covered before they purchase this module.

Users then enter the drainage area and other parameters called for by the module on a query-and-answer basis. A graph of 2-, 5-, 10-, 25-, 50-, 100-, and, in some cases, 500-year floods can be displayed. Points from historical flow records can be checked to verify the validity of this graph.

HYDROGRAPH generates a unit hydrograph, based on certain basin hydrologic parameters. Then input rainstorm values are used with the unit hydrograph to generate a basin hydrograph.

The module calculates the unit and basin hydrographs in 5-minute increments, and the user may specify any output time interval which is a multiple of 5 minutes. It is designed for basins under 50 square miles. Results may be inaccurate for larger basins.

SCS standard storm data for 6- and for 24-hour storms are built into the module. If users want other storm lengths, they have to input their own storm data through the keyboard. This manual entry process involves some restrictions. For example, cumulative rainfall must be entered for time intervals that are evenly divisible into the overall storm length. The module may not produce accurate results for storms with duration longer than 24 hours.

Time of concentration can be calculated either by the curve number method (for smaller basins) or the upland method. Computer-stored data aid the user in selecting input for the upland method. The maximum time of concentration the module will handle is 100 hours.

RESERVOIR ROUTING routes a hydrograph through a reservoir using the storage indicator (modified Puls) method. Hydrographs calculated by the HYDROGRAPH module can be used from disk storage, or new ones can be entered through the keyboard. A stage storage discharge curve must also be inputted. This module handles storms with up to 1000 data points.

Entering data from storage is simple, but if an incorrectly-formatted file is used the module will abruptly terminate, forcing the user to restart the package from scratch. The module includes a procedure for editing the hydrograph data.

For stage storage discharge (SSD) data entry, three numbers, each in correct units, must be entered for each point. These are input in triplets. Stage and storage values must increase monotonically or the module will not accept them. Keyboarding mistakes can be corrected by using the backspace before each number is entered. Entries can also be edited in a separate procedure. Once an SSD curve has been entered, it can be saved on disk for future reuse.

STREAMFLOW GAGE ANALYSIS makes three methods available to determine flood peaks for periods of more than a year. These are the Extreme Value Type I (Gumbel) method, the Log-Pearson Type II (LP) method, and the Log-Normal (LN) method.

The module takes yearly peak flood data as input. A minimum of 10 years of data is required by the module. These data can be read from an existing disk file or entered from the keyboard, and the module provides for editing the data as well. With the LN and LP methods, historical data points can be used along with the yearly data.

The user selects the number of desired flood peaks to be calculated and the desired recurrence intervals. For the LN and LP methods, the module checks for high and low outliers. These can be deleted or retained at the user's option. For the LP method, a calculated skew is displayed, and the user can modify this if desired. Users must also provide a K value (from Bulletin 17B of the Water Resources Council) for the calculations.

CHANNEL performs normal depth analyses on triangular, rectangular, trapezoidal, circular, pipe-arch, or user-defined channel shapes. It is only for channels that are flowing free.

The user enters, in response to screen-displayed prompts, the channel slope and Manning's n-factor. The calculation can either use an input depth or a flow (the flow option is not available for pipe-arch channels). A channel geometry description is also entered. For user-defined channels, up to 50 points can be used to describe an irregular or natural configuration.

HYDRO PLUS III

This package analyzes drainage systems and produces storm water detention reports. It gives the user a choice of five different design methods.

Three of these generate inflow hydrographs and route them through storage facilities. There are also two "bowstring" methods usually used with smaller basins.

HYDRO PLUS III runs on IBM/PC and compatible computers and on HP Series 80 computers. The package sells for $2250 from Plus III Software, P.O. Box 88276, Atlanta, GA 30338 [(404) 394-5886].

A main menu gives the user access to the five design methods, to an outflow calculation routine, and to a routine that generates a rainfall data base. The basic inputs to each of the design methods are a basin area, storm frequency, either time of concentration or lag, either rainfall intensity or 24-hour precipitation, and either runoff coefficient or curve number based on ground cover.

The DEKALB COUNTY RATIONAL HYDROGRAPH method uses the hydrograph constants from the Dekalb County (Georgia) Drainage Procedures Manual. The hydrograph generation procedure consists of a series of eight screen-displayed queries for data, which the user enters from the keyboard. Drawing on a user-selected rainfall data base, stored on disk, the package then calculates a hydrograph, stores it in one of ten available "bins," and prints the results in report format.

Calculation of the runoff coefficients for a given basin area, needed for hydrograph generation, is accomplished by a separate eight-step procedure.

Provided they have been generated using the same time of concentration, a hydrograph in one bin can be combined with that in another, and the package provides a three-step query and answer procedure to accomplish this.

Storage routing is accomplished by a five-step procedure. Once a set of pond parameters has been entered, using this procedure, it can be stored, recalled from memory, and revised as needed. The continuity equation (outflow = inflow + or − storage) is solved iteratively, with intermediate values of the routing curve obtained through linear interpolation. Results are printed in tabular format, with maximum elevation, storage, and discharge identified. Graphs of inflow and outflow can also be printed. If desired, several hydrographs can be generated and routed through a single area and storage segment.

Reruns with revised data are eased by the ability to change basin area, runoff coefficient, storm frequency, and time of concentration and then immediately generate new output.

The UNIVERSAL RATIONAL HYDROGRAPH method follows virtually identical procedures but is designed to make use of data from published curves for rainfall-gauging stations throughout the United States.

For the BOWSTRING MASS STORAGE method, the user selects a rainfall data base and keys in data for runoff coefficients and impervious, landscaped, and natural areas. The package then generates a report that includes basin areas, composite runoff coefficients, and bowstring calculation sheets.

The user enters pond parameters, and the package calculates corresponding pond volumes. The pond data can be stored, retrieved, and revised by the user. These data can then be used by the package to print a storage summary.

Up to six storms can be entered, and the package will print basin areas, composite runoff coefficients, and bowstring calculation sheets for each of these. Graphs can also be printed.

Where bypass ponds are used, the BOWSTRING WITH BYPASS MASS STORAGE method is used. It follows procedures similar to those just described.

The SOIL CONSERVATION SERVICE HYDROGRAPH method follows calculations established by the U.S. Department of Agriculture Soil Conservation Service. It is for medium-size basins with areas generally between 200 and 1000 acres.

For this method, the user is provided with a routine to calculate predeveloped and developed curve numbers for a basin area. When the appropriate curve number and other basic data are entered, the package calculates input hydraulic length and input basin lag, and the user is given a chance to substitute revised values for these parameters. A hydrograph is then generated. Four storage "bins" for hydrographs are provided. Two hydrographs can be combined, provided they use the same time base.

Like the previous methods, this one provides for entering, storing, revising, and retrieving pond parameters and for routing the hydrographs through pond storage. Hydrologic reports are generated, and several hydrographs can be routed through a single area and storage segment.

To facilitate repeat calculations with revised parameters, users can revise the basin area, curve number, 24-hour precipitation, or basin lag and then get a revised hydrograph. They can also enter a new 24-hour precipitation and input storm frequency and route a revised hydrograph through a selected pond.

The FLOW RATE CALCULATION module calculates stage-discharge relationships for broad-crested vee-notch, rectangular, Cipolletti, and trapezoidal broad-crested weirs, and for circular standpipes, circular orifices, and trapezoidal channels. The calculation methods used restrict the application of the package to inlet control operation for these structures; that is, to situations where a weir is not affected by downstream conditions or a standpipe feeds into a structure with greater water carrying capacity.

To run the calculations, the user selects the desired structure, then enters several items of input data in response to screen-displayed queries. The package then prints a stage discharge curve for the selected structure.

The RAINFALL DATA BASE GENERATION module takes in user-keyboarded data and produces a stored file that can be used to calculate hydrographs. There are some restrictions on the data that can be entered. Rainfall intensities for 2-, 5-, 10-, 25-, 50-, and 100-year storm frequencies, and for 27 different times of concentration between 5 to 1440 minutes, must be used. That means a total of 162 intensity entries must be made to fill out a single rainfall file.

The package provides for entering all these values in one step. The data that have been input can be printed and proof-read. Then a separate editing step allows the user to correct any erroneous entries.

HYDROSIM: HYDROGRAPHIC SIMULATION

HYDROSIM is used to model drainage basins. It can calculate and use up to 145 hydrographs for combinations of subareas, channels, diversions, reservoirs, and inflows.

The package includes three modules. Module I ($295) performs all package functions for one stream branch (but will not retrieve a diverted hydrograph). Module II ($495) will model up to five stream branches and stores four hydrograph diversions. Module III ($595) models up to 10 branches and stores seven diversions. HYDROSIM runs on IBM/PC/XT/ AT and compatible computers. The vendor is HYDRASOFT, P.O. Box 194, American Fork, UT 84003 [(801) 756-8313].

HYDROSIM can compute a hydrograph for a subarea of a drainage basin, based on rainfall-runoff relationships. It can accept user input hydrographs, divert any portion of a hydrograph from the system, and retrieve a previously diverted hydrograph. The package can also route a hydrograph through a reservoir or detention basin or down a channel. And it can combine hydrographs from different branches at a confluence.

These capabilities can be used to model a watershed, provided it can be subdivided into stream network components. The overall conceptual procedure is to divide the drainage basin into subareas, based on the purpose of the study. The subareas are then linked using the various component capabilities of this package to form a watershed model.

To instruct users on constructing this kind of model, the manual gives a single example with a sketch of a drainage basin, together with a network model that shows a reservoir component, six subbasin runoff components, and three hydrograph combination points, all interconnected by channel routing segments.

The general procedure for the computation is to follow this model starting at the uppermost subarea in the drainage basin and following the first branch of the model down to the first combination point. Then start at the top of the next branch that goes to that combining point, and the next, until all branches that enter that point have been calculated. The inputs to the combination point are then combined, and the computation proceeds downstream to the next combination point where a similar procedure is followed. Eventually this procedure will complete calculations for all branches of the model.

Along the way, the user is required to enter a good deal of data, with somewhat different parameters for each component of the model. In general, this is the same kind of data that would be required for hand calculation of similar results. The manual does not indicate the extent to which the package is designed to facilitate this data entry, nor the extent to which the package has built-in checking provisions to help insure the accuracy of the input data.

Users are also expected to make some computation choices. For example, for the subarea component of the model, the package allows use of either the SCS Dimensionless Unit Hydrograph, a user-supplied hydrograph, or a kinematic wave computation. These design choices will probably have to be based on experimentation on the part of the user, since the manual gives no indication of what tradeoffs are involved.

Options of this kind add considerably to the flexibility of the package. Thus the user is given a choice of specifying an SCS curve number for storage loss rates or specifying an initial loss plus an infiltration rate. For the reservoir component, the package includes built-in calculations for spillways that are trapezoidal and for broad-crested weirs. For the channel routing components, trapezoidal, rectangular, triangular, or circular channels can be selected, or a table of storage-discharge data can be entered for channels with irregular cross section.

The manual gives the user no details on package procedures, relying entirely on the presumption that the software displays will be self-defining. An annotated list of error and caution messages is provided. Samples of printouts produced by the package are given. The manual has no index, presumably because it is not intended to serve the user as a reference tool for use when problems arise.

SDNET: BACKWATER CALCULATIONS IN GRAVITY-FLOW PIPE NETWORKS

This Storm Drain Network analysis package handles both full and partially full pipes. Minor losses and headwater effects can be included. The package uses an orderly and easy-to-follow entry procedure that simplifies the difficult job of correctly keyboarding extensive network data.

SDNET runs on IBM/PC and compatible computers and on CP/M computers. It sells for $375. Disco Tech Microcomputer Products, 600 B Street, P.O. Box 1659, Santa Rosa, CA 95402 [(707) 523-1600].

SDNET works from a main menu. Data entry is started by selecting the "Create New Job" option. A data entry screen is displayed and the cursor moves to the next entry position as the user completes the previous one. When the entries on a screen are complete, the user can review what has been entered and make changes before entering the entire screen.

A Minor Loss screen allows the user to select calculations for sudden enlargement or contraction, entrance, bend, angle, junction, manhole, or catch basin losses, for inclusion in the computed results.

Working with a hand sketch of the pipe network, the user consecutively numbers each pipe and node, then keys in the total number of pipes. If the Manning number for all pipes is the same, that number is then entered.

A data entry screen is then displayed for the first pipe in the system, and the user enters upper and lower node numbers, length, diameter, flow, and Manning number (if different Manning numbers are used) for that pipe. Similar screens are then filled out for each of the other pipes in the system.

When entry of pipe data is completed, a General Node Data screen is displayed. The user enters the design HGL at the low end of the system, indicates whether the entrance loss coefficient is to be constant, whether headwater is to be considered in the computations, and whether the package should check for maximum HGL at each node.

An entry screen for the first node is then displayed. The user enters the node type (round, rectangular, angle, or junction), then diameter, width, and angle, as appropriate. The node elevation is entered and, if needed, an entrance loss coefficient, maximum design HGL, and headwater value. If bend and losses are being considered, the user must enter deflection angles between pipes entering that node. A similar screen is then displayed for each of the other nodes of the network. When all the node screens have been completed, the package calculates the slopes for each pipe in the system. These can be viewed at the user's option.

The entered data are automatically stored on disk and can be retrieved as needed, by entering a user-assigned job number. Since numbers are easily forgotten, the package displays a user- entered description of the stored data to verify that the desired job is being retrieved. This is a clumsy procedure, which could have been improved by using names rather than numbers, to identify the job files.

Once retrieved, the input data can be viewed on the display screen or printed. This provides ample means for rechecking the data for errors, and if any are found, editing procedures allow the user to go to the data screen in question and make the corrections. Changes made in this way may include adding or deleting pipes from the system

When all the input data are complete and correct to the user's satisfaction, a flow analysis can be called for. During the calculation process, which may be lengthy for larger systems, the package keeps the user informed of its progress with messages. If HGL is being checked, the package will inform the user when and how much the calculated value of HGL exceeds the maximum design value at a given node. The user is then given the option of aborting or completing the calculation process.

A restriction on the systems that can be handled is that they must be simple "tree" network with a single system outlet.

USA-STORM: SEWER SYSTEM HYDRAULICS

This package calculates hydraulic properties for pipe culverts, box culverts, and open ditches for systems with up to 100 separate reaches.

USA-STORM runs on IBM/PC, TRS-80, and CP/M computers. It sells for $300 from Universal Software Applications, 13001 Cannes Dr., St. Louis, MO 63141 [(314) 878-1277].

Working from a hand sketch of the system, the user designates a new file name for the input data and then enters a description for each reach. This is done on a query-and-answer basis. Instruction text for data entry is followed by the entries themselves, all packed onto adjacent lines of displayed text in capital letters. The screen display is difficult to read and seems to have been set up with little thought for ease of entry and for checking the accuracy of the entries.

The first query asks for the type of reach (Pipe, Box, Culvert, or Ditch). Then a series of appropriate parameters are requested to describe that particular type of reach. Many of the queries ask the user to supply a string of four different parameters, and these are to be keyboarded on a line, separated by commas. This format is compact but makes it difficult to read the entries and check them.

When the user has entered data for all the reaches in the system, the command END is typed in response to the next request for a reach-type. This stores the entered data and brings up the package master menu. Stored data can be edited by deleting or adding. The data are reviewed one reach at a time. If a change is made, it involves all the data for that reach. Since only data are displayed for review, the identity of each data item may not be immediately apparent, making the checking process a potentially difficult one. There seems to be no provision for identifying a single number that needs to be changed and then making that change without reentering the other numbers that relate to that reach.

When the input data are correct to the user's satisfaction, the main menu choice of processing the data is invoked. The package then goes through its paces and turns out reports. The main report includes results for culvert and ditch slope and hydraulic capacity, runoff tributary to each inlet and quantity of flow in each culvert, depth of flow, friction loss, velocities and velocity heads, turn losses, and hydraulic grade line. All this is presented in a form that conserves paper but makes it a chore to interpret the numbers that appear. A separate report shows calculated backwater results in the form of lists of distances upstream with corresponding water surface elevations for each reach.

WATERFLO/PLUS

This package calculates water surface profiles for flow through a natural channel such as a river or stream. The calculations are valid only for tranquil (subcritical) flow. However, the package is designed to take account of the effects of bridges and culverts. And there is an encroachment feature to assess the effects of levees and fill areas.

WATERFLO/PLUS runs on IBM/PC and compatible computers and on HP 86, 87, 9816, and 9836 computers. It sells for $2000 from Plus III Software, 4380 Georgetown Square #1018, Atlanta, GA 30338 [(404) 451-5358].

The main task for the user of this package is to enter data describing the cross sections of the channel. This input is done from the keyboard in response to sequences of screen-displayed queries.

Sections may be natural or for a bridge or a culvert. In each case the queries will call for somewhat different data inputs. Formats for these three types of cross sections are shown in the manual. What the user has to do is prepare cross sections for the channel being studied that conform to these formats. For example, the profile of a natural section may include up to 50 points, and an input distance and elevation for each such point must be entered.

Instructions in the manual tend to get a bit vague. Thus, the user is told to enter data pairs for all the points in a natural cross section but is not told what spacing or punctuation to use during this keyboard entry process. An example of some entry data would be helpful here, but unfortunately, none is given. The explanation for entering Manning's n values and corresponding ground points seems completely incomprehensible.

For bridge sections, the maximum number of points that can be entered is 20. From one to six culverts can be accounted for in a culvert cross section, and these may be either box or circular culverts.

Procedures for revising, deleting, inserting, and adding data points are provided. There seems to be no uniform revision method. Each particular type of section has its own procedures to follow.

For checking purposes, the package allows the user to print out the data that have been entered for any selected cross section. If any mistakes have been made in the data entries, the user can cycle once again through the input process for any cross section where errors are found.

When data entry has been completed and the data have been corrected and stored, the user can proceed to computation of the water surface profile. Here the user has the option to run all the cross sections in the file or to select only certain of those sections and omit others.

For friction slope calculations, the user is given a choice of four different methods, and a reference is given that discusses the merits of each of these methods. The package even allows different calculation methods to be applied to different cross sections. The user supplies expansion and contraction coefficients, and these can be different for different sections. Other user options include computation of normal and critical depths at each natural section, and calculation of a rating curve for the stream profile at any natural section.

Printed results can be in the form of a summary table to which a detailed listing of pertinent data at each section can be added. If desired, the user can also have a printed record of the computation process, showing the number of iterative trials and intermediate solutions. Also available are plots of cross-sectional data.

Chapter 5
Surveying and Cartography Packages

In attempting to meet the need for the very large number of different calculations that surveyors have to perform, surveying packages become collections of many diverse computation routines. For example, Survey System I.I includes a selection of routines for coordinate geometry calculations for traverse entry and reduction, topographic reduction, and stakeout, as well as a sunshot routine, and calculations for specific surveying applications to such areas as sewers, earthwork, roadways, and public lands; there is even a legal description routine.

The cost of surveying software does not seem to be related to the number of functions a package will perform. Thus the Sun Valley Surveyor's System package, which performs almost as many different calculations as Survey System I.I, sells for a much smaller price, while PC CAD, with fewer functions sells for only slightly less than Survey System I.I.

Cartography packages

Computer manipulation of map information involves, in the first place, putting basic map data into computer format. With the MultiMap package, input data can be entered using a separately purchased digitizing pad. An alternate way of getting the data into the computer with this package is by purchasing already prepared files of computer-style map information. The vendor makes a variety of such files available, at a price. For users of the ATLAS 2.0 package, the digitizing option is not yet available (but is planned), so its users rely on the map data the vendor can provide in computer-file form. Once the basic map data are in place, personal computer users can annotate the maps, shade and color map areas, and display and plot the results. Both packages provide these capabilities. In addition, MultiMap allows users to restructure the map boundaries and calculate areas within a map.

The Digital Paintbrush System was designed as a general- purpose graphics package, but it includes some features that are very useful for cartography applications. The package comes with its own digitizer, which can be used as a planimeter as well as a point-inputting device. The drawing features of this package are quite flexible, allowing sketching as well as input of lines and areas defined by points. Created figures can be stored, retrieved, and "dragged" into place on a drawing.

Ease of operation

Other nice features of the Digital Paintbrush package include a pop-up command menu and a movable data window. Calibration of the digitizer is simplified by a well-designed procedure. Commands can be given to the package through the digitizer pen as well as from the computer keyboard.

Such features are not luxuries. They can make the difference between efficient work and slow going for users who may have to spend hours in front of the computer screen. That is really the measure by which the operating techniques employed by all these packages should be judged.

The MultiMap package also allows users to give commands with their digitizing pen. The other packages all operate from keyboard commands. Most of them use menu displays, but the Atlas package has users press function keys instead of making menu choices.

Survey System I.I uses a well-organized tabular data-entry arrangement. Unfortunately users are restricted to line-at-a-time entry and do not have full-screen freedom to input and edit the data. This package also offers another convenience feature. Up to 30 bearings can be stored, then readily accessed by number from a special file.

Coordinate geometry

Coordinate geometry calculations have long been handled with the help of computers. Users of minicomputers and mainframes for such calculations are likely to be familiar with the COGO coordinate geometry language. The USA-COGO package makes that language available for personal computer use. Like human languages, computer languages have to be learned, and COGO is no exception. So its use is restricted to those who are willing to make, or have already made, the considerable investment of time and study needed to master and apply this language.

Many of the calculations that USA-COGO makes available in a general form are provided by the other packages as menu-selectable procedures. For example, the coordinate geometry module in Survey System I.I has a menu with over 30 choices. There are routines for traversing radial stakeout, calculating angles right, calculating inverses, finding bearing-bearing distance-distance, and bearing-distance intersects, and another for right-of-way intersects on both sides of straight-line segments. There are also trilateration, resection, and triangulation routines, and area and circular curve calculations, among others.

The coordinate geometry portion of the Sun Valley Surveyor's System offers a menu with 16 choices. Users work from displayed prompts that ask for specific information. When all needed information has been entered, the package immediately calculates and displays the answers and will print them as well, if desired.

PC CAD has 13 menu-selectable coordinate geometry routines with accompanying graphical displays that can take shape as the input information is keyboarded. For example, in the TRAVERSE routine, the display adds each new point and its connecting line to the previous point, as each entry is made.

ATLAS 2.0

This mapping package works from already-constructed boundary-outline files. Users can label the maps, using data files for annotation. They can shade-hatch and color map areas as well as display, print, and plot the resulting maps. Available boundary-outline files cover census tracts and other areas of the United States.

ATLAS 2.0 runs on IBM/PC computers and sells for $449 from Strategic Locations Planning, 4030 Moorpark Ave. #123, San Jose, CA 95117 [(408) 985-7400].

Function keys on the IBM/PC keyboard are used to invoke most of the procedures in this package. F1 is the Help key. F3 operates a map-display zoom function, and the zoomed displays can be saved. F4 provides for storing and retrieving maps and legends. F5 is for data file handling; an accompanying Data Ranges Assign Menu allows ranges of data to be defined and also displays statistics on the data. F7 allows the user to place assigned numbers of colored dots into map areas; it can also be used to display maps with hatched areas. F9 retrieves and saves map files. F10 is the quit button.

F8 is for assigning hatch patterns to map areas that represent assigned data ranges. Pressing this key displays a Hatch Assign display with 15 rows, each a different color, and 20 columns, each a different hatch pattern. The lowest assigned data range is displayed and the user positions a blinking white rectangle, using the arrow keys, over the desired pattern-color location. When the enter key is pr ssed, the next lower data range is displayed and the procedure is repeated for each succeeding data range. This completed, the package displays the title and legend of the map, so the user can check for correct hatch assignments. If these standard hatch patterns are not sufficient, the package has a provision for loading in additional patterns.

F6 allows users to label features of a map. Label characters can be large, medium, or small. The labels can be the feature names that are already part of the boundary-outline file for the map. They can also be taken from the data file for the map. Once such labels have been automatically entered, they can be moved or deleted (but not added or rewritten) using an editing procedure. There is also a comment procedure for inserting added labels.

F2 controls plotting and map configuration. The Plot Configure Options Menu reached via this key provides for setting up the contents of the legend and title for the map as well as for selecting overall colors, hatch density, and other features of the map. A Plot Configure Device Menu lets the user set up for the plotting equipment being used. Plotters directly supported by the package include Hewlett-Packard 7470A, 7475A, 7220, and 7550A. This key also provides for initiating the actual plotting.

A POSTPLOT routine allows other plotters, including Hewlett-Packard 7580, 7585, 7586, 7221, Amdek Amplot II, Houston Instruments DMP29, DMP40, and IBM XY749, XY750, to be used.

No digitizer input

There are no practical means for users to construct their own boundary-outline files using this package. The only suggested method is to keyboard formatted description files. However, a supplementary Boundary File Editor package is being prepared by the vendor. This will allow creation of such files from digitizer input.

The package does accept annotation data files prepared by users with the help of spreadsheet and other packages, provided these are in standard flat-ASCII or DIF format. An ATLAS 2.0 routine called DataForm is then used to convert these to a form useable by the package. However, to get a match, the names assigned to areas on the boundary-outline file must be identical with those used in the data file, and a number of rules for the formats of the files must be observed.

A SKELETON routine provides users with a file that lists the area names derived from a boundary-outline file. This skeleton file can then be edited, with the user's own spreadsheet, word processor, or editor package, into the format required by ATLAS 2.0.

When a completed data file is matched to a boundary-outline file, AT-

LAS 2.0 will show the user which areas on the map remain without assigned data and which data items cannot be matched to any map areas.

THE DIGITAL PAINTBRUSH SYSTEM

This is a graphics symbol-manipulation package rather than one specifically designed for cartography. It is limited in resolution and in the map size (just over 8 by 10 inches) it can handle. But it does have a digitizer and can easily create boundary outlines and calculate areas. The price is reasonable.

The Digital Paintbrush System runs on IBM/PC/XT/AT computers. It sells for $495, including the digitizer, from Jandel Scientific, 2656 Bridge-way, Sausilito, CA 94965 [(415) 331-3022].

The Digital Paintbrush digitizer connects to the computer through an IBM Game Control Adapter. At startup the user is prompted to calibrate this equipment. This is done with a calibration template. Six marked points are entered by touching and pressing the pen; the user follows a sequence displayed on the computer screen, gets visual and audible response, and a prompt indicating whether the calibration was sucessful or needs repeating.

A main menu display offers Graphic Design and Measurement-Estimation programs. There is also a Graph-Chart program, and menu choices include some utility operations. Selections can be made either from the keyboard or by moving the pen so the screen cursor is on the chosen menu item, then pressing the pen.

Digitizing procedure

Measurement-Estimation is the program that allows the pen and pad to be used for digitizing and planimetry. The main display here is a drawing area, with a pop-up command menu and data window (the data window is moveable).

The drawing is scaled by responding to prompts with the unit of distance to be used, then by placing the pen on two points. The distance between them is defined as any number of units the user wishes.

In similar fashion, x,y-coordinates can be set up. Once this is done, the data window will display the correct coordinates each time the pen is pressed.

The DIST command allows the user to enter two points, then see the distance between them displayed in the data window. A similar function is performed by the AREA command. These measurements can be added by the SUM command. The LABEL command lets the user assign a name to any of these data measurements.

There is a PEN command that lets the pen continuously enter data points as an outline is traced. With this command and DIST, the pen becomes a planimeter; trace a path after entering these commands, and the total distance is displayed in the data window at the SUM command.

The LINE command creates a line between two defined points. There is a choice of four colors for drawing and data display. Information in the data window can be printed on command.

Statistics display

The STATS command shows a statistics screen. On the left is a columnar display of data on point coordinates, distances, and areas that have appeared in the data window. About 20 lines of data are shown, and the user can scroll to see items on longer data sets. The limit is 200 values per data oot. Computer-stored data sets can also be examined.

Math transformations can be applied to the data sets, and a number of standard statistical procedures can be performed on the original or transformed data sets. The results can be displayed in graphical form by the Graph-Chart portion of the package, which allows users to easily create bar, line, and pie charts

Graphics design

Although freehand drawing can be done through the Measurement-Estimation program, it is the Graphic Design program that is best set up for this kind of activity. Here lines can be created by pressing the pen at the endpoints; then the line can be dragged to any desired location. Rectangles and ovals of any size can be similarly created and dragged into place. Points can be entered, then connected by a smooth curve, using the CURVE command. A FILL command allows areas to be filled with selected display colors; the cursor is placed in the desired area and the pen pressed. There is also a ZOOM command for accurate drawing in specific areas.

Text can be added to drawings with the ALPHA command. The package comes with one text font in place, and others can be loaded from a utility disk.

An Edit menu provides CUT (select area to be edited), MOVE, SIZE (change size), and other commands. SWAP allows images from stored symbol libraries to be brought into the current drawing. Any image created by the user can be stored in such a library.

Presentation and printout

Drawings created with this package can be displayed one at a time, or in sequence, like a slide show. In fact, Polaroid Palette equipment can be used to generate 35mm slides of the drawings.

A number of different color and black-white printers can be used with this package. Currently, no plotting equipment is supported. This seems appropriate for the relatively low-resolution drawings that are produced.

MULTIMAP

This package allows users to digitize existing maps, then restructure and annotate them, compute and shade areas, and display and plot the results. Files of already-digitized maps of areas of the United States and some other countries are available, at prices ranging from $100 to $750 each, for use with the package.

MultiMap runs on IBM/PC/XT computers and sells for $495 from Planning Data Systems, 1616 Walnut St. #2103, Philadelphia, PA 19103 [(215) 732-1300].

The various routines in this package are stored in named files on the package disk, and they must be called, by name, from the computer's DOS system software. Map data are also stored in named files. The manual for the package assumes that the user is familiar with IBM/PC file manipulation methods. Once a routine is called, the user is prompted by the package for any needed information

Digitizer input

Input data can be entered from a digitizing pad, which must be purchased separately. As coordinates are entered, boundary lines are displayed on the computer screen. To digitize a point, the user moves the cursor or stylus to it and presses the cursor button or stylus to enter the point coordinates.

There is a menu at the top of the digitizer pad, with seven boxed functions: Enter, Add Boundaries, Remove Boundaries, Save and Resume, Save and Exit, Quit without Save, and Erase Current Boundary. The same function boxes are displayed at the upper left of the computer screen. These functions are invoked by pointing to them with the cursor or stylus; the computer responds with a tone and lights the corresponding box on the screen display.

Fussy alignment

Aligning a map on the pad can be a fussy business. The procedure is to line up the bottom edge in a preliminary manner, then to enter two points on that edge and see if they have the same y-coordinates. If not, the map is slightly rotated and points entered again, and again until, for a 10-inch map, the coordinates are within 0.015 in. of one another.

Coordinates may be expressed in latitude-longitude terms if these are known for the four corners of the map (as on USGS quadrangles). Otherwise inch coordinates are used, and the user must measure and enter the x,y- coordinate locations of the four map corners in decimal inches, starting from the lower left-hand corner at 0,0. Users also tell the package what map scale, in units per map-inch, is being used.

Polygon by polygon

Add Boundaries is the command used to set up digitizing data entry. As each point is entered, a small dot of light is displayed, a tone sounds, and a displayed-point counter is incremented. When points describing a complete boundary have been entered, the user gives the Enter command, a low tone sounds, the point counter returns to zero, and a boundary counter is incremented.

The package includes some built-in checks on the accuracy of the input data. If the beginning- or endpoint of a boundary is very close to one that has been previously entered, the package will query the user as to whether the two points are meant to be identical and will snap them together if told to do so. If the data for a point depart greatly from those of the preceding points or digitizer signals are unclear, the package will query the user for repeat entry of that point.

The user manual suggests entering boundaries to make up one map polygon at a time and giving each polygon a name-label. The package has a boundary analysis routine that assembles boundaries into polygons and notes any digitizing errors. The polygons are also displayed for comparison by the user with the original map and for user approval or rejection. The boxed functions can be used to store boundaries and to replace erroneous boundaries.

Adjacent polygons can be grouped together using a POLYAG routine. This routine also converts files of digitized data into a form that can be handled by the package's plotting routine. To group polygons, users must write a formatted command file with the help of their own word processing or editing software.

The TPLOT routine is used to display a map on the computer screen. If the map is to be annotated with attribute data that appear in its polygons, a formatted data file must be prepared in advance, using word processing or editing software. TPLOT itself has a menu display, which allows the user to set up desired map parameters (borders, resolution, plot size, etc.). One of the choices is a submenu for selection of shading patterns for polygons. The keyboard function keys are used to make changes while the map is displayed and to recall the pop-up menu display if parameter changes are desired. The arrow keys control movement of the display cursor, so changes can be made at specific desired map locations. TPLOT also provides for dividing up attribute data into categories and for a histogram display of these categories.

Plotters that can currently be used with the package include the Houston Instruments HIPLOT DMP series; Hewlett-Packard 7470 and 7475; and IBM 7371 and 7372. Digitizers include the Houston Instruments HIPAD series; Summagraphics ID, BIT PAD TWO, MICROGRID series, MM series; Hitachi HDG series, and Tiger.

PC CAD

PC CAD offers a baker's dozen of coordinate geometry routines plus programs for handling points, area, and curves. There is an intersections program as well as one for cul-de-sac calculations, and also a variety of useful field calculation routines. With a hard disk, this package will handle up to 32,000 points.

PC CAD runs on IBM/PC/XT/AT and some compatible computers and also on the Macintosh computer; it sells for $1450. An optional Plotting Program for HP7400 Series plotters sells for $1000; a Plotting Program for HP7500 Series plotters sells for $3000. The vendor is Houseman & Associates, Allied Cypress Bank, P.O. Box 474, Cypress, TX 77429 [(713) 890-5160].

The main menu for this package offers 12 options. Eight of these lead to further menus that are used to operate the main programs offered by the package; the other four are utility commands that change data file numbers, turn a batch processing mode on and off, and call for printing or help.

Coordinate geometry

This program offers 13 menu-selectable routines for performing specific computations. In each case, the user follows a short interaction with the computer to enter data and receive results. A graphical representation of the results can be displayed as the input information is keyboarded.

For example, a TRAVERSE routine calculates the coordinates of a point when the user inputs its bearing and distance from a starting point. The user enters the starting-point number, then keys +1 to display that point. Then the bearing, distance, and number of the next point are entered. Succeeding points are entered in the same way. The display adds each new point, and its connecting line to the previous point, as each entry is made. These items may each be corrected before pressing the Enter key, and the program allows the user to rescind an entry for further correction. An AUTO-TRAVERSE routine calculates coordinates of equidistant points along a straight line, given the starting point, bearing, and distance between points.

Sideshots and their inverses can be added by a SIDESHOT routine. An INVERSE routine calculates the bearing and distance between two points of known coordinates. CURVE COMPUTATIONS calculates points on a circular curve given the P.C., radius point, and the radial bearing from the P.C. to the radius point. INSCRIBE CURVE calculates centerline and right-of-way P.C.s and P.T.s, and the radius point. An OFFSET TRAVERSE routine calculates the coordinates of a point on a line parallel to a defined line, given the offset, starting point and bearing, and the distance of the unknown point.

Intersection routines include those for BEARING-BEARING, BEARING-DISTANCE, and DISTANCE-DISTANCE. A RIGHT-ANGLE INTERSECTION routine calculates the point of tangency of a circular curve, given a point on the tangent line, the radius point, and the curve radius. PARALLEL INTERSECT calculates the coordinates of a point, given the coordinates of three known points and the offsets of two lines formed by the three points.

The area and closure of a tract can be calculated with a MAP CHECK AND AREA routine. The tract may include curves, deflection angles, or angle-rights.

Points, areas

A Points program includes a routine to ASSIGN POINTS, which provides for entering and storing coordinates, elevations, and point descriptions. REASSIGN POINTS allows the user to duplicate a set of coordinates under new point numbers. A POINT-COORDINATE TRANSFORMATION routine converts points to and from Traverse Mercator, Lambert, UTM, or Alaska coordinates and latitude-longitude. All the needed constants come with the package, stored on disk.

The ENTER N&E routine is used to enter northings, eastings, and elevations of points. There is also an ENTER LONGITUDE AND LATITUDE routine. RECALL N&E prints elevations and grid factors for entered points identified by number.

A SEARCH routine will list the numbers of all points that have a given description. Point values can be deleted with CLEAR POINTS. Sequences of points can be plotted with POINT PLOT. The ROTATE AND TRANSLATE routine moves a sequence of numbered points around a reference point to a specified bearing.

An areas program offers the user several different ways to work with areas. A POINT-TO-POINT routine has the user enter a one-line sequence of point numbers, with codes for angle and radius points, then calculates the enclosed area. HINGE POINT calculates the coordinates of a point, given two other points, the bearing of a line, and an enclosed (triangular) area. PARALLEL SIDE calculates the area of a trapezoid, given two points and the directions of lines from the points. AREA OF A CUL-DE-SAC calculates the coordinates of two points on a radial lot line, given two points on the opposite lot line, the radius point, rear lot line bearing, and the enclosed area. ARC-HINGE calculates the coordinates of a point on a curved lot line, given two points on a lot line, the radius point, and the enclosed area. ARC-LINE calculates the coordinates of two points on a lot line parallel to two points on the opposite line, given the opposite line and rear line bearings and the enclosed area. LOT calculates tract areas.

Curves, intersections, cul-de-sacs

The CIRCULAR CURVE routine calculates the field staking information for a circular curve. The user has a choice of the deflection angle or the tangent offset method. The delta angle, radius, street width, and station of the P.I. or P.C. are entered; then the routine produces the staking data. SPIRAL CURVE calculates the data needed to lay out a spiral curve. The user enters the length of the spiral, its radius or degree of curve, the P.I. station, I angle, and the desired interval between stations on the curve. VERTICAL CURVE calculates elevations along the entrance grade and curve, a vertical curve of desired length (if one exists), and the exit grade. CURVE MATHEMATICS calculates a set of curve elements, given any two of the elements. The CIRCLE THRU 3 POINTS routine calculates the radius point, given three points on the curve.

The Intersections program has two routines for calculating the P.C., radius point, and P.T. at each block-corner of an intersection. CURVE-CURVE does this for two curved streets, STRAIGHT-CURVE for a straight and a curved street. There is also a STRAIGHT STREET intersection routine. OFFSET INTERSECTION calculates the intersection of two offset lines. RIGHT-OF-WAY defines lines parallel to a centerline at given offset distances.

OPEN CUL-DE-SAC calculates the P.C., radius point, and P.T. of the entrance and exit curve of an open cul-de-sac. Similar results are calculated by BULB CUL-DE-SAC and OFFSET CUL-DE-SAC routines.

Field calculations

POINT-TO-POINT ANGLES calculates the angle defined by an occupied point, a backsight point, and a foresight point. RADIAL STAKE-OUT calculates angles and distances needed to set survey points, given the instrument point and a backsight point. TRIANGLE SOLUTIONS calculates angles and sides given three sides, two sides and an angle, or one side and two angles.

STAR SHOT calculates the azimuth of a line from hour-angle observations of a star. The routine includes a procedure for interpolating between parallels of lattitude and longitude to determine the location of the current point. Alternatively, users can enter exact longitude and latitude. Then time-zone time and watch correction data are entered, and finally repeated circle readings for the star and the reference mark. The routine then does its azimuth calculation. A SUN SHOT routine offers the user a choice of the altitude or the hour-angle method, and requires users to enter constants from the nautical almanac.

STATIONING calculates the stationing and offset of a point, given its coordinates, the baseline bearing, and the base point on the baseline. RE-SECTION calculates the coordinates of an instrument point, given three known coordinate points and the angles between them, measured from the instrument point.

FIELD TRAVERSE takes field angles or bearings and slope or horizontal distances as input. It computes and adjusts the traverse. Three-dimensional traverses can be handled. SECTIONAL SUBDIVISION calculates the coordinates of the center of a section or of the 1/16th section corners. STADIA SURVEY calculates the northing, easting, and elevation of a point, given the location and height of the instrument, a benchmark elevation, stadia readings, the vertical angle, and the horizontal angle or azimuth. CONTOUR MAPPING creates and draws contours.

SURVEYOR'S SYSTEM

This package is a collection of 12 programs that can be useful to surveyors. The Surveyor's System runs on IBM/PC and CP/M computers. It sells for

$295 from Sun Valley Systems, 844 Sun Valley Rd., Birmingham, AL 35215
[(205) 853-8440].

The main menu for the package lists all twelve available programs for the user's choice. When one of these is chosen, another menu appears with additional choices to make use of that particular program.

Coordinate geometry

For example, the coordinate geometry (COGO) program in this package has a menu with 16 choices. This program operates with just two or three points at a time. The user starts by entering the northing and easting of the first point. Then enough information can be entered to allow the program to calculate the coordinates of a second point. Or the northing and easting of two points can be entered and enough information added (bearings, distances) to allow the program to calculate the coordinates of a third point.

Users work from displayed prompts that ask for specific information. When all needed information has been entered, the package immediately calculates and displays the answers and will print them as well, if desired.

This COGO program also has a routine that will calculate the bearing and distance between the given points. Another routine will calculate an area, given the coordinates of a series of points; the last point in the series must have the same coordinates as the first.

There is a routine that allows users to follow a traverse by starting from an original point, then calculating the coordinates of the next, and of succeeding points, from their bearings and distances. If the coordinates of a series of traverse points are entered, a Meets and Bounds routine will calculate bearings and distances as each succeeding point is entered. Then when the figure is closed by entering the first point once more, it will calculate the area. A similar calculation can operate from a stored file of traverse point coordinates; in this case the user has only to enter the number of each succeeding traverse point to get bearings and distances.

Traverse building and balancing

A Traverse program allows users to build and store a traverse file. Up to three sideshots can be entered from any traverse point. Bearings are each entered on a single typed line with commas between the distance, angle, and direction quadrant. Points may also be entered by typing their northing, easting coordinates. The program prompts the user for each entry. Slope angles can be included in the bearing information. The user chooses at the beginning whether to use vertical or zenith angles. Coordinate descriptions of points must then include elevation numbers.

The Traverse program will calculate and print the closure, area, perimeter, and angular error of a traverse. Selection of these computations and appropriate displays and printouts is made from a computation menu. If the computer is equipped with a color-graphics card, a plot of the traverse can be displayed.

Once a traverse file has been created, it can be balanced by a program that uses Crandall's method or by another that uses the compass rule.

Triangles, curves, volumes

A triangle solution program finds unknown sides, angles, and areas for triangles with five combinations of known sides and angles. A circular curve program calculates all the components of a curve; the user inputs two components selected from a choice of the 12 pairs of components the program can accept.

A horizontal curve layout program calculates the data needed to stake out a circular horizontal curve. The user sets up the instrument on the P.C. and sights along the tangent. The program calculates the deflection angle and chord distance to each station around the curve. Where there are offset curves, the program can do its calculations for both the primary and offset curves at the same time.

Another program calculates the elevations of stations along a vertical curve or grade. For grade calculations, the user must give the elevation of the P.C. and the grade in percent and for curves, the curve length and the beginning and ending grade in percent.

Cut and fill areas and volumes can also be calculated. The inputs to this program are elevation and offset (from a centerline) coordinates that define cross-section outlines. The program determines which part of the cross section is cut and which is fill and calculates the area of each. It also calculates the cut-fill volume for each cross section and for the whole job.

A borrow pit program calculates volume by adding up the areas of rectangles and triangles. The user describes the borrow pit surface in terms of the dimensions of these areas and specifies a depth of cut for the pit.

Coordinates, reductions

A coordinate transformation program allows points on a map in one coordinate system to be transferred to a map in another coordinate system. The user chooses scaling points and enters the coordinates of at least two such points in both systems. The program calculates translation factors. Then, as each point in the first system is entered, it will calculate the northing and easting of that point in the second system.

A stadia reduction program has the user input instrument elevation and height, rod reading, rod interval, and vertical or zenith angle. The program then calculates the horizontal distance and elevation of the rod.

SURVEY SYSTEM I.I

This package is a collection of many calculations and aids that could be helpful to users of personal computer surveying software. The collection is more diverse than found in most other surveying packages.

Survey System I.I runs on most personal computers, including IBM/PC/XT/AT, TRS-80, and CP/M machines. It sells for $1800 for 8-bit computers and $2200 for 16-bit computers. Separate packages for Data Collection ($500) and Plotting ($1000 for single-pen, $1500 for multiple-pen) are available. The vendor is C&G Software Systems, 3300 N.E. Expressway #8-R, Atlanta, GA 30341 [(404) 451-6203].

Included on the main menu for this package are over 20 choices of input, calculation and output options, and of further menus. For example, by selecting the TRAVERSE INPUT/EDIT option, the user calls up a short menu with options for manually entering a traverse file and editing or printing the file. Users are warned to end each procedure properly, else the data disk being used "may become jumbled."

Tabular data entry and editing

Screen-displayed queries for the manual entry of a traverse file ask the user for such general items as the name and date of the job. These then appear as header information above a tabular data entry display. Lines in the display are numbered and the user enters them one at a time.

The first column in the manual entry display is for the instrument point number. If the user enters a number, the reverse-video cursor will move on to the H.I. column (unless the user opted to omit elevation data), then to the Horizontal Angle column. If the user merely presses Enter, instead of an instrument point number, the package assumes that foresight data are to be entered. The cursor then moves to the appropriate columns to have the user enter rod height, horizontal angle, slope distance, vertical angle, foresight number, and a brief eight-character description of the foresight.

In this way, all the data for a traverse can be entered. When finished, users can opt to store the data on disk, store and immediately begin editing, or discard what has been entered.

Editing, like data entry, is done one line at a time. There are keyboard options, displayed on the main editing screen, to delete the current line, insert a new line, change the current line, move up or down to the next line, or end the editing procedure. During line editing, there is a current line display with column positions numbered. The user selects a column position that is to be changed and enters a new value. When all desired changes to that line have been made, pressing Enter instead of another column-position number returns the user to the main editing screen.

This editing procedure is easy to use and methodical, but it lacks the speed and freedom that full-screen editing of the entire data display could offer.

When a traverse file has been completed, the user can opt to have it printed out, a very useful feature for rechecking the data before or after calculations take place.

Diverse traverse calculations

Once entered, the data can be massaged by a traverse reduction routine to reduce distances to the horizontal, calculate elevations, average angles, and point coordinates. This routine has separate procedures for closed-loop traverses, traverses beginning and ending at known points, and open traverses with sideshots. Users choose which of these procedures to follow and are then queried for appropriate information.

In the closed-loop procedure, the user can enter interior-exterior angles, deflection angles, or azimuths. Bearings are entered in numerical format with a quadrant number preceding the degree numbers, then a decimal point followed by minute and second digits. The package calculates angular error per point and total angular error. If desired, this procedure can also automatically adjust the angles. Users can also elect to balance the traverse and, if they do, to adjust the coordinates using their choice of the Compass, Transit, or Crandall's rules. A table of the points in the traverse and another of the sideshots will be printed.

If users have a first instrument point and backsight, and a last instrument point and foresight, they can use the procedure for traverses with known endpoints. No entry of angles and bearings is needed, but this procedure does the same calculations as the closed-loop one just described.

When the user does not want do deal with closure information, the procedure for open traverses can be followed. Here, the result is a stored and printed table of coordinates, elevations (if desired), and point descriptions, useful for reducing sideshots, entering topo notes, or picking up a point from a previously calculated traverse.

Coordinate geometry features

A coordinate geometry module offers the user a menu with over 30 choices. The first of these is a Traverse routine that uses previously stored coordinates. Users begin this one by entering the point number from which they wish to begin traversing. Then they select which type of input is wanted: angle, deflection angle, bearing, or azimuth. Data for traverse points are entered one point at a time. The user sees a display that shows data for the previous point (bearing, distance, northing, easting, and elevation) along with queries for angle, distance, and vertical for the current point. Use of descriptions is optional. Another option in this routine is to create points spaced along a line from the last occupied point. Another routine calculates points on a curved line at given arc distances.

A Radial Stake-Out routine calculates angles, distances, and azimuths from a given instrument point and backsight point to all stored points within a given radius. A Calculate Angles Right routine finds distances, angles to the right, and a foresight azimuth from a given backsight and instrument location to specified points. There are inverse routines for calculating the inverse between two points or between sequences of points. Bearing-bearing, distance-distance, and bearing-distance intersects can be calculated. A bearing-bearing intersect can also be calculated for two lines specified by their offsets from two points. And a right-of-way routine calculates intersects on both sides of straight-line segments.

A Trilateration routine calculates coordinates for an unknown point, given its distances to three known points; a Resection routine turns angles between the three known points; and there is also a Triangulation routine. There is a routine for calculating the perpendicular distance from a point to a line. From a circular curve radius or a central angle, together with either an arc length or chord length or tangent, the remaining parameters can be calculated by a Circular Curve routine. From the chord and middle ordinate another routine will calculate curve and radius data. Areas of closed figures, lots and tracts, can be calculated and summed.

A powerful routine allows coordinates of a data file, or blocks of coordinates within a file, to be translated, rotated, moved, or adjusted to grid coordinates. Elevations can also be translated. An area cutoff routine will do cutoff both by hinged point and by bearing.

Users can store up to 30 bearings in an "Assigned Directions" file. These can then be accessed by number, as needed, instead of having to keyboard the full bearings. A suffix can be used with these numbers to indicate increments of 90 degrees off the filed bearing. Bearings can also be defined by citing two points; the package will then calculate the bearing from the first to the second point.

Plat checks

A Map Check module, designed for running plat checks, takes bearings and horizontal distances as inputs. Curved property lines are handled by inputting central angles, arc lengths, or chord-bearings. When all data are entered, the user gets a printout of the closure information. If this proves disappointing, data for specified points can be corrected. Coordinates can be adjusted using the Compass, Transit, or Crandall's rule.

Topo reduction

There is a routine here for reducing stadia notes of a radial topo. It is designed to accommodate the various types of instruments used in the field. For example, vertical angle input can be by zenith (0 degrees up), nadir (0 degrees down), or horizontal angles (+ and − for up and down, or 360 degree).

Computer-based calculations can aid this kind of work. For example, if the user is set up on a point of unknown elevation, it is feasible to shoot a benchmark using a vertical angle and simply assume an elevation for the instrument location. The coordinate geometry features of the package can later be used to translate all the elevations to the correct level.

Other routines are for reducing both EDM topo notes and grid topos. A stadia profile routine allows users to profile from instrument and backsight control points without actually placing stations on the ground. Coordinates of each shot are calculated and inversed to a reference point (a point on the profile line with a known station). Then the distance is added to the station of the reference point to get the station of the shot. There is a similar routine for EDM profiles. Another routine is used for topo interpolation.

Other routines

There is more. A Solar Observation routine calculates azimuths for true north and grid north from solar observations. Users must make use of data in The Ephemeris published by the U.S. Department of Interior Bureau of Land Management.

A horizontal circular curve stake-out routine caters to users of unidirectional theodolites. It calculates the angles-right to each station along the curve and thus eliminates the need to subtract deflection angles from 360 when staking a left-handed curve. Another routine calculates coordinates for field stake-out of stations along a spiral curve.

There is also a routine that calculates grades on vertical curves and gives the station and elevation of the high/low point, as well as one that prints a boundary-call table suitable for placing on plats.

A sewer design routine is for use after coordinates for manhole covers have been calculated (using coordinate geometry). It produces point numbers, stations, deflection angles, distances, bearings, and percent slope between manholes, invert elevations, and descriptions.

An earthwork routine takes data on offset distances, from a baseline to existing contours, and on elevations for each section. The routine calculates section areas and cuts and fills. It provides for corrections, additions, and deletions in individual sections.

A public lands section subdivision routine calculates 1/16th-section corners, producing a chart of point numbers of the 1/16th corners and a bearing-distance-area printout of each 1/16th section.

A legal description routine works from coordinates in a data file. The calls come from inversing between point numbers, thus eliminating transposition errors. Curvilinear property lines can be handled.

With a station routine, users can enter point numbers to define the center of a roadway, then get a station and offset to a point number. Alternatively, they may enter a station and offset to create coordinates for a point.

Dot and pen plotting

The package will point-plot coordinates or profiles at any scale, using wide-carriage dot matrix printers. Optional plotting software can drive Numonics plotters Series #5400 or #5600.

USA-COGO

The COGO language has been in use for some time, mainly on minicomputers and mainframes. This package deliberately makes use of commands that will be familiar to those who have previously used COGO on larger computers.

Up to 999 point coordinates and 25 curves can be stored for retrieval as needed. Additional sets of points and curves can be stored on disk for future use. The package handles calculations using up to 16 significant digits.

USA-COGO runs on IBM/PC, CP/M, and TRS-80 computers. It sells *for $500 from Universal Software Applications, 13001 Cannes, St. Louis, MO 63141 [(314) 878-1277].*

When started up, this package presents the user with a menu that allows for input or for running output, CRT, or plot programs. On the input option, the user provides a file name for what is to be entered or calls for an existing file that is to be changed.

For input file entry, the query ENTER COMMAND = ? appears, and the user is expected to key in an appropriate command designation, such as STR, the command used to enter point coordinates. The package provides little sequences of prompts to help along with completion of the commands. For example, with STR a prompt asks HOW MANY POINTS? (are to be entered), then prompts for each point with ENTER J,Y,X = ? thus asking for the point number and its coordinates. To return to the main menu, the user must enter the EOJ (End Of Job) command.

Existing files can be displayed or printed, and edited. They appear in a programlike format with each line numbered. A command line is typically followed by several associated data lines. Single-letter keyboard commands allow the user to move from one command line to another, adding and deleting command and data lines as needed, or to scan the file and stop at desired points.

An output program produces printouts or displays of coordinates along with computed quantities like areas and distances. A plot program will produce elevation-distance plots with points shown as numerals and lines between them traced out by sequences of separated points.

The manual lists descriptions of 73 COGO commands. At the beginning of this section there is a single-page list of command names and three-letter codes. There is, however, no alphabetic listing of the codes or the names, so users will be hard pressed when they wish to look up any of the commands.

Chapter 6
Finite Element Analysis Packages

As long as finite element analysis was done only on large computers, the applications it found in engineering were necessarily limited. Today many finite element packages run on personal computers. By bringing this capability to the desk of virtually every engineer, these packages open the way to much more widespread employment of finite element techniques. More important, they challenge the inventiveness of engineers to find new uses for these techniques in tackling design problems.

This chapter is not the only one in which finite element packages appear. A number of these packages, specifically designed to deal with beams, trusses, and frames, are discussed in Chapter 3, "Structural Design and Analysis. Packages covered in the present chapter are those that offer a variety of elements intended to model many different types of objects. Because of their interesting features, the special-purpose CAEPIPE and CAE-FRAME packages are also discussed in this chapter.

There may be some misconceptions about using personal computers for finite element analysis. Because these computers are physically small does not mean that they cannot handle large problems. Today's minicomputers and mainframe computers are faster than personal computers, and their capacity to store data is generally greater. But the differences between the small machines and their larger cousins usually amount only to about an order of magnitude.

Later in this chapter we will take a close look at the actual capacities and speeds offered by personal computer finite element packages, but let us begin by considering the question of computing speed.

How important is speed?

A personal computer like the IBM/PC generally does its computational "number crunching" more slowly than a mainframe computer or a minicomputer like the DEC VAX or a Prime machine. That means that a small problem that runs for 10, or 20 seconds on the PC might be completed in just 1 second on a larger computer. A large problem that could run for an hour on the larger machine might grind away for 10 or 20 hours on the PC.

In terms of inconvenience and disruption of work activity, the differences in these situations may not be very significant. Seconds of waiting time will not make a significant difference. Where long minutes or hours of computing are involved, the user will probably turn to other tasks while the problem runs.

The difficulty with computer runs that last for hours is that an analysis might have to be repeated several times, with changes incorporated each time, before the needed design information is obtained. Then runs that take 10 hours each can easily add up to a week of design time, and the larger machine may be needed.

One of the main advantages of a micro/personal computer is that the user has complete control over what the computer is asked to do and when it is used. There is no waiting for programmers or data processing managers, and no need to compete with other users for shared resources. In many situations these advantages will override the drawback of slower computational speed for the small machine.

A side benefit of the personal computer is that it virtually forces the vendors of software packages to make their packages easy to learn and to use. Personal computer packages are expected to be self-explanatory, allowing users to sit down at the computer keyboard and interact with screen-displayed questions and instructions to accomplish whatever they desire.

As we shall see, the extent to which the packages described in this chapter manage to reach the goals of easy learning and use varies. But overall their achievement is impressive, reducing the user's chores dramatically compared to what most mainframe and minicomputer finite element software has demanded.

To help users evaluate the personal computer packages intelligently, some explanations of what they do and what they offer are in order.

Finite Element Equations

Finite element packages usually have to solve second- order differential equations in order to find the static and dynamic properties of structures and systems. The general form of those equations includes an unknown vector with acceleration velocity and displacement components. Known quantities include mass damping and stiffness matrices and a vector of applied forces and moments.

To obtain static solutions, only the equations involving the stiffness term have to be solved. Dynamic analyses involve the solution of the other terms as well.

Structures and systems that are to be analyzed by the finite element method are represented by node points interconnected by elements. An element is defined by its deflection capacity, which is expressed in terms of nodal deflections (degrees of freedom). In a three-dimensional structure, these can be thought of as translations along the three axes and rotations about these axes. So there can be six degrees of freedom at a given node. If an element is restrained from movement, one or more of these degrees of freedom will be removed (zeroed).

The number of equations that have to be solved to analyze a given structure corresponds to the active (nonzero) degrees of freedom. The number of rows and columns in the matrix that represents those equations will also correspond to the active degrees of freedom. So degrees of freedom are a measure of computation time since larger matrices will take longer to solve.

Generally the nonzero elements of the stiffness matrix will tend to cluster near the main diagonal. The distance of the furthest nonzero element from that diagonal is termed the "semi-bandwidth" of the matrix. A matrix with a small semi-bandwidth can be solved relatively fast, and with the use of a relatively small memory space. Thus the limits on problem size will depend on the semi-bandwidth of each problem as well as on the number of nodes or degrees of freedom involved.

Various techniques are used to simplify the needed matrix calculations. As much advantage as possible is taken of symmetry; this allows half the stiffness matrix to be immediately discarded. Zeros in the main diagonal of the matrix can also be discarded. Other programming techniques strive to optimize the speed of disk or memory access. Some of these techniques are fairly standard, others may be the individual inventions of software package designers. Depending on the ingenuity with which such techniques are applied, different packages may run similar problems more or less rapidly.

In some packages the ability to handle large problems can be limited by the precision of the arithmetic the computer employs. When so-called single-precision arithmetic is used, roundoff error can produce answers that are increasingly inaccurate for larger problems.

Main memory and disk storage

One way to solve the system of equations that will yield the key answers is to place all the necessary information in the main memory area of the computer. This memory is directly, rapidly accessed by the central processing circuits of the computer, and the solutions can therefore be completed at the maximum speed the computer can muster. The drawback to this use of main memory is one of size. Even the 640 thousand bytes of main memory (a byte is approximately the amount of memory required to store one alphabetic character) allowed as a maximum by the IBM Personal Computer is not sufficient to accommodate and process solutions for larger finite element problems.

A second approach makes use of the computer's disk storage. This storage can be substantially larger than the main memory. For instance, a so-called hard disk unit may provide 10 million or more bytes of storage. In this approach, the solutions are computed in blocks, taking one block of equations at a time from disk memory into main memory for solution. Then the size of problems that can be handled is limited only by the size of available disk memory and the time the user is willing to wait for a solution to run. Although finite element software is designed to minimize use of disk storage space and to speed access to and from the disk, disk-based solutions are much slower than those based on main memory.

The essential tradeoff is a fast but limited-size main memory solution vs. a much slower disk-based solution that can handle very large problems. In an attempt to get the best of both these approaches, at least one vendor (COADE) has structured its packages so they will run smaller problems in main memory but will automatically shift to a disk-based solution when larger problems are presented.

Finite element packages that run on personal computers often place limits on the number of nodes, elements, and degrees of freedom that can be handled. Most of these limitations refer to main-memory based solutions. They are simply the limits on the equations that can be handled within the computer's available main memory space. Problems that fit within these limits may run in a few seconds or in a matter of minutes.

Easing data input

Most finite element packages for micro/personal computers use interactive dialog between the computer display and the user to shape the way information is entered and package capabilities are employed. With this kind of interaction, the user is prompted to provide all the data the package requires and to make all the alternative choices the package provides. Interactive input of data and commands is useful not only to the beginning user but also for those who do finite element analysis only occasionally and are likely to forget commands and procedures between sittings at the computer. However, the step-by-step format imposed by interactive use can become confining for the constant user who soon becomes very familiar with the necessary procedures, is looking for the most efficient way to do problem solving, and may prefer to issue direct commands. It is possible to offer users the best of both worlds by providing interactive menus with the option of using direct commands. The SUPERSAP package approaches this kind of operation by offering menus as an optional feature.

Some of the packages continue to use the "batch" entry procedures familiar to users of finite element programs that run on larger computers. For these, the user must prepare the necessary input items in correct format, then enter them into the computer as a group. At least one of the personal computer packages allows for the use of word processing to set up this kind of batch input.

One notion promoted by some finite element package vendors is that the user can come to the computer keyboard with just a rough sketch of the system that is to be analyzed. However, as we have already seen, dealing with truss and beam elements requires the user to come prepared with data on cross-section properties, and various material properties are also required as input to many analyses. These can include such properties as Young's modulus, Poisson's ratio, weight and mass densities, and inertias. Where anisotropic behavior is to be represented, elastic constants are needed. For heat transfer calculations, inputs may include convection and radiation properties. Thermal stress analysis requires thermal expansion coefficients and stress-free temperatures.

Built-in computer files can ease the input burden on the user by collecting and storing this kind of information. The storage capability is often referred to as a library or database. In some packages, data the user puts in for one element can be drawn from the database for use with other, similar elements. When packages are directed to very specific types of design, a lot of very useful information can be kept in the database. For example, the CAEPIPE package from SST carries complete descriptions of standard parts in its database. From this database, pipes and piping components, complete with all dimensions and properties, are supplied at the user's request. The SUPERSAP A Beam module returns all the geometric and area properties contained in Rev 7 and Rev 8 of the American Institute of Steel Construction manuals and calculates those area properties not contained in the manuals.

The units of input and result quantities are an important concern. For correct results, units of input parameters must be not only correct but also consistent with one another. Most of the personal computer finite element analysis packages rely on the user to monitor correctness and consistency of units. However, the packages from SST (CAEPIPE and CAEFRAME) prompt the user for the right units for input data and display the correct units for the output data. Users can elect to input either in English units (based on inches or feet) or in metric units (based on centimeters or meters). But regardless of what input units are used, the packages will display results in whatever units the user selects, making all necessary conversions internally.

Another way that computers can ease the laborious process of entering data is by providing internal controls or checks on the accuracy of the input.

Both logical and typographical errors can be checked in this way. Packages may, for example, refuse to accept negative values for area or for Young's modulus. In connection with the entry of nodes and elements, the package can check to see that there are no isolated nodes. Visual checks of a graphical display of the input model are especially valuable in uncovering errors such as missing or misplaced elements.

Generating nodes, elements, and meshes

To simplify the process of inputting node and element data, some of the packages allow the user to input data for nodes and elements, then replicate that data to reproduce those nodes and elements as needed to form the desired structure. For example, if a beam is to be defined by six identical nodes with interconnecting elements between them, the user has only to input data for the first element and the first and last node locations. The package will then replicate the data for all the desired nodes and elements.

Objects to be modeled by these packages can be defined in a very general way by placing nodes on the object's surface and interconnecting them with appropriate elements. The process of setting up this network of nodes and elements is called mesh generation. In micro/personal computer packages, as in similar software for larger computers, automatic mesh generators for specific types of objects are frequently contained in "preprocessors" that come with the packages.

Of the packages discussed in this chapter, only two provide a variety of preprocessors. The SUPERSAP package has ten and the MSC/pal package has seven. In the case of the SUPERSAP package, these preprocessors are selected so the shapes they produce can be used individually, or combined with one another (this is called substructuring), to serve as models for all the mechanical and structural problems the package designers could envision.

Looking at graphics

The packages described in this chapter come with various graphic capabilities. Some packages provide no graphics at all, or would have the user rely on an external computer-aided design (CAD) package to provide graphics.

Nevertheless graphics are an important feature for a finite element analysis package. In the first place they provide a valuable check on the correctness of the model the user inputs into the computer. Sometimes the user may leave out a node or misplace an element. Even if many nodes and elements are generated automatically, the user will still want to see that the desired shape has actually been generated. It is therefore almost essential to view the shape that results from the input data, and to note how that shape is covered by nodes and elements. Errors in the input data, even gross errors, are not easily recognized in numerical form, but they can be dramatically obvious in a graphical view.

To examine the graphical display of the model from every aspect, a number of packages, particularly those that deal with three-dimensional models, allow the user to translate and rotate the image. In addition it is helpful to be able to view images larger than the screen area, to "zoom" in on details of the model and to "pan" across to reveal off-screen portions.

To connect the actual data to what the user sees on the graphical shape, some means of correlating the two is needed. This is usually provided by displaying node and element numbers on the graphics. Some packages also provide the reverse capability. While viewing the complete model, users of packages from SST can ask to see material properties on a certain element. The desired data will be displayed and the indicated section of the model graphics will be highlighted.

It is convenient to have both graphics and data shown on the display screen at the same time. One way of doing this is to provide a split or windowed screen with separate areas for graphics and data; this is provided in the Images 3D package from Celestial Software. Packages from SST use two separate display monitors: a monochrome monitor for data and a color monitor for the graphics.

Display of the deformed model, after loads have been applied, is another valuable feature. This allows the user to see where the largest deflections take place and to observe the overall way the model responds to the loads. Although the same information is included in the output data listings, one picture can be worth a thousand lines of numbers. Some packages provide magnified viewing of the deformed portions of the model so these changes can be viewed more easily.

Animated graphics display is a desirable feature. It can lead to a clearer understanding, for the designer, of such characteristics as the vibrational response of structures.

Color display can also be used to advantage. For example, in the CAE-PIPE package, result values that meet code limitations are shown in yellow, while those that exceed the code are shown in red. In the Images packages, colors are used to distinguish between element and message types. The SUPERSAP C-Plot module draws stress, deflection, and temperature contour plots in multiple colors.

Data at the output

Because all the packages described in this chapter use the finite element method, they produce similar basic output data. For static analyses, the basic outputs are deflections, reaction forces, strains, and stresses. For dynamic analyses, the basic outputs are more varied: resonant frequencies and mode shapes, transient responses, and frequency responses.

The usefulness of these packages can be enhanced by giving users control over combinations and selections of the basic output variables. For example, maxima and minima can be sorted out and listed for displacements and stresses. Results can be compared to relevant standards, deviations from allowed values can be listed, and outputs for different load cases can be compared.

Graphics can be used to present these output data as well as to show views of the models. The Finite/G package from COADE, for example, provides contour plots of stresses, displacements, and variables of heat transfer analysis.

Transfers to and from larger computers

In several cases, the packages described in this chapter are versions of software originally designed to run on larger computers. Thus both the SAP-86 and SUPERSAP packages are derived from the SAP IV software that has been in use on mainframe and minicomputers for several years.

As long as the files of input data built up in the personal computer versions are identical in format to those used with the larger computers, there is little difficulty in transferring models input on a smaller machine, to be run on a larger one. This can be particularly valuable where large models are to be run repeatedly.

Even when there is no version of the package that runs on larger computers, it is possible to transfer models from micro/personal computers by translating the model data files into formats that can be accommodated by the larger computers. Thus for the Images 3D package from Celestial Software, there are translation routines that allow the user to move models built on a personal computer over to larger machines that run such finite element programs as Strudl, Nastran, Ansys, and Stardyne.

Becoming a user

Most of the packages described in this chapter operate on an interactive basis. That means that when data are needed from the user, a request for them is displayed. If a command is needed, the user is notified by the software and is usually presented with a choice of available alternatives. This interactive dialog between user and computer eliminates the need for the user to memorize procedures and command names, and speeds the process of learning to use the package. Some packages also provide screen-displayed help messages to aid the learning process.

For those users who are generally familiar with finite element analysis, vendors who have interactive packages estimate it will take from 20 minutes to a few days to begin to run practical problems. In contrast, estimates for time to learn from vendors of those packages that do not provide interactive dialog range from several days to two weeks.

Most of the packages provide sample problems to help the new user understand how the packages work. These are helpful, particularly if problems similar to those sampled are what the user wants to run, but they are no substitute for a well-written manual.

Beyond learning the mechanics of package operation, users should be aware that the finite element method is not as straightforward as we are sometimes led to believe. It is an approximation method that allows users to easily generate bad models as well as good ones. The object is to create models that reasonably represent the mechanics of the objects that are being analyzed.

There can, for example, be differences in the way mass is distributed, depending on the number of nodes and elements used in a model. Thus it may be possible to model a given structure using 20 nodes and get answers that correspond closely to what would be measured in an actual, physical structure. However, if the same structure is modeled with 10 nodes, the answers may be inaccurate.

Many universities offer short courses in finite element analysis that provide excellent perspective on the pitfalls that may be encountered in using these models.

Hand holding and updating

All of the package vendors will field questions from users over the phone. In some cases the vendors encourage users to send in printouts of their input and results so problems that present difficulties can be rerun and further analyzed. Experience with the responsiveness of a vendor is the only way to gauge the extent to which they will actually prove helpful so, if this is a matter of concern, prospective users would do well to discuss it with colleagues who are already using the package under consideration.

Finite element packages, like any other software, are subject to continued change and improvement. Several of the package vendors indicated that they issued update disks every six months or once a year. The cost to users for these updates ran from the cost of disk and postage to about 10 percent of the purchase price.

CAEPIPE, CAEFRAME: RICH IN FEATURES

These packages solve static problems for 2D and 3D structures and systems. CAEPIPE analyzes networks made up of standard piping elements andfittings. CAEFRAME analyzes truss and frame structures. User-oriented features include a graphics display that utilizes color to highlight results, stored libraries of standard elements, and the ability to automatically convert units and monitor their consistent use. The specialized nature of these packages permits fast operation, with larger problems running only a minute or two to completion

The one-time license fee for CAEPIPE is $6900; for CAEFRAME the fee is $4900. The packages run on IBM/PC and compatible machines. Required equipment includes 640K main memory, 8087 math chip, monochrome adapter and display, Techmar Graphics Master board, color graphics monitor, and a graphics printer. The packages are available from SST Systems, 335 W. Olive Ave., Sunnyvale, CA 94086 [(408) 773-1171].

With the CAEPIPE package, up to 450 elements can be used. In piping systems with many branches, only about 200 nodes can be used. The limitation is in the available computer main memory size, a maximum of 640K in the case of the IBM/PC. With CAEFRAME, 2700 degrees of freedom can be accommodated for a beam problem, or half that number for a plate or shell problem, depending on the bandwidth of the stiffness matrix.

Elements for CAEPIPE include the piping itself, elbows, standard fittings, elastic supports, and hangers. For CAEFRAME, the elements include beams (six degrees of freedom per node), trusses (three degrees of freedom per node), plate elements (six degrees of freedom per node), and spring elements (six degrees of freedom).

Standard pipe components

The packages have built-in libraries of standard components. CAEPIPE has standard piping materials and the ITT-Grinnell pipe hanger catalog. The program automatically selects the appropriately sized hanger once it's location on the pipe network is specified. It also checks for conformity with ANSI standards.

CAEFRAME has stored libraries of standard AISC structural sections, pipe sections, standard pipe, and structural material properties. The package checks for conformity of the structures to AISC codes.

Types of loads for CAEPIPE include sustained dead weight and pressure, seismic G loads, thermal expansion, and anchor movement. These can be applied in any combination permitted by ANSI standards.

The CAEFRAME package handles applied displacements, seismic G loads, nonuniform distributed loads (triangular, trapezoidal, etc.), thermal, loads, and concentrated loads at the nodes or at any location along the elements. Up to 99 loads and 99 load cases can be used with either package.

According to the vendor, speed of operation for CAEPIPE running a complex piping problem with many branches and 200 nodes was under 2 minutes per load case. More typical problems with about 50 elements run about 25 seconds per load case. CAEFRAME runs a problem with 30 elements in about 25 seconds for the first load case. Problems with 100 elements run in just under 2 minutes per load case.

Packages take care of units

The user can elect to have input and output either in English or metric units. The input and output selections are independent. Thus the user can elect to have the package prompt for input entries in English units (based on inches or feet) or in metric units (based on centimeters or meters). But, regardless of what input units are used, the packages will display output results in whatever units the user selects, making all necessary conversions internally.

CAEPIPE can automatically generate series of runs and elbows. CAE-FRAME includes automatic node and element generation. Both packages include numerous checks to detect inconsistent input data. If, for example, the user attempts to input a pipe element and connect it to an incorrect fitting, the CAEPIPE package will immediately bring that discrepancy to the user's attention.

Color: dual screen display

Two display screens are used, one for interactive text and data display, the other for color graphics and data. As the user enters the input data on the text monitor, a graphical representation of the resulting model takes shape on the color screen. In this way the user can see immediately when obvious input errors are made and can verify that the data represent the model that is desired.

The graphic display can be rotated. Users can also "pan" across images larger than the display area and "zoom" in on display details. The color display also highlights the node or element the user is currently inputting or examining.

Information on the model is coordinated with the display, and is available for user inquiry. For example, with the CAEPIPE package, the user can ask to see material properties on a certain 6-inch section of pipe. The desired data will be displayed and all the sections of the model that use that 6-inch pipe will be highlighted on the graphics screen. This provides an added method for checking on the correctness of the model.

Deflected shapes of models can also be displayed on the color screen along with result data selected by the user. Thus the user can elect to view all pipe elements that are subjected to stress above, say, 7000 psi. The model will then be shown with these elements highlighted and with the calculated pressure numbers displayed next to these elements.

The user can control a magnification factor on deflections so that, if too small to be seen clearly, they can be emphasized as needed. On the display of the deflected model, maximum values are highlighted. The highest stress value is shown in a box.

There is a Browse command that allows the user to call for selected results to be displayed on the text screen, while corresponding elements of the model are highlighted on the color screen. For instance, the user can ask to see the forces on element number 33. These will be listed on the text screen while element 33 is highlighted on the color graphics screen.

Output data include stresses, displacements, forces, moments, spring forces, support loads, and stress ratios (calculated over allowed values).

The vendor finds that users familiar with piping or frame design can learn to use these packages in about four hours. To supplement the manual and the interactive procedures, help information that guides the user with screen-displayed messages is provided.

Support is available from the vendor by telephone. It is provided with the packages, along with updates, for 90 days. After that time, the monthly charge for further updates and support is about 1.5 percent of the license fee.

EASI4: FOR STRUCTURES AND TEMPERATURES

EASI4 performs static analysis and will shift automatically from a main memory based analysis to one based on disk access. The package also has thermal capabilities. For example, those who want to analyze welding stresses can enter the differential temperatures and thermal coefficients, and the package will do that analysis.

EASI4 sells for $500; an improved version that uses the MegaBASIC computer language sells for $600. Both packages are available to run on computers that use the CP/M-80, CP/M-86, and MS-DOS (that includes the IBM/PC) operating systems.

Floppy disks used with these packages must have capacities of at least 150K bytes; 128K main memory is required, 256K if the MegaBASIC version is used. The vendor recommends that users have their IBM/PCs equipped with the full 620K of main memory, so as to handle as many problems as possible within that memory. The package is available from EASI Software, 2891 Livonia Center Rd., Lima, NY 14485 [(716) 346-2022].

EASI4 uses main memory based finite element solutions and can solve typical plane frame structures having about 160 nodes on an IBM/PC. On so-called 8-bit personal computers, like the Apple II, structures having about 80 nodes can be handled. EASI versions written in the MegaBASIC language can solve structures with 2000 or more degrees of freedom.

Any problem that is too large to solve within main memory is automatically shifted to a disk-based solution. Then the equations are brought into main memory a few at a time for solution. This is considerably slower, but the complexity of the structures that can be handled is limited only by the available disk storage space. With a hard disk, very large structures whose solutions may run for 20 or 30 hours can be handled.

EASI4 has rod elements, three-node and four-node membrane elements, and three-node and four-node plate elements.

Interactive data entry

To prepare data for input to the package, the user has to break down the structure into coordinates, then enter the materials properties. Data entry is interactive. The user enters data in response to questions from the program. After entry is completed, the user can go back and edit what has been entered. There is no built-in checking of the input data, except for a graphical check on the shape of the input structure.

The package can produce simplified views of the input and deformed structure, with elements represented by asterisks. The displays can be rotated and reproduced on a printer.

There is a stored table of materials. For each material type the user enters cross-section and material properties. Then when the structure is defined, the user references the entries on this table. When applying loads, the user has to calculate the moments for point loads. There can be uniform loads on the rod elements.

Some of the larger aircraft companies have put their engineers on these packages to get them familiar with finite element analysis. The main reason for this choice has been the ease of use. According to the vendor, it usually takes engineers about 20 minutes to begin running problems on this package.

EASI Software takes phone calls from users who have problems. About once a year they issue an upgrade of the packages. The current upgrade includes a new manual and disk, at $50 for current users.

FINITE/GP: FOR A VARIETY OF PROBLEMS

Finite/GP handles static analysis for heat transfer and fluid flow as well as for structural problems. The package includes mesh generation and substructuring capabilities. It also provides carpet plots of output data for the heat transfer and fluid flow analyses.

There is a $3500 one-time charge for the package and a lease arrangement for those who wish to try out the package. Sections of the package are offered separately. For example, a section is offered on axisymmetric analysis, another on 3D frame analysis.

Finite/GP is for use with the IBM/PC and compatible computers. Added equipment required is an 8087 coprocessor chip, 512K main memory, color graphics adapter, and a dot matrix printer. The package sells for $3500 from COADE, 8552 Katy Freeway #320, Houston, TX 77024 [(713) 973-9060].

Finite/GP solves for plane stress, plane strain, axisymmetric stress, plane heat transfer (convection or conduction), axisymmetric heat transfer (convection or conduction), flat plate bending, potential fluid flow (Poisson equation solving), and will also find 3D beam and truss solutions.

Structural elements available include the beam, three-noded and four-noded quad elements, also a six-noded triangle and an eight-noded quad.

The package uses a disk-based solution technique and will handle up to about 2000 degrees of freedom. Problems using 2000 constant strain triangles have been sucessfully run by the vendor. The same problems can be run using six-noded triangles, and fewer elements would be required.

The vendor finds that the average problem will run under 10 minutes on this package. Problems that are so complex as to be near the limits of the package are said to run about 20-30 minutes.

All the input data are stored in the same allocated memory area. Node, element, and load data all compete for the same space, so the number of load cases that can be handled depends on the size of the problem. Like nodes and elements, the number of loads and load cases is limited only by available memory.

For heat transfer calculations, the required inputs are convection, con-duction and thermal expansion coefficients, and stress-free temperature.

Data input is interactive, so it can be performed by answering screen-displayed questions. An alternative batch-mode input, using a word pro-cessor to format the input data, is also provided.

Graphical and data output

The mesh generation technique used is a conformal mapping. The user can start with a simple sketch of the object that is to be represented and use the mesh generation facility to get a useable model. Substructuring is provided so different shapes can be attached to one another for analysis.

Both input and deformed structures can be graphically displayed. In heat transfer analysis, graphical output includes contour curves and surface (car-pet) plots of temperatures, and gradients. Numerical data output for heat transfer includes temperature, potentials and gradients.

Fluid flow analysis yields velocities, potentials, and pressures. Structural analysis produces the usual stress and displacement information. Carpet plots of these results can also be displayed. The user chooses from a menu which plots are to be shown.

The package provides no built-in transfer of files to larger computers. However, a file is reserved by the package for handling the formats, and users able to do so can specify the necessary reformatting.

User questions are taken over the phone. With the package purchase the user gets one year of updates. That includes two major updates plus several minor ones. After the first year, users must make a separate support agree-ment with the vendor.

FRAME 2D, AND SAFE: SIMPLE AND EASY

Frame 2D is for static analysis of two-dimensional structures. Similar anal-ysis of three-dimensional structures is done with the SAFE package. Both are quite simple to learn and to use. Only one type of element, a beam, is available for Frame 2D. SAFE offers a larger variety of element types and can handle models with up to 600 nodes and 600 elements. The capacity of Frame 2D is only about half as great. The packages allow fairly complicated loading and run reasonably fast.

Frame 2D costs $495. SAFE costs $795. The packages run on IBM/PCs and compatible computers, require 128K main memory, two disk drives, *packages are available from Engineering Software Co., 1405 Porto Bello, Arlington, TX 76012 [(817) 261-2263].*

Frame 2D uses straight-line beam elements. These have been used to model such structures as airplane wings, frame structures, and even C-clamps, since curved surfaces can be approximated by straight-line segments. It will handle up to 75 to 150 nodes and about 300 elements.

A larger variety of elements is offered to the SAFE user. These include both plane and space elements for trusses and frames, a pipe/shaft element, plane stress triangle and rectangle, a rectangular plate for bending applications, and elastic foundation elements for beams and slabs.

Models with up to 600 nodes and 600 elements can be handled by SAFE. Up to 25 sets of different element characteristics can be used in any model.

Types of loads in Frame 2D include those at node points (x, y, or moments) and distributed pressure loads perpendicular to the surface of the elements. The package will accommodate as many load cases as can be handled in disk storage.

Frame 2D uses main memory based solutions. A structure with 36 nodes and 55 members ran for about 3 minutes to a solution.

Frame 2D is interactive, cueing the user on the data items to enter. If the geometric data are entered in incorrect format, the package will not accept them. As with most finite element packages, users must come to it prepared to input a number of characteristics of the structures beyond the geometry. For example, to represent the cross-section properties of beams in Frame 2D, the user enters a flexural inertia quantity (I) and a section modulus (I/C). The flexural inertia is used to calculate the element stiffness for the matrix computation. The section modulus is used to calculate the maximum bending stress following the matrix solution. Frame 2D will handle 30 different cross sections within one structure.

Using the graphics

Once users key in the data, they can view a graphics representation to see if everything has been correctly entered. The package will run without a graphics card, but to view the models a graphics card must be used. In fact, if there is no graphics adapter installed in the computer, the package will sense this fact and the interactive dialog will not even offer the user the option of viewing graphics displays.

The package also provides displays of the deformed structures, after loads have been applied. There the user can see the deformation and get an idea of where the largest deflections take place.

SAFE has some added graphics capabilities. It allows the user to specify a desired viewing angle, then display the structure as seen from that angle. It also includes panning of images and zooming in increments of 20 percent increase or decrease in size.

The Frame 2D package includes a calculation of the factor of safety for each member. The user can input a stress allowable. Then the stress in each member is compared to that stress allowable and a factor of safety is calculated. All that is tabulated. Then at the end of the process, the worst-stressed elements are pinpointed and identified so the designer can take remedial action if needed.

Frame 2D data results include displacements and rotations at the nodes with maximum and minimum node deflections noted. For the elements, axial and shear forces, bending moments, maximum stress, and factor of safety are listed. Maximum and minimum stress, moment, shear, and force in the structure are noted.

Easy to learn and use

The effort needed to learn to use the packages is minimal. The vendor has had few requests for assistance from users who seem to be able to run the package after about a half day of experience. The package disk includes sample problems, and many users start by going directly to these sample problems to learn how to use the program.

The vendor's policy is to try to answer all users' questions the same day they call. To this point, there have been no upgrades on either package, but when and if there are they are, to be made available to all users at nominal cost.

IMAGES 2D, 3D: DYNAMIC ANALYSIS WITH A SPLIT SCREEN

These two packages provide static and dynamic analysis of 2D and 3D structures and systems. A variety of different elements is available. There is no mesh generation, but facilities for replicating nodes and elements are quite flexible. Many internal consistency checks of data input are provided to aid the user. Complex loading cases can be handled easily with these packages. The 3D package has a convenient split-screen graphics capability.

The 2D package costs $500 for the static analysis version and $1300 for the static plus dynamic versions. The 3D is $1500 for the static version, $3900 for the combined version. A companion program that performs AISC/ASME code checks of structural members sells for $200. The packages will run on the IBM/PC, XT, AT, and IBM compatibles. A color graphics adapter is required. For the 3D version, the 8087 math chip is *required; it is recommended for the 2D package. The vendor also recom-mends a hard disk for the 3D package. Images 2D requires 256K main mem-ory. Images 3D requires 512K main memory. Images 2D and 3D are available from Celestial Software, 125 University Ave., Berkeley, CA 94710 [(415) 841- 7175].*

Images 2D will handle structures with 100 nodes, 150 beam elements, or 50 triangular plate elements. The total degrees of freedom it can accom-modate is 300, with three degrees of freedom per node. Images 3D will handle 300 nodes; elements handled can include 300 beams plus 300 plates plus 300 springs with a total of up to 1800 degrees of freedom for both static and dynamic analysis.

Six types of elements are available for the 3D package: truss, beam, mem-brane plate, membrane plus bending plate, a single-node spring, and a two-node spring. The 2D package has all the above elements except for the membrane-plus-bending plate and the two-node spring. Up to 50 different cross sections are available for each package for use with the beam and truss elements.

There are five different types of loading: concentrated loads or moments, gravity loads that can be automatically generated on request, enforced or specified displacements, temperatures for calculation of thermal expansion, and distributed loads. Both the 2D and 3D packages have these. In addi-tion, the 3D package has pressure loads and tapered distribution loads.

Five separate load cases in 2D and up to 99 in 3D can be built up and used for each design. Those can be summed and factored as desired. A built-in routine sums and applies factors to the load cases.

Generating nodes and elements

In Images 2D there is node and element generation. The user specifies the endpoints, and the package will interpolate to fill in elements on a straight line. Users can also specify an element and then replicate it by spec-ifying the nodes to which it will be attached.

The 3D package generates nodes and elements using pattern, repeat, and fill capabilities. And there are many other preprocessing features built in. A complex model such as a piping elbow can be generated from a single node without need for the user to calculate any coordinates. There is the ability to rotate and offset and do scaling factors in any direction.

The user can input nodes in any convenient fashion. Then a minimization routine will renumber the nodes for calculation purposes, so as to shrink the size of the calculation that will be needed. If the structure should prove unstable, or for any other reason changes are desired, the package provides a cross-reference list that allows the user to find the node location of any particular degree of freedom.

The package also checks to see that the model the user inputs can run. It will detect user input errors such as failing to specify a needed material property or creating a node and not connecting it to anything.

Split-screen graphics

The original geometry in complete form, or with nodes-only, or elements only, can be displayed. There is zoom capability to focus the display on specific areas of complex models.

The 3D package has a split-screen capability. As the data for the model are entered in response to prompts on one side of the screen, the user sees a graphics representation of the model growing on the other side.

In static analyses, plots can be displayed of the deflected shape. For dynamic analyses, mode shapes can be plotted and animated.

The data output repeats the input geometry, stiffness information, and load cases. Output static analysis data include deflections, global loads, local loads, beam stresses, and restraint reactions. Dynamic results include natural frequencies and mode shapes, along with participation factors for seismic analysis.

For the 3D package there are translation files that allow the user to build a model on a micro/personal computer, then run it on larger machines that run Nastran, Ansys, Strudel, and Stardyne.

Both packages are menu-driven so the user has virtually nothing to memorize in the way of commands. Pressing an H will display help instructions when users are puzzled.

According to the vendor, someone who understands the basics of finite element analysis modeling techniques can sit down and be running problems on these packages within an hour.

Program updates are provided free of charge for six months. After that, users can get an annual maintenance agreement. Support is by telephone. Often problems that come in over the phone are run by the vendor to check so that proper advice can be given to the user.

MSC/PAL: STRESS AND VIBRATION ANALYSIS

MSC/pal performs both static and dynamic analysis on structures that can be modeled by beams, plates, and associated elements. Among its features is the ability to handle tapered beams. Several preprocessors are included to ease the input of some common structural problems. The package comes with a comprehensive manual and a dozen assorted sample problems.

MSC/pal sells for $995. The package will run on the IBM/PC with two disks and a color graphics monitor, or on a Compaq computer. The analysis (but not necessarily the graphics) will run on virtually any IBM/PC compatible machine. With an 8087 math chip the package is said to run about five times as fast, so it is highly recommended. The package is available from The MacNeal-Schwendler Corp., 815 Colorado Blvd., Los Angeles, CA 90041 [(213) 258-9111].

Up to 300 nodes can be used to define the geometry of an MSC/pal problem. In static analysis, depending on the problem, there can be up to 1800 degrees of freedom overall, but for most structures, the allowable overall degrees of freedom will be substantially lower. In dynamic analysis, 250 flexible degrees of freedom are allowed. Those have to be reduced by the package to 125 dynamic degrees of freedom for normal modes and transients. For frequency response, the package is limited to 225 flexible degrees of freedom that are then reduced to 100 dynamic degrees of freedom.

Static and dynamic elements

Beam elements can be pin-ended rods whose neutral axes do not have to be coincident with the grid-point locations of the structure. There are constant cross-section beams that can be defined by their cross-sectional areas. Tapered rectangular beams can also be defined, with a different cross section at one end than at the other. And pipe-type beam elements can be defined by their inside and outside diameters. If the user defines spring constants at one end and the connectivity of the element, the package will generate an equivalent beam. There is a triangular plate element that can act either as a discrete (Kirchoff) triangle or as a membrane element.

For dynamic analysis there is a damping element that can represent three-dimensional viscous damping. The same element can also be used for single-axis damping. A link element functions as a rigid link with six scalar springs at each end. There is a single-axis spring element for lumped parameter vibration studies, which can be extended to act as a 3D stiffness element.

All loads are applied to nodes. There is no provision for distributed or gravity loads. As many load cases as desired can be set up.

Users have to know the material properties of the structure. Isotropic material is handled. If the user provides E and G or E and Nu, the program will calculate the third value. The user must also provide a mass density value for dynamic analysis problems.

Preprocessors and graphics

There are specialized preprocessors to help the user input data for transverse beam bending problems, torsional shaft systems, four types of roof trusses, planar frame problems, and three different types of plate analyses.

The package has a built-in capability that allows similar nodes and elements to be replicated in a single dimension. But there is no mesh generation and no substructuring capability.

MSC/pal is basically run from commands that the user must know and use. However, there is some interactive input connected with the specialized preprocessors.

Input geometric data can be given either in cylindrical coordinates, or in rotated rectangular coordinates as well as in the basic rectangular coordinates. The package does not provide internal checking on the correctness of the input data.

The package will display the input geometry, allowing the user to rotate and examine it. It will also diplay the deformed geometry, and most appropriate for a dynamic analysis package, it also provides animated views.

An MSC/pal input file can be translated into an MSC Nastran file, to be run on a larger computer.

The MSC/pal manual covers not only installation and operation of the software; it also explains the method of analysis used and the options available to the user. An applications section of the manual goes through 12 sample problems step by step and compares classical analysis results to those of finite element analysis.

SAP86: MAINFRAME-STYLE ANALYSIS

SAP86 does both static and dynamic analysis of 2D and 3D structures and systems. It is a personal computer version of the SAP IV software used on mainframe computers. Files can be uploaded and downloaded from mainframes that use SAP IV.

SAP86 data input is not interactive (but an interactive version is planned). Users prepare the input in batches, mainframe computer style. It has no built-in graphics, requiring the use of an external CAD package for graphics display.

The package sells for $995. It runs on the IBM/PC and compatibles. Required equipment includes 384K main memory, the 8087 math chip, and two floppy drives or one floppy with a hard disk. SAP86 is available from Number Cruncher Microsystems Inc., 1455 Hayes St., San Francisco, CA 94117 [(415) 922-9635].

Elements for use with SAP86 include 3D beam and truss, thin shell/thin plate, 3D solid, 3D pipe, and 3D thick-shell, 2D plane stress and plane strain, 2D membrane, and 2D axisymmetric. There is also a boundary element.

Groups of elements can be combined in only limited ways, due to floppy disk storage limitations. One grouping includes 3D beam and truss, 2D elements, the thin shell and plate elements plus the boundary element. Another group that can be combined is the 3D solid, thick shell, and the boundary element. A third grouping is the 3D beam and truss, pipe elements, and the boundary element. Types of loading provided by the package include pressure, gravity, and thermal loads in addition to concentrated loads.

The limit on nodes is 600 to 800, depending on the type of problem being run. Elements, degrees of freedom, and load cases are limited only by the available storage.

Dynamic analysis capabilities include computation of modes, frequencies, and a response spectrum. There is also computation of time histories by modal superposition or by direct integration.

Static analysis of a thin-shell structure with 55 nodes and 52 elements was run by the vendor in about 3 3/4 minutes. Mode and frequency analysis of a plane frame composed of 3D beams with 110 nodes and 189 elements ran in just over 23 minutes.

Batch input files

The package uses batch input. The user prepares a data file, and that file is then read by the package. Along with geometry information, the package requires input of fairly standard properties. For some elements, the stress matrix has to be input. But generally what is required is Poisson's and Young's moduli and the shear modulus. For beams, the inertias and cross-sectional areas are required.

SAP86 provides node and element generation. The user specifies desired beginning and end points, and the package fills in between. There is no substructuring capability.

There is a check mode that verifies that needed node-point data have been entered and that the limits of the program have not been exceeded, but no internal checking to see that entered values are within reasonable ranges.

External packages for graphics

SAP86 has no graphical display capabilities. These are provided by an interface to the MicroCAD and AutoCAD graphics packages. Input and deformed structures can be displayed. There is no animation capability.

Outputs include stresses, stress histories, displacements, nodal forces, moments, mode shapes, frequencies. Time history response can be obtained using modal superposition, or with direct integration of the equations of motion. The package will also do response spectrum analysis.

The file input is identical to that used in the public domain SAP IV code. There is no communications facility in the SAP86 package, but users can upload and download files from larger machines that use SAP IV. Files can be downloaded and run on the personal computer, or larger problems can be uploaded to run more rapidly on the larger machine.

If the user has a general knowledge of finite element analysis, it will probably take about two weeks to begin to run simple problems. The package has no interactive capability and therefore no built-in teaching facility.

Telephone consulting is provided to get users started and to help solve any problems with the software which may arise, but not for continuing consultation on finite element analysis. Minor updates are provided at the cost of postage and floppy disks.

SUPERSAP: PLENTY OF ELEMENTS AND PREPROCESSORS

The SUPERSAP package solves both static and dynamic finite element problems using a disk-based solution method. It makes a wide variety of elements available to the user.

There are ten preprocessors, each with its own mesh generation facility, and structures prepared with these can be combined to form many different model shapes. Input data can be stored for convenient use. Output data can be flexibly combined.

The complete SUPERSAP package sells for $5000. Users can purchase the processor unit only, without preprocessing, graphics, or postprocessing, for $850. It runs on IBM/PC with 640K main memory, 8087 coprocessor, and a 10-million-byte disk. It will also run on the Pixel computer. SUPER-

SAP is available from Algor Interactive Systems, Essex House, Essex Square, Pittsburgh, PA 15206 [(412) 661-2100].

Using a 5-million-byte disk memory, SUPERSAP can handle problems with 2000 and more degrees of freedom. A beam problem with 800 degrees of freedom, containing about 350 elements, and a 3D problem with about 400 nodes were run by the vendor; each took about 2 hours to reach a solution. A small truss problem with only 12 degrees of freedom ran in about 2 minutes.

A large variety of element types are available, including 3D beam, pipe, and truss (with 2 nodes) membrane, plate/shell (with 3 to 4 nodes), brick (with 8 to 21 nodes), boundary, rigid link, and direct stiffness elements, 2D axisymmetric and plane strain and stress elements (with 3 to 8 nodes). 2D solid and 3D brick heat transfer elements are also available.

Beam area properties are defined by an area that resists axial force, two areas that resist shear deflection, a constant to represent the torsional moment of inertia, and two moments of inertia to represent the two directions of flexure. Beam orientation can be arbitrarily assigned by the user.

With most of the elements, orthotropic material behavior can be represented; the truss, beam, pipe, and brick elements are isotropic.

Loads can be point, pressure, constant acceleration, critical buckling, centrifugal, weight, center of gravity, or thermal. Number of load cases is limited by available disk memory.

Material property inputs for the elements include Young's modulus, Poisson's ratio, weight density, and mass density. Truss and beam elements require cross-section area properties.

Comprehensive preprocessors

Ten different modeling preprocessors are provided. For example, the RADGEN preprocessor produces shapes like pressure vessels and containers. Models can be constructed in parts by these preprocessors, then manipulated to match one another and be joined together to form more complex models. The concept is to provide enough of these preprocessors so that they can serve for models of all the structural and mechanical problems the package designers could envision.

An Edit feature in the package is used to construct and edit the models. Data entry is on an interactive basis. Once entered, the data for an element or a configuration can be recalled from storage, modified, and reused, as needed. For example, stored data relating to elements include material properties, area properties acceleration constants, and base load constants, as well as the element data.

There are a number of built-in data checks. The package will, for example, refuse to accept negative values for area or for Young's modulus. Both logical and typographical errors are checked.

Graphics and postprocessing

Graphic display includes both input and deformed models. The user enters and sets up the model and then can view it to verify the setup process. The user can then make spot checks at various points to further verify its correctness. To correlate the graphic display with the data, node and element numbers can be shown on the graphics. No animation is provided; that capability is planned for future versions.

Postprocessing provisions allow the user to create various stress deflection, and load case combinations. These results can then be displayed graphically.

Problems can be transferred to and from larger computers, like DEC VAX and Prime machines, that run versions of the SUPERSAP package.

Users experienced with other finite element packages will likely be able to use this one with just a few days of practice. With interactive data entry and selection, the user does not have to memorize commands, and this simplifies the learning process.

User questions are handled by telephone. An update disk is supplied every six months at added cost.

Chapter 7
Simulation Packages
For Personal Computers

There are several different types of personal computer simulation packages. Most of them seem to expect that users will be willing to train themselves to become simulation programmers. None have gone to the trouble of fully using the interactive capabilities of personal computers so as to provide simulation facilities that can be handled by the occasional user, equipped only with an engineering knowledge of the work at hand.

GPSS and SLAM are simulation languages that have been used on large computers for some time and are now available in personal computer versions. These languages are general-purpose in the sense that they can be used to model a wide variety of systems. To model with one of these languages, the user has to juggle perhaps a hundred different functions and routines understanding many special rules for employing and combining them.

The large computer versions of these languages were written under the assumption that the user would put together a set of input instructions, then enter these into the computer for a "run", receiving output material at the end, in an essentially batch-processing environment. For the most part, the personal computer versions of these languages, GPSS/PC, GPSSR/PC, and SLAM II/PC, seem to carry on this same assumption. These packages do have some PC-oriented features, but these are add-ons to what continues to be a basic batch-processing approach.

Programmed objects and routes

PCModel is also a simulation language, but of a more specialized sort. In the simulations carried out by this package, objects are moved through processing stations. Each stop takes a defined length of time, and the whole process follows a defined route. That limits the applications to manufacturing, transportation, and other situations where what is to be simulated can be described by the particular capabilities this package offers. PCModel displays are spectacular, giving the user a moving picture of the objects of interest as they pass from one position to another.

To get PCModel into operation, the user has to write a routing file, with commands drawn from a set of over 40 directives and instructions. As with any computer language, there are formats and syntax rules to learn. One of the example simulations shown in the manual involves the movement of objects through two testing stations and one adjustment station. Setting up this simulation required the writing of over 100 lines of statements in the PCModel language. So, to use this package, one has to become a PCModel programmer and put in the study and practice time needed to attain this status. While many engineers would find it helpful to run and use one of these models, few are likely to be willing to go through the apprenticeship required to be able to build their own models.

Systems that can be described by formal state and output equations can be simulated with the help of the Psim package. Actually, Psim might be more accurately described as consisting of pieces of a package that the user has to assemble in order to do a simulation. First, two procedures have to be set up to express the particular equations being used. Second, the Psim main program, including these procedures, has to be compiled and linked to other Psim calculation and graphical display routines. Then the user can begin to run the simulation.

Tutsim is a package that makes analog computing available on personal computers. What users of this package have to know is mainly how to put together analog-block models.

PC-oriented features

The GPSS/PC package makes good use of the IBM/PC keyboard. With this package, selected keys take on some new or added functions. For example, a most useful feature is the ability to easily set up function keys so they will produce whatever package operations the user desires. There are also audible signals, various beeps, that tell the user when the package is ready to take input, is finished with its current computation, and when there is a syntax error in the input. The package displays single-character prompts. These cue users on when to enter such items as labels, verbs, and different types of operand fields. The package checks each statement for correct format, when it is entered. There is also a HELP facility; by pressing the ? key while typing any part of a statement, the user can get a display of the valid options available for that specific part.

The GPSSR package includes interactive debugging facilities, designed to help the user locate problems while a model is running. The package also has an interactive report mode through which the user can decide what output information is to be displayed.

SLAM II/PC has trace reports, shown during execution, to reveal errors that are connected with individual events in the model.

Large computer compatibility

One of the advantages of having a personal computer package derived from software originally designed for larger computers is that the two may be "compatible," so that input from the personal computer can be run on larger machines and vice-versa. For example, GPSSR/PC is designed to be a "substantial" subset of the versions of the GPSS simulation language used on larger computers and is said to be compatible with the descriptions of the GPSS language found in most textbooks.

When it comes to compatibility, more can be less. The authors of the GPSS/PC package have gone to pains to add features that are not available in large computer versions of GPSS. This gives experienced users added flexibility, but it also means that models set up with other versions of the language cannot simply be read and run by this package.

Graphics displays

Most of the simulation packages have limited, if any, graphics capabilities. Thus GPSS/PC has a PLOT command that allows users to view selected variables as the simulation proceeds, and the GPSSR/PC package allows users to see a histogram display of any selected variable.

An exception is the PCModel package with its excellent visual depiction of the processing systems it simulates. The objects in these systems are represented as little reverse-video rectangles, each containing a single symbol designating the type of object. These objects move on the screen along user-defined paths and between user-defined graphical symbols. The speed of movement can be adjusted in fine steps by the user, to view what is happening or to let the process run at full speed to accumulate statistics on the system. Meanwhile, at the bottom of the screen, a digital process clock runs, and there are also ongoing displays of process counts and statistics.

The art of simulation

To use personal computer-based simulation packages like GPSS/PC, GPSSR/PC, and SLAM II/PC, those who are not already familiar with the large computer software from which they are derived will need to learn a completely new language. Competent use of the package also requires some background in statistics, needed to validate models and interpret results. But those will just be first steps for neophytes in the art and practice of computer simulation.

The real challenge is not simply to set up and run models. It is to use these packages so that the models bear a useful resemblance to the real situations that are to be simulated. Above all, users need considerable experience in working with the models before they can handle the kind of verification, validation, and modification needed to come up with meaningful results.

GPSS/PC

This package is an adaptation of the GPSS General Purpose Simulation System software which has been in use for several years on larger computers. It processes models at the rate of about 300 simulation block-entries per second.

GPSS/PC runs on IBM/PC and compatible computers. It sells for $900 from Minuteman Software, PO Box 171, Stow, MA 01775 [(617) 897-5662].

Although GPSS/PC has interactive capabilities not found in the large computer version, it is still essentially a special-purpose computer language. There are 11 general commands to initiate overall package operations, 16 control statements, and 44 statements used to create specific types of simulation blocks.

Users must learn how to program in this language by mastering its commands, statements, and procedures. This includes some special use of the keyboard. Selected keys take on some new or added functions beyond those familiar to IBM/PC users. A feature that can be most useful is the ability to easily set up function keys so they will produce whatever package operations the user desires.

Some of the features of GPSS/PC are additions to what was available in large computer versions of GPSS. This gives experienced users added flexibility, but it also means that models set up with other versions of the language cannot simply be read and run by this package.

Building a model

To build a simulation model, the user writes sequences of GPSS/PC statements, in much the same way as statements in BASIC or other computer languages are written. These models, and the processing statements that accompany them, can be used immediately or kept in disk storage for subsequent use.

Statements are made up of parts, called fields, that must be correctly sequenced and formatted. There are statement-number, label, verb, operand, and comment fields. And there are expression fields, in which mathematical and logical expressions can be handled. Some 26 operations and functions can be used in these expressions. There are also over 45 system numerical attributes (SNAs). These "state variables" can be used to control and keep track of the course of a simulation.

Editing a line

The EDIT command allows users to alter a statement called up by its statement number. Keys and key combinations take on special editing functions when this command is given. Like other operations, these functions can be set up as single F-key actions. There is a separate DELETE command to remove unwanted statements.

Built-in controls and help

GPSS/PC is supplied with a number of mechanisms with which the package spots potential problems and reports them to the user. There are audible signals, various beeps, that tell the user when the package is ready to take input, when it is finished with its current computation, and when there is a syntax error in the input.

To guide the user in correctly entering statements, the package will display single-character prompts. These cue users on when to enter labels, verbs, different types of operand fields, etc. Of course, users must learn the meanings of these prompts as part of learning to program in GPSS/PC language. The package checks each statement for correct format, when it is entered.

There is a HELP facility. By pressing the ? key while typing any part of a statement, the user can get a display of the valid options available for that specific part.

When the package runs out of memory during a simulation, it will notify the user, who then has to know how to take appropriate action and avoid the loss of important data.

Error messages are mainly understandable phrases, and those that may be puzzling can be translated by referring to the user manual section where they are explained.

Plotting and reporting

The package has a PLOT command that allows users to view selected variables as the simulation proceeds.

A standard output report can be produced by the REPORT command at the end of a simulation. This displays but does not print the information. To get printed results, users must run a separate GPSSREPT program that comes with the package.

GPSSR/PC

GPSSR/PC is designed to be a "substantial" subset of the versions of the GPSS simulation language used on larger computers and is said to be compatible with the descriptions of the GPSS language found in most textbooks.

GPSSR/PC runs on IBM/PC and compatible computers. The package can make use of, but does not require, an 8087 math chip. GPSS/PC sells for $750 ($250 to educational customers) from Simulation Software, 760 Headley Dr., London, Ontario, N6H 3V8 Canada [(519) 679-3575].

The user's manual has a nice introductory section that discusses a model of a car wash as an example of how the GPSSR/PC language works and tells how to interpret the formatted printouts the package produces. In the course of this discussion, the reader gets a sense of the difficulty and intricacy involved in setting up a simulation so that it bears some resemblance to the real situation that is supposed to be simulated.

Users of this package who are not already familiar with the large computer GPSS software from which it is derived, will need to learn a completely new language. But that will just be the first step for those who are neophytes in the practice of computer simulation. Competent use of the package requires some background in statistics, needed to validate models and interpret results. And they will need considerable experience in working with the models before they can handle the kind of troubleshooting needed to come up with meaningful results.

Fortunately, a number of textbooks are available from which beginners can learn to use the GPSS language and thus be in a position to start to use this package. There is no listing of such textbooks in the package, however.

Setting up a simulation

Users first write a set of GPSSR/PC language statements to describe the model they wish to run. This is done with the user's own text editor or word processing package. The resulting file is then run by the GPSSR/PC package, which includes interactive debugging capabilities. These allow the user to stop a simulation and step through any designated number of blocks, checking the simulation results there. This facility does not seem very easy to use, nor do the results seem simple to interpret. The package itself provides no means to edit the language statements; this must be done by going out to the external text or word editing software.

GPSSR/PC makes use of about 39 block-creation statements, 6 control statements, and 17 definition statements. And there are some 57 different standard numeric attributes (SNAs) that can be used with the package. When variables are defined, about 12 logical and mathematical operations can be used to set up the expressions.

There are two versions of the software; both are included in the package. One uses 16-bit addressing and is designed for use with computers that have 128Kbytes of main memory. The other version, for handling larger models, is designed to access up to 1024K. The 128K version is said to be more memory-efficient and to run faster.

The package allows users to see a histogram display of any selected variable. GPSSR/PC also allows users to select which statistics will be displayed and what information on the final state of the model will be included in the report the package shows.

PCMODEL

In the simulations carried out by this package, objects are moved through processing stations. Each stop takes a defined length of time, and the whole process follows a defined route. The display screen can show the movement of the objects in simulated time. The simulation typically runs 100 times faster than real time.

PCModel runs on IBM/PC/XT/AT computers. It sells for $450 ($200 to educational customers) from Simulation Systems Software, 2470 Lone Oak Dr., San Jose, CA 95121 [(408) 270-2300].

This package is designed to model the movement of manufactured items through an assembly process. It can also be used to model traffic movements, distribution, and similar situations where objects move along routes. Users build a graphical model of the process that will show the motion of the objects in their surroundings. They also write a sequence of flow statements in the PCModel simulation language that will bring the model into action.

In action, the objects are represented as little reverse-video rectangles, each containing a single symbol designating the type of object. The objects move on the screen along user-defined paths and between user-defined graphical symbols. At the bottom of the screen a digital process clock runs, and there are also ongoing displays of process counts and statistics.

The route can be quite complex, involving bypasses, crossovers, and loopbacks, and there can be conditional branching. The package can anticipate collisions of the objects and will automatically avoid these by delaying object movements. A limit to model size is that there cannot be more than 32,000 grid points in the graphics model of the process. Up to 100 jobs with 65,000 objects per job can be defined. Failures can be simulated by inserting blockages in the route.

Statistical data are collected by the package on the processes that are modeled. These include figures on the number of active objects being simulated the number completed and utilization statistics at up to 21 points along the route.

Users can control the simulation process by putting the simulation clock into a second-by-second mode or into one where the clock advances immediately to the next time when there is an object movement. The speed of simulation can be varied from maximum to real-time speed in 35 steps and users can also halt the simulation or single step it one clock cycle at a time.

Models, statistical data and screens showing the simulations at any desired point can be saved in disk files.

Setting up the routing

Overall operation of the package and control of the simulation display is exercised through a main menu aided by use of function keys for such matters as speeding up or slowing down the simulation.

To get the package into operation the user has to write a routing file with commands drawn from a set of over 40 directives and instructions. A typical simulation will require a routing file containing 10 to 20 thousand characters so a considerable amount of keyboarding is involved. The user must know how to use the commands and as with any computer language there are formats and syntax rules to learn. One of the example simulations shown in the manual involves the movement of objects through two testing stations and one adjustment station. Setting up this simulation required the writing of over 100 lines of statements in the PCModel language.

To use this package, one has to become a PCModel programmer, and put in the study and practice time needed to attain this status. While many engineers would find it helpful to run and use one of these models, it seems to this reviewer that few are likely to be willing to go through the apprenticeship required to be able to build their own models.

PSIM

Psim provides pieces of a package which computer-wise users must put together if they wish to simulate. Only those systems whose operation can be described by state and output equations in required form can be simulated.

Psim runs on Apple II computers equipped with UCSD P-system software. It sells for $35 ($40 overseas) from Prof. A.Galip Ulsoy, College of Engineering, University of Michigan, 2250 G.G. Brown, Ann Arbor, MI 48109 [(313) 764-3312].

The first thing users have to do is to set up the necessary equations that describe their system. The state equations must be of the form $dx/dt = f(x,u,t)$ where x and u are vectors of state variables and of input functions, and t is the time variable. The output equations must be of the form $y = g(x,u,t)$. After appropriate algebra to put equations into required forms, the user can turn to the software.

Users are expected to start by setting up two formatted procedures, which express the particular equations being used and which become part of their operative version of Psim. The Psim program must then be compiled and linked to two other programs, Psimpack (calculation routines) and Plotpack (graphical display routines), before the package is actually ready to run. Each time new equations are used, this setup, compilation, and linking procedure must be followed anew. The Psim manual assumes that users are familiar with all the necessary computer procedures and therefore gives no guidance in these matters.

When the operative version of Psim is executed, a menu is displayed that leads users to view or change parameter values or initial conditions, to run the simulation, view the results, and quit the package.

After setting parameter values from the state equations and setting initial conditions, the simulation run option can be taken. Users are then presented with another menu that allows them to set initial and final times and a display interval for the run. After this, the main menu run option is again taken, and the simulation is run.

To see results, users take the main menu display option. They can see or print a tabular display of T, $y(1)$, and $y(2)$ values. If they opt to see a graphical display, the package queries for the variables to be plotted. Then a menu with plotting feature choices is displayed. At this point the manual cops out and advises the user to look through the program listing of the Plotpack routine to find out how to make the appropriate choices.

There are some printing glitches in the plotting feature. Users are warned that getting a printout of a plot will take about 10 minutes. There is a choice of a smaller or larger display format, but a printout of the smaller will be blessed with some missing points.

Returning to the main menu, users can set new parameter values and initial conditions, and then rerun the simulation.

SLAM II/PC

SLAM II/PC is a personal computer adaptation of a simulation language originally designed for larger computers. The PC version of the language includes about 100 different functions and subroutines. Both continuous and discrete simulations are handled. Users have to learn the language and be proficient in the use of PC-DOS software; a knowledge of FORTRAN is also a requirement for serious use.

SLAM II/PC runs on IBM/PC/XT/AT and compatible computers. It sells for $975 ($200 to academic customers) from Pritsker and Associates, 1305 Cumberland Ave., PO Box 2413, West Lafayette, IN 47906 [(317) 463-5557].

SLAM II/PC is a competent package for those who are willing to become programmers and to learn this specialized programming language. It is open-ended in that FORTRAN routines can be incorporated into almost any aspect of its operation. This means that those who are competent FORTRAN programmers can enlarge the operations of this package, adding any features they wish. And there are many features that could and should be added to take advantage of the possibilities offered by personal computers.

Like many other translators of packages from large computers, the authors of the SLAM II/PC package have made relatively little use of the direct interactive capabilities of personal computers. There is no provision in the package for preparing the input files that describe the models. Users must turn to their own text editing or word processing packages for this. Nor is there any use of menu displays or interactive dialog between the user and computer to enhance the simulation process. There is no interaction allowed during simulation itself. All the user can do is submit an input file, run it, and get an output file. If any changes are to be made, the input file is revised (outside the package) and resubmitted for another run, just as if the PC were a mainframe computer.

Using the package can be a time-consuming process. Before any simulation can begin, the user has to load the package, and that takes about 15 minutes when floppy disks are used. Then the simulation itself is run, and the time depends on the complexity of the model. The package displays a trace report during execution that informs the user of the current simulation time.

SLAM II/PC has no provisions for storing or printing error messages. This means that it is difficult to interactively edit a model to iron out its imperfections. The trace reports shown during execution reveal errors that are connected with individual events in the model. Unfortunately, these reports move across the display screen too fast to allow the user to absorb what they contain.

Output reports can be displayed, but printing requires that the user resort to their own computer system's (DOS) software. The displayed and printed output is where the user has ready access to reports of errors discovered in the input file, and to the trace reports. In addition, output reports include statistics on variables and on simulation activity.

A big book

There is a 600-page textbook that includes an introduction to simulation and a description of the SLAM II language. However, this textbook is not organized as a user's manual, nor is it set up as a tutorial on the language. The result is that it is difficult to learn the language, even for those who set out to do so. Perhaps this creates an opening for tutorial courses in the language.

The package offers no on-line HELP facilities, no tutorial, no explanatory displays. It comes with some sample models recorded on disk, but these are not discussed in any printed material, nor is there any displayable explanation of their functions.

TUTSIM

This package runs analog simulations on a personal computer. It makes a large number of different analog blocks available to the user and provides for hard copy output on a plotter or dot-matrix printer.

Tutsim runs on IBM/PC and CP/M-based systems. The package sells for $300, from Applied i, 200 California Ave., Palo Alto, CA 94306 [(415) 325-4800].

Before the word "computer" became completely taken over by the digital machines that so dominate the field today, there was another kind of computer that seemed, at least for a while, destined to share the future on equal terms. In these analog computers, functions such as integration were performed by circuit blocks plugged together to model processes that the engineer wished to simulate.

However, the integral and differential equations that are handled by an analog computer can also be solved digitally. The Tutsim package takes advantage of this capability to use a personal computer to simulate the operation of an analog computer.

The various analog functions, such as pulse formation, attenuation and integration, are brought into play through Tutsim commands such as PLS, ATT, and INT. The package allows the user to set up a number of such analog functions (blocks) and interconnect them into a model of some larger process.

A variety of function blocks are available in the package. These include: addition, multiplication and division, cosine, sine, exponent, square root and logarithm, Boolean logic functions, and a block that will generate arbitrary piecewise-linear functions. There are also resistance and conductance blocks, as well as blocks for constants, delays, gain, maximum and minimum, and white noise, among others.

For each Tutsim block, the user is required to supply appropriate parameters. In the case of a pulse-forming block, for example, the on-time, off-time and "gain" of the block must be supplied. Users must also specify the minimum and maximum values that the output of each block can assume, as well as the step size and total simulation time for the model.

Each block is specified by a single-line Tutsim instruction. Once a simulation has begun, it may be interrupted at any time the user wishes to change the block or system parameters. Unfortunately, this editing process is laborious because it must be done on a line-by-line basis, rather than allowing the user to view and edit a screenful of simulation instructions.

Compared to the instantaneous response that analog computer users get, this package can grind rather slowly when presented with complex simulations. Simulation results can be preserved by outputting them on a printer or a Houston Instruments HiPlot plotter.

Chapter 8
Drafting Packages

There is a close relationship between personal computer packages that provide for graphics display and those that can be usefully employed to perform drafting tasks.

Basic graphics capabilities may include the ability to create drawings by freehand sketching, to replicate and mirror-image drawings or "symbols" that can be used to make up drawings, to move symbols and sections of drawings, and to join items together to make up an overall drawing. Many graphics packages also provide for creating text annotations and moving or manipulating them to appropriate positions on drawings.

Basic drafting features

Personal computer drafting packages build on these features offered by graphics packages. But computer-based drafting could offer little or no improvement over manual drafting methods unless it also allowed engineering drawings to be conveniently and rapidly created. Thus a capable drafting package like VersaCAD provides lines, arcs, circles, rectangles, fillets, and regular polygons as primitive drawing elements. These can be placed on the screen at any location, in any desired size. There is also a cross-hatch function that works automatically to fill closed areas.

Dimensioning is another essential feature of conventional engineering drawings. To make the use of drafting packages efficient, varying degrees of automatic dimensioning are offered. For example, a package like RoboCAD will automatically annotate lines and other features with dimension text, but dimension lines, arrows, and reference marks have to be drawn by the user. In the CADKEY package, once the distance between two designated points is computed, the user may choose to dimension the horizontal, vertical, or parallel distance. After the location of the dimension text is selected, the package automatically creates the text, arrowheads, and associated lines. Size and font of the text, arrowhead size, and other parameters can be adjusted as desired. Dimensioning of arcs, circles, and angles is carried out in a similar manner.

The ability to handle both English and metric units, when calculating dimensions, is a useful one offered by several drafting packages, as is the ability to translate automatically from one system of units to the other. Some drafting packages make dimensioning an optional feature. Thus CADPlan offers an optional automatic dimensioning program, but it costs an added $250.

In personal computer drafting packages, control over text can be quite flexible. For example, with the Drawing Processor II package, the user can define the size, slant, and ratio of width to height of the text, as well as it's location on the drawing. And in 3D drawings, the text will remain attached to the proper plane when the image is moved or tilted.

The ability to handle drawings sufficiently complex to represent the actual objects with which engineers have to deal is another essential capability for drafting packages. For example, the EnerGraphics package is a very capable graphics tool that comes close to being useful for general drafting applications. However, the package limits drawings to 800 line segments and 200 arcs and symbols. At that level of complexity, many simple layout drawings can be put together, but detailed and complex objects cannot be properly represented by engineering drawings. In contrast, capable drafting packages are able to handle thousands of elements in a single drawing.

Speed of operation is another very important characteristic of capable drafting packages. Most of the presently available packages are slow, particularly when they redraw displayed objects. The panning process, in which the user shifts the displayed view of a drawing that is larger than the computer screen, involves time-consuming redrawing. For a complex drawing, a single panning move may take over a minute to complete, and that is a time delay large enough to try the patience of most users.

One way of speeding up the redrawing process is to simplify the calculations that it involves. Thus the CADPlan package attains its relatively speedy operation by using integer arithmetic, instead of the more accurate floating point arithmetic used by most other drafting packages. For many applications, the slight distortion introduced by this approach may not be significant. For example, a rectangle 10 feet long will expand about a quarter of an inch when it is rotated 30 degrees by CADPlan, and it will continue to expand each time it is rotated. This growth is due to the arithmetic rounding that takes place.

Ability to create drawings in layers is an important feature for many applications of drafting packages. The layers can be used to portray such items as overlapping plumbing, electrical wiring, and other details in a building design, or to plan the levels of a layered printed circuit board. Some packages provide for only a few layered drawing levels, others for many. Thus the VersaCAD package allows each drawing to include up to 250 layers of material and each layer can be shown in a different background color to help keep track of layer location.

A variety of features

Personal computer drafting packages offer users many different kinds of features which may be more or less important depending on the uses to which the package will be put.

Most packages will offer the user choice of a number of different types of lines for drawing. These can include solid lines of several widths, as well as dashed, dotted, and combination lines. Similarly, a variety of different text styles and fonts may be available.

Special editing features can be helpful. For example, the CADKEY package provides some very specific selection functions. When editing a drawing, the user can choose to affect only points, or lines, or arcs, or other specific types of items. If, for example, the user chooses to edit and delete points, the package will not allow adjacent lines to be inadvertently deleted.

Being able to easily create lines that are accurately horizontal or vertical is a helpful feature. In the AutoCAD package, an orthogonal mode of operation converts all lines at less than 45 degrees to the horizontal, and all those at more than 45 degrees to the vertical. If they wish, users can define the angle from the vertical and horizontal at which this orthogonal "snapping" will take place.

Another useful drawing aid is a displayed background grid. Many packages provide the ability to "snap" points on a drawing into alignment with the crosspoints of this kind of grid. And they also allow the user to specify the spacing between grid dots.

A powerful feature, which seems to be offered only by the AutoCAD package, is to provide nonprogrammers with the ability to customize package operations. Users who want tailored package functions will appreciate the ability to define their own display menu choices and also the ability to create "macros," special command sequences to get the package to perform customized tasks.

Stretching and distorting basic drawing shapes can be a valuable drafting asset. The CADPlan package, for example, allows rectangles to be pulled into squares, or long thin shapes, with size changes as desired. With the Design Board package, a circle can be stretched into a keyhole shape, using a function that causes parallel motion of selected points.

3D capabilities

The beauty of 3D packages is their ability to create a computer-stored representation of a three-dimensional object. The stored image can then be turned about and examined on the display screen and conventional engineering drawings can be readily created from two-dimensional views of the stored data.

Some 3D packages, like CADKEY and MicroCAD, provide both object-creation and 2D drawing capability. Others, like Design Board 3D, just allow the user to set up and store 3D objects, leaving the production of engineering drawings to other compatible packages.

For viewing 3D objects, a desirable feature is automatic hidden-line removal. Without it, displayed views of 3D objects can often be confusing, and it is difficult to recognize whether objects are complete in all details. Unfortunately, automatic hidden-line removal is a feature still under development and not always completely satisfactory. Thus the MicroCAD package has a hidden-line removal feature that works on only one object at a time. If one object is in front of another, the package will not remove all the lines in the area where the two overlap. The vendor of this package believes that, at present, the most efficient way to remove hidden lines is to have the user do it manually. The CADKEY 3D package provides no automatic-hidden line removal at all. Manual editing functions can be used to remove such lines. However, if the display of the object is then rotated, it will have to be reedited to correct these lines.

Drawing elements, like lines and curves, are plentiful for 2D drawing, but few vendors offer any similarly convenient 3D drawing elements. One exception is the optional 3D program offered with the VersaCAD package, which includes a 3D "box" as a primitive element. The Design Board 3D package provides meshlike spherical and elliptical "dome" elements and allows mesh-formed 3D surfaces to be flexibly defined.

Curve fitting is a feature made available by some 2D drafting packages. The VersaCAD package has a Bezier curve-fitting feature that allows drawing segments to be connected by smooth curves. Drawing Processor II allows curves to be fitted to any selected points, then stored and used as defined drawing elements.

Curve-fitting capability is extended into three dimensions by the Design Board 3D package. Here, surfaces are defined by first fixing four corner points which the package uses to set up a rectangular mesh. The user then sets the position of some of the desired points of the surface above or below the plane of the rectangle; using a Bezier curve-fitting procedure, the package then forms a curved surface that goes through these points. Depending on the fineness of the mesh that is used, quite complex curved surfaces can be formed.

The EnerGraphics package, which has been mentioned as having near-drafting capabilities, also provides an example of partial 3D capabilities. It creates 3D surfaces, but only as representations of mathematical functions or sets of points in three-dimensional space. 3D objects may also be created, but these can only be made up of planar panels which are copied and moved about to form the 3D forms. And there is no ability to use views of the 3D images as 2D drawings.

Viewing images and drawings

Most personal computer drafting packages provide a variety of viewing capabilities. As has been mentioned, panning across a drawing tends to be slow because of the massive calculation and manipulation involved in the redrawing process. Zooming features usually work more rapidly, and to some extent, these can be used in place of panning.

A feature which has been artfully employed by some packages is the ability to display several different images, views, or items at the same time, by dividing the screen up into display "windows." For example, on the CAD-KEY package display, in addition to an area or window where the current part is shown, there is a status window that indicates such parameters as the current level, color, line type, pen number, working scale, and depth, while a third window displays the currently-available menu choices. Other information on the screen display includes the current coordinates of the drawing cursor and prompts to aid the user in choosing menu options.

In a similar manner, the Design Board 3D package presents the user with a display screen divided into four windows which show a perspective view, along with top, bottom, and right side views of the object being modified.

Storage features

More than any other feature, the ability of personal computer drafting packages to retrieve predrawn "symbols" and sections of drawings from storage has contributed to their productivity. For example, users of the VersaCAD package can make up parts which are then stored in "pages" containing up to 100 parts each. The stored parts can be called up and placed where desired in the currently active drawing. The user simply points to the desired part with a graphics tablet stylus and presses the Enter key. The vendor makes about 5000 predrawn part symbols available.

Some packages allow entire drawings to be retrieved from storage and added to the currently active drawing. A point to watch for here is that, while the retrieved drawings can be displayed and printed or plotted, there may be no capability to modify them or to connect them to lines on the currently active drawing.

As stored files of drawings and symbols continue to grow, locating the desired item from all those that are stored can become a problem. Packages that allow drawings to be filed under descriptive names can help to ease this problem, but it is mainly up to the users to take care to keep proper track of what they have stored. Some packages allow objects within drawings, as well as the drawings themselves, to be named for retrieval from storage.

Computer-stored information can include data about the items that are drawn as well as the graphical data. Such information can be very useful when it comes to compiling bills of material, cost estimates, and other documents related to drawings. Some packages allow written specifications, costs, and other information to be filed for each object in a drawing. To create a bill of materials, the package may automatically identify all the appropriate objects in a drawing and print a summary showing such information as the vendor, order number and cost for each item. Compiling a bill of materials in this way is generally a slow process but can nevertheless be a convenient one.

One storage problem that can be most annoying arises when the capacity limits of the computer's disk files are reached. What is needed is a procedure that can avoid any loss of information entered into the computer but not yet stored on the disk. This problem is not too well handled in some packages. For example, when an AutoCAD drawing gets too large to be contained on a single storage disk, the display is turned off and the user is asked whether the drawing should be retained or abandoned. However, either answer produces the disheartening message "AutoCAD gives up."

Generating computer output

When the user has finished creating objects and drawings with one of these packages, the next order of business is generally to produce plotted output, or some other form of useful output.

One of the main problems encountered with plotters is that each drafting package is able to utilize only certain models of plotting equipment. If a prospective purchaser of a package already has a plotter, it is important to find out if the package being considered is designed to accommodate that plotter and, if not, what it will cost to get an appropriate interface.

It can be useful to exchange drafting information between one computer and another. Often a personal computer may be used to do drawings which are to become part of a larger set of drawings stored on a larger computer. AutoLINK is a package designed to transfer information between personal computers using AutoCAD software and larger computers using INTER-GRAPH software. In the near future more packages performing this kind of communication function can be expected to appear.

Some packages make it convenient for the user to display objects and drawings one after another as in a slide show. An extension of this, providing animation of drawings, is achieved in the AutoCAD package by a feature that saves images in a special file, then allows them to be played back in rapid sequence.

An active art

Developing drafting packages for personal computers is an active art. What is available today is only a prelude to the tools that will be available in the near future. This is evident in the continuing changes and updates to the best of the existing packages. That means that the best choice is probably a package that is open to such improvements, makes them frequently to keep up with the state of the art, and passes the improved versions on to their users at reasonable cost.

AutoCAD: A SEASONED AND VERSATILE DRAFTING PACKAGE

Among 2D drafting packages that run on popular personal computers, AutoCAD is widely regarded as a standard of comparison. It is certainly the best-selling package. AutoCAD supports a wide variety of input and output equipment, has most of the features available in such packages, and is well designed. Storage operations are particularly well-handled.

AutoCAD is designed to run on several computers, including the IBM/ PC, IBM/XT, Victor 9000, Zenith Z100, NEC APC, Colombia, Eagle PC, Digital Microsystems, TI Professional, DEC Rainbow, Compaq, and many CP/M computers. Price of the package is $1000. Semi-automatic dimensioning costs an added $500. It is available from AutoDesk Inc., 150 Shoreline Highway #B20, Mill Valley, CA 94941 [(415) 331-0356].

AutoCAD provides a choice of easily invoked drawing elements. In addition to straight lines, there are circles, arcs, trace lines, and solid, filled-in areas.

Once created, objects can be nested within other objects. For example, identical doors in a drawing of a building can be produced by calling for the door shape and specifying the locations at which it is to appear. Shapes can be placed, stretched, shrunk, scaled, rotated, and repeated. Materials within a screen-display window, defined by its four corner points, can be moved as a group.

Flexible drawing features

An orthogonal mode of operation converts all lines at less than 45 degrees to the horizontal and all those at more than 45 degrees to the vertical, or the user can define the angle from the vertical and horizontal at which this orthogonal "snapping" will take place. As an optional drawing aid, an alignment grid may be displayed, and the user can specify the spacing between the grid dots.

For dimensioning, the package will compute the distance between any two points and also the area enclosed by a set of points. An optional semi-automatic dimensioning feature is available.

A zoom feature allows a selected small area to be enlarged to fill the screen or a portion of a drawing to be reduced to fit into a larger context. A portion that is to be viewed in this way can be defined by simply pointing to the upper right and lower left corners of the rectangular area that is desired.

Internal data are maintained in "floating-point" format. The package allows a ratio of a million to one, or better, between the largest and smallest objects that are represented.

Drawings can be stored in overlays, a convenient feature for multiple layer designs. With a 640K main memory in the computer, AutoCAD can handle up to 127 such layers. However, once a layer is created it remains an active part of the drawing. Material displayed on all such layers will continue to be scanned, eating up processing time, even when they are not being used.

Animation of drawings can be achieved by a feature that saves images in a special file, so they can be played back in rapid sequence.

Other features include: partial deletion of drawing elements, such as breaking an existing wall to inset a window; a cross-hatch command that can draw from a library of 38 pre-defined patterns or invoke user-defined patterns; a freehand sketch mode of operation; automatic creation of fillets; automatic closure of polygons; the use of circular/radial arrays; alternate text fonts; units that can be decimal, or in feet and inches.

Speed of operation

Like other personal computer drafting packages, AutoCAD is slow, particularly when it is redrawing. The package takes time scanning all drawing layers in the redrawing process. Panning a displayed drawing requires redrawing; for a complex display the panning move may take over a minute to complete.

As the drawing in progress gets larger, program operation gets slower. However, use of the 8087 coprocessor can help speed up zooming, editing, and panning. Another feature used to speed up operation is the ability to temporarily eliminate filled areas, thus speeding up image regeneration after panning or zooming.

When a drawing gets too large to be contained on a single storage disk, the display is turned off and the user is asked whether the drawing should be retained or abandoned. However, either answer produces the disheartening message "AutoCAD gives up." To avoid this situation, the floppy disk user must keep in mind that, because of work and backup files, only about a third of the disk space is available for storage of the actual drawing file. In general, it is wise to assign only one drawing to a floppy disk.

Wide choice of peripherals

The package offers excellent peripheral support. A light pen, touch pen, or a mouse, as well as the keyboard or a digitizer pad can be used for input.

AutoCAD is designed to be run using two display screens simultaneously, one for graphics, the other for text. If only one screen is used (this can be done when it is connected to the IBM Color/Graphics Adapter), the user has to constantly switch back and forth from text to graphic mode. If higher resolution than that provided by IBM displays is desired, the package can be used with a Hercules Graphics card that provides 640 by 400 pixel resolution.

The package provides for use of electronic tablet input. In tablet mode, however, no reference cursor is displayed on the screen to indicate the user's position. A nice tablet input feature is the ability to make menu choices by pointing to tablet areas, instead of having to refer to the display screen.

Use of a plotter for output is required by the package. Maximum plotting resolution is 0.025mm. Paper from size A to E may be used, provided the chosen plotter will accommodate it. Multiple plotting pens with different colors and line types can be supported.

Customizing and communication

Users who wish to customize AutoCAD operation, or have it customized for them, will appreciate the user-defined menus and the ability to create "macros," special command sequences to get the package to perform customized tasks. The package is designed to be customized by nonprogrammers. For example, previously created shapes or drawings can be recalled by pointing to a single item on a menu display. Drawing sessions can be initiated from a command file that sets up the custom commands that are to be used in that session. This kind of customizing may also include special prompts to remind the package user of how to proceed. And these can be conveniently set up using a text editor or word processing program.

For those who use digitizers with multiple buttons, menus can be customized to show button numbers, so menu choices can be conveniently made from the digitizer.

Communication with central drawing files, or other computers, is handled by storing drawings in a standard-code "ASCII" format for transmission or reception. This allows drawings to be easily sent over telephone line connections.

The package is well supported. The vendor claims that it now has over 1500 users. It is written in the "C" computer language, which can easily be moved from one type of computer to another, so improved performance on more capable machines than the IBM/PC can be expected in the future.

AUTOLINK: TRANSLATES BETWEEN AUTOCAD AND INTERGRAPH

It is sometimes desirable to transfer drafting work done with a personal computer over to a larger computer, or to move work in the other direction. This package allows such transfers to take place between a personal computer using the AutoCAD package and a minicomputer or mainframe using INTERGRAPH software. These transfers take place over wire or telephone connecting lines.

The AutoLINK package resides on the larger computer and includes communications software. Both computers must be equipped with serial asynchronous communications equipment. AutoLINK costs $10,000 and is available from Interactive Graphic Services Co., 200 South Meridian St., Indianapolis, IN 46225 [(317) 638-5057].

CADAPPLE: SEE REVIEW OF VERSACAD

CADKEY: DRAWINGS OF WIREFRAME PARTS

CADKEY is a well-organized two- and three-dimensional drafting package. The user creates three-dimensional objects or parts, which appear in wire-

frame form. Drawings can then be displayed or plotted to represent projected or isometric views of the part.

The package runs on IBM/PCs and compatible computers. It sells for $1895; a yearly upgrade package is available for $200; the vendor is Micro Control Systems, 27 Hartford Turnpike, Vernon, CT 06066 [(203) 647-0220].

CADKEY users choose the operations they wish to perform from a well-organized sequence of screen-displayed menus. The menu options can be chosen from the keyboard or from the user's digitizer board. Experienced users can bypass the menu sequences, invoking CADKEY functions directly by entering command codes.

The screen display is also well-organized. In addition to an area or window where the current part is displayed, there is a status window that indicates such parameters as the current level, color, line type, pen number, working scale, and depth. These parameters can be changed immediately, as desired, by entering special keyboard commands. A third window displays the currently available menu choices. Other information on the screen display includes the current coordinates of the drawing cursor and prompts to aid the user in choosing menu options.

Creating lines

Drawing can be done by making a "string" of lines, in which the next line begins where the last one left off. Or lines can be defined by making them parallel to, or perpendicular to, existing lines. In a more general way, a line can be created by defining its endpoints.

Because of the difficulties that can arise in placing lines accurately on a three-dimensional drawing space, CADKEY provides nine different ways to define the endpoints of a line. These range from positioning the cursor to indicate the desired endpoints, to locating them at endpoints or center-points of existing lines or arcs, to entering the exact endpoint coordinates on the keyboard.

In addition to lines, the package provides for the creation of points, arcs, circles, rectangles, and fillets.

Transforming shapes

Once a basic shape, like a square, has been created, it can be transformed by translating, rotating, shrinking, or expanding it. Shapes can also be replicated or copied. The material to be copied can be defined by surrounding it with a box. Or the type of item to be copied can be chosen and then the particular item to be copied can be spotted by placing the cursor on it.

Created items can be viewed from the top, front, back, bottom, and left or right sides, and there are also two isometric views that can be chosen. Each of these views can be used as drawings to be displayed or plotted.

Viewing manipulations provided by the package also include panning and zooming. A two-dimensional grid can be set up, with spacing selected by the user. Drawing points can be forced to align with the grid to a snap resolution selected by the user.

Specific and wholesale editing

Editing functions allow the user to trim or extend lines and arcs, and to delete items that have been drawn. The package provides no automatic hidden-line removal. The editing functions can be used to remove such lines. However, if the part is then rotated, it will have to be reedited to correct these lines.

To aid in handling complex drawings, the package provides very specific selection functions. Thus the user can choose to select only points, or lines, or arcs, or other specific types of items. If, for example, the user chooses to edit and delete points, the package will not allow adjacent lines to be inadvertently deleted.

Sections of a drawing can also be deleted in a wholesale manner by first surrounding the desired material with a defining box, then deleting it. If desired, the specific selection of types of items to be deleted can be combined with this box deletion technique.

Dimensioning automatically

Automatic dimensioning is accomplished by having the package compute the distance between two designated points. The user may choose to dimension the horizontal, vertical, or parallel distance. After the location of the dimension text is selected, the package automatically creates the text, arrowheads, and associated lines. Size and font of the text, arrowhead size, and other parameters can be adjusted as desired. Dimensioning of arcs, circles, and angles is carried out in a similar manner. In addition labels, with witness lines, leaders and arrows, can be created and positioned as desired.

Filing parts, shapes, and drawings

When work on an object has been completed, it can be stored as a "part" under a file name selected by the user. Other stored files may contain information on shapes, and notes that can be retrieved whenever needed to be added to the part that is being created or modified. Views (drawings) that are to be plotted are stored in special plot files.

Plotting itself is carried out as an operation quite separate from the rest of the package functions. This has the advantage that, provided the computer is capable, plotting can proceed while the user turns to other CAD-KEY tasks.

CADPLAN: FAST AND FLEXIBLE

CADPlan operates rapidly, faster than many other personal computer based CAD packages. It has a good supply of primitives, good editing features, and good support of peripherals. CADDraft is a junior version with smaller drawing-size capability.

Written for the IBM/PC, it requires 320K main memory, two floppy disk drives, IBM Color/Graphics Adapter, plotter or printer. List price of the package is $1200. An optional database feature sells for $350. An autodimensioning feature costs $250. An abbreviated version of the package, called CADDraft, is available for $95. The vendor is Personal CAD Systems, 981 University Ave., Los Gatos, CA 95030 [(408) 354-7193].

Package operation and documentation are designed to make CADPlan easy to learn, and they do their job well. The prompts, menus, and other displayed information items are easily and quickly understood.

There is an initial menu of 18 commands. These are supplemented by added subcommands. Drawings are filed and can be retrieved by name; no provision is made to allow added displayed notes in case the user should fail to remember the name assigned to a given drawing.

Primitive elements available for drawing include lines, arcs, circles, and rectangles, as well as predefined symbols and text. Available line types include solid, dashed, and dotted in three different colors. Line width and text size can be defined by the user. Symbol libraries can be created for frequently used drawing items.

Initial use of the package is quite easy, but in order to take full advantage of its capabilities, the user has to employ the package commands with considerable skill and knowledge.

The package allows shapes to be stretched as desired to modify or create a drawing. Rectangles, for example, can be pulled into squares, or long thin shapes, with size changes as desired. There is, however, no provision for automatically changing the scale of an entire drawing.

Editing can be performed on any stored drawing. This is somewhat complicated by the fact that shapes created by different techniques have to be edited differently. For example, if a rectangle was originally created by constructing four separate lines, each can be separately edited. However, if it was created as a program-generated rectangle, it must be edited by overall commands. There is no way to tell, simply by looking at a drawing, just how its shapes were created.

Like other similar packages, CADPlan makes libraries of ready-to-use symbols available.

The price of speed

CADPlan attains its relatively fast operating speed by using integer arithmetic instead of the more accurate floating-point arithmetic used by most other drafting packages. For most applications, the distortion introduced by this approach may not be significant. For example, a rectangle 10 feet long will expand about a quarter of an inch when it is rotated 30 degrees by CADPlan, and it will continue to expand each time it is rotated. This growth is due to the arithmetic rounding that takes place.

Layering, zooming, windowing

Drawings can be layered, with up to 10 layers allowed on an IBM/PC with a 320K main memory and up to 65 layers with a 640 K memory. The layers can be used to show overlapping plumbing, electrical wiring, or other detail in a building design. Or they can be used to plan the levels of a layered printed circuit board or any other type of drafting that lends itself to layering.

With several layers in simultaneous use, the operation of CADplan may slow down. However, the user has the option of switching off layers not in current use to speed things up again.

A zoom command works together with a pan command that allows the user to move a screen display over the entire surface of a drawing larger than the screen. The package must redraw the screen each time the pan moves outside the presently viewed area, and that greatly slows down the panning process. Zoom operates in steps of 2X magnification

The windowing feature is a helpful one. Up to five separate windows, each showing a different drawing area, can be simultaneously displayed. And the user can quickly switch back and forth between these areas, thus avoiding the need to use the slower panning feature.

Two helpful options

There is an optional automatic dimensioning program ($250) that measures the distance between any two selected points and draws a dimensioning line with accompanying dimension text. This feature is quite flexible. Text can be placed as desired.

Another optional program module is a database feature which is designed to ease the process of creating a bill of materials from a finished drawing. This feature allows a library of useful information related to shapes and objects to be maintained. For example, written specifications, costs, and other information can be filed under each object, a very important feature for many types of design.

To create a bill of materials, the package counts the number of objects in a drawing and prints a summary showing the number of each object along with the vendor, order number, and cost, automatically taking these items of information from the database. Compiling a bill of materials in this way is a slow process but nevertheless a convenient one.

The package is designed to work with a three-button "mouse" input device, but it also accommodates at least three different brands of input tablet devices. Input via digitizer tends to be slow.

About a dozen different plotters can be used with the package, as well as IBM and Epson dot-matrix printers. A recent addition is the 8-pen Model 84 plotter from Calcomp in Anaheim, CA.

CADDraft limitations

The low-cost version of CADPlan, called CADDraft, comes with considerably smaller drawing capacity. It can handle only 10 drawing layers and a 500-point database, while CADPlan can handle up to 65 layers and 67,500 points. Features of CADPlan missing in CADDraft include: copy, step, and repeat commands; vertex highlighting; absolute and relative coordinate input; view recall and fit commands; area and volume calculations.

DESIGN BOARD 3D: CREATING 3D OBJECTS

Design Board 3D is a capable package for creating computer-stored representations of three-dimensional objects, including hidden-line perspective views. Although it can produce plotted versions of various views of the created objects, it is not a full-fledged drafting package since it lacks the ability to dimension and annotate the drawings. The package vendor pro-

vides optional software to convert Design Board views into input for the AutoCad drafting package.

Design Board 3D runs on IBM/PCs and compatible computers equipped with a math chip and mouse input device. It sells for $750. Software to convert its output for use with AutoCAD sells for $295. The vendor is MEGA CADD, 401 Second Ave So., Seattle, WA 98104 [(206) 623-6245].

This package is remarkable, if only for the fact that the keyboard goes dead as soon as the software is powered up. Users had better get familiar with using a mouse for input, for it, and the display screen, will be the only means of communication they have with Design Board 3D.

This means that when words like file names are to be entered, they have to be picked out, one letter at a time, by moving crosshairs around on an alphabet display; the same is true for numbers. Since the Design Board package does not include any capability to add annotation or dimensions to drawings, this limited means of alphanumeric communication is adequate to the task at hand. When it comes to entering lines and points, the mouse is far easier to use than a keyboard. Nevertheless, why the keyboard had to be completely dead is something of a mystery.

Polygons plus

The basic shape created by this package is the polygon. Any polygonal shape with up to 17 sides can be formed in a plane and then extended in the third dimension to create a building block shape. These blocks can then be combined, as desired, to form more complex 3D objects. In addition to polygons, the user can also play with three "net" type forms: a spherical dome, an elliptical dome, and a saddle-shaped curved surface. Each of these are formed by an open mesh of intersecting curved lines.

While the user is creating an object, the screen shows a large "creation space" complete with backgound grid, a smaller perspective view space, and small menu rectangles that contain the various commands that can be mouse-chosen. As the object is created, its perspective view will take shape automatically. Included on the perspective space is a little x,y,z-axis orientation figure and a numerical reading of the current location of the drawing cursor along these axes.

To create a square, the user defines the endpoints of one side by moving the crosshairs with the mouse, then places one more point to show on which side of the line the square will lie. The package does the rest. To form a rectangle, a similar procedure is followed, but the distance from the line to the opposite side must be specified. Arbitrary plane shapes can be formed by specifying their vertex points. To turn these plane figures into parallelopipeds, all the user has to do is specify a top and a bottom point in the third dimension. The principle of this package seems to be to have the user do only the minimum necessary to achieve the objective, an admirable approach.

Spherical domes are created by defining a center and radius points. In addition the user must indicate the degrees of the dome, that is, the angle from the center of the sphere that defines the extent of the dome. For a hemisphere, that angle would be 180 degrees. A similar angle must be chosen for elliptical domes, along with major and minor axis dimensions.

Surfaces are defined by first fixing four corner points; the package uses these points to set up a rectangular mesh. The user then sets the position of some of the desired points of the surface above or below the plane of the rectangle; using a Bezier curve-fitting procedure, the package then forms a curved surface that goes through these points. Depending on the fineness of the mesh that is used, quite complex curved surfaces can be formed. However, the package will not display grids if more than 1800 grid points are to appear on the screen.

The user has a lot of control over the object creation process, including the ability to rotate, move, or scale the objects, repeat parts or whole objects, mirror-image, snap to the grid or turn off the grid, connect one object to another, and pan and zoom.

Perspective viewing

If the creation-mode views of the objects are not sufficiently enlightening, the user can view the model in perspective and move the viewing around to expose all sides. Creation produces a wire-frame version of the object, but automatic hidden-line removal can be invoked for better viewing. Curved surfaces and domes are not affected by this hidden-line removal process. They continue to appear in mesh form. There are also some hidden-line imperfections that may show up where different objects intersect.

Pulling and twisting

Once objects have been created using Design Board, they can be modified to take many different forms. For example, one face of a cylinder can be collapsed into a single point to pull it into a conical shape. Or a circle can be stretched into a keyhole shape, using a function that causes parallel motion of selected points. In a similar fashion, an entire face of an object can be moved in parallel fashion, stretching all the lines that connect it to the rest of the object as it moves.

During these modification procedures, the user is presented with a display screen divided into four windows which show a perspective view, along with top, bottom, and right-side views of the object being modified. This allows added insight into the results achieved by the various changes the user makes.

Printing and plotting

Views displayed on the screen can be printed on a dot matrix printer, or plotted, provided your plotter is a Hewlett-Packard or Houston Instruments model supported by the Design Board package. The simplest way to get hard copy is to dump the screen, that is, have the printer reproduce exactly what is displayed on the screen. If the user wants to get a scaled drawing, including a perspective drawing with hidden lines removed, these too can be produced.

DRAWING PROCESSOR II: SOME NICE DRAFTING FEATURES

This drafting package is designed for digitizer pad input. It has a curve-fitting feature and easily generates ellipses, but line handling can sometimes be awkward. There is no panning.

The package is for the IBM/PC and compatible computers. It requires 256K of main memory, and the use of the 8087 math coprocessor chip is recommended. It also requires use of a color graphics adapter. The IBM color adapter or graphics cards from several other vendors may be used. If a second display screen is available, the package will support two-screen operation.

List price of the package is $995. A version that lacks overlays, computer-aided dimensioning, command file input, and component menu extension is available for $495. Program revisions for a period of one year cost $100 extra. It is available from BG Graphics Systems, 824 Stetson Ave, Kent, WA 98031 [(206) 852-2736].

Unlike most other drafting packages, this one does not operate from screen-displayed menus. A digitizer pad is the preferred form of input. Drawing commands are selected from the digitizer pad by spotting them on a menu strip (at the top of the digitizer) with the drawing stylus or puck. Editing of on-screen drawings can be done in a similar manner so, if desired, the computer keyboard can be ignored and all drawing tasks, including ordering of output plots, can be conducted from the digitizer pad. However, commands can also be keyboarded.

Unless instructed otherwise, the package ordinarily assumes the user is drawing straight lines. Pressing the stylus to define a point, then moving elsewhere and pressing the stylus again will result in a line being drawn between these two points. If the user does not want this to happen, the "pen up" command must be given. If not, the user runs the danger of drawing unintended lines while moving from one part of the drawing to another.

Handling lines, can sometimes be awkward. The package does not include rubberbanding of lines, and there is no automatic creation of orthogonal lines. When the stylus is moved across the digitizer, the cursor on the display screen does not follow it.

Control over text is quite flexible. When text is incorporated in a drawing, the user can define the size, slant, and ratio of width to height of the text, as well as its location on the drawing. In 3D drawings, the text will remain attached to the proper plane when the image is moved or tilted.

The Drawing Processor has a useful curve-fitting feature. In addition to creation of lines, arcs, circles, and ellipses, curves can be fitted to any selected points, then stored and used as defined drawing elements. Components, such as these curves, can be manipulated by stretching, shrinking or rotation and can be added as choices on the digitizer menu strip.

Lines drawn close to the horizontal or vertical can be automatically adjusted so they become orthogonal. The package allows a tolerance to be set for this correction process to take place. The package will also report on distances between points, areas enclosed by lines, and angles between lines.

Pan by zoom

There is no panning facility provided with the Drawing Processor. To get a view of portions of a drawing beyond the immediately displayed area, the user has to zoom out for a wider view, then zoom back in again on the desired area.

Operation of this package depends on use of the 8087 math coprocessor chip, which is capable of dramatically speeding up calculation. Nevertheless, the package tends to run rather slowly compared to some of the other CAD packages for personal computers.

Like most packages, this one is supported by telephone-based technical support. Unfortunately, there seem to be only a few support people available, and users have found the support number is often continuously busy. The vendor has also been found to be slow in delivering replacement disks when they are needed.

ENERGRAPHICS: CHARTS AND DRAWINGS WITH LIMITED 3D

This is a multipurpose graphics package for creating charts, simple 2D drawings, and displays of some 3D objects. It is almost but not quite suitable as a drafting tool since there is no ability to use essential tools like graphics tablets, nor is attention paid to providing dimensioning.

EnerGraphics runs on the IBM/PC and compatible computers. It sells for $250. A plotting option costs an additional $100. It is available from Enertronics Research, 150 North Meramec #207, St. Louis, MO 63105 [(314) 725-5566].

Extensive use is made of the ten function keys on the IBM/PC keyboard. These keys are used to implement ten different modes of operation. Some attempt was made to make their use consistent across all the modes, but this is only partially sucessful, so the same key may have several different uses. However, users are reminded of the key functions by menu displays.

Charts and slide shows

There are separate, but similar, procedures for creating bar, pie, and line charts. In each case, after the chart is set up, it can be edited to meet user requirements. Data inputs to these chart creation procedures can be in equation form, or in the form of (DIF) files derived from spreadsheet packages, as well as from direct keyboard entry.

Completed charts can be displayed one at a time, and they can also be shown in sequence, presenting a sort of slide show. In addition to its displays, the package can produce printed and plotted outputs.

Simple 2D drawings

The package provides for 2D symbols, made up of line segment, arc, and dot elements, to be created by the user, stored, and then placed as needed on drawings. The symbols can be rotated, reduced, and enlarged, as well as translated to any position. When creating these 2D drawings, the same elements can be used along with the symbols, and text can be added from the keyboard as desired, with a choice of font styles. LIke elements and symbols, text can be rotated, translated, reduced, and enlarged.

The drawings are limited in complexity by two restrictions. Overall, a 2D drawing may not contain more than 800 line segments and 200 arcs and symbols. In addition, other "overlay" drawings can be added from storage to the working drawing. Up to ten such overlays can be added. However, once added they cannot be altered.

Two-dimensional drawings can be scaled, and the scale of a drawing can be changed as needed. There is a zoom feature that allows portions of a drawing to be enlarged up to 1024 times. Sections of a drawing can be defined, and these sections can then be rotated, translated, enlarged, and reduced.

Limited three-dimensional capabilities

Energraphics allows users to create three-dimensional surfaces that represent mathematical functions or sets of points in three-dimensional space. Given the function, the package will calculate the data points to be displayed.

3D objects made up of planar panels can also be constructed. Points and lines can be copied and rotated, to quickly construct these panels in a variety of shapes. The panels can then be oriented in 3D space, copied, and rotated to form the 3D objects. In turn, these 3D objects can also be rotated.

Perspective, isometric, and oblique drawings of a 3D object can be displayed, and the zoom feature can be used with these displays.

There is an automatic hidden-line removal feature that functions with some restrictions. If 3D objects are not constructed with careful attention to the hidden-line removal rules, this feature will not operate satisfactorily.

No 3D hard copy

Graphs and 2D drawings can be printed and, with the help of a separate optional program, plotted as well. However, there seems to be no way to print or plot the 3D creations of EnerGraphics. These drawings can be stored, and they can be included in the slide shows the package provides for, but the package provides no way to produce hard-copy versions.

ENTRY LEVEL: SEE VERSACAD REVIEW

MICROCAD: 3D FOR DESIGN

This is a 3D package, directed more to design and modeling than to drafting. It runs on the IBM/PC and requires 128K main memory, two floppy disk drives, and a color monitor board. List price is $500, from Computer-Aided Design, 764 24th Ave., San Francisco, CA 94121 [(415) 387-0263].

With MicroCAD, wire-frame shapes can be created, rotated, and viewed in isometric or perspective. Shapes defined by mathematical functions can be plotted. The package draws lines and arcs, insets text, edits drawings, and stores symbols that can be retrieved and inserted into the drawings.

A particularly pleasing feature is the ability to use the display cursor to represent the observer's eye, when producing varying views of an object. The cursor can be moved to the desired viewing position; then the new perspective can be generated at the push of a button.

There is a hidden-line removal feature that works on only one object at a time. Thus if one object is in front of another, the package will not remove all the lines in the area where the two objects overlap. There are other restrictions as well. If lines connecting planes are not drawn twice, they will disappear in some views. The vendor believes that at present the most efficient way to remove hidden lines is to have the user do it manually.

The main weakness of the package is its slowness in redrawing. This becomes more obvious when large or complex drawings are being handled. Text and curved lines are easily added to drawings, but they add measurably to the time needed to redraw. To reduce the need to redraw, a zoom function can be used to get close-up or distance views.

Input and output devices

The package can be used with keyboard, display, and dot-matrix printer. Use of a plotter is not required by the software, but the HP 7470A plotter is supported. To supplement the keyboard, a light pen can also be used, and several digitizers will work with the package. Operation is through a series of menus. Points can be entered numerically through a coordinate menu. There is also a main menu, an edit menu, and a plot menu for getting hard-copy output.

Other features

Plan and elevation views are available for all drawings. Both are ordinarily isometric views, but perspective views are available at the press of a key. A quick rotation feature allows a 3D object to be viewed from each of four sides (90 degrees apart) by sucessively pressing a two-key combination.

Component shapes can be stored, rotated, and scaled. Although components can also be joined to each other, attaching lines must be moved separately when the components are moved.

An optional rotatable character set feature ($150) allows text to be attached to any of the three plancs, so that it will move or rotate as the images are moved. Another option is an automatic dimensioning feature. Callouts, arrowheads, dimension lines, and strings are generated. There is also an optional bill of materials module that reports on quantity, unit, and extended cost for assemblies of parts that have been appropriately prepared using MicroCAD.

The package will find the area size, center of gravity, and moment of inertia for any selected area of a displayed object. It will also find the volume of solid objects. Circles and arcs can be generated. The user must define a point on the arc, the center of the arc or circle, and the angle of the arc.

An obtuse manual

The manual is somewhat peculiar. It reads like a calendar rather than a book, and the introduction section begins on page 56. This section is preceded by a discussion of software and equipment requirements phrased in computer talk that may be unfamiliar to many engineers. And it is followed by a listing of a BASIC routine for reading MicroCAD files. In short, the manual seems to have been written for the convenience of the vendor rather than of the user. However, once it begins to describe actual package operation (on page 84), it is quite easy to follow.

PC-DRAW: DRAWING BUT NOT FULL-FLEDGED DRAFTING

This package supplies a number of tools for drawing but not a full-fledged drafting capability. Shapes can be created, stored, and placed as desired in the drawing area. The documentation is good.

The package runs on an IBM/PC with 128K main memory, two disk drives, and a color graphics adapter. Use of a light pen is optional. Price of the package is $250. It is available from Micrographx, 8526 Vista View Dr., Dallas, TX 75243 [(214) 343- 4338].

PC-Draw provides for using stored sets of prepared icons or drawing elements. Current versions come with symbols for software flowcharting, logic diagrams, and electrical drawings. Users can create their own stored symbols as desired, and this can be done while a drawing is in progress. When selected from the symbol display, with cursor or light pen pointing, a symbol can be placed at any location on a drawing, expanded or compressed, and rotated using keyboard commands. For most of the manipulations a single-key command is used.

The optional light pen can be used to make selections from any PC-Draw displayed menu, to control cursor movement, to produce freehand line drawings, to locate circles, and to perform many combination-key functions.

Resolution of the drawings is poor, and all lines that are not horizontal or vertical suffer visibly from the "jaggies." While these jagged angled lines are quite easy to draw, they are difficult to erase.

Drawings can be divided up into pages, where several screen displays can be component pages of a larger drawing. Printouts allow two screens to be shown on a single printed page; with condensed printing, four pages can be squeezed onto one printed page. Larger drawings must be made up by pasting together several printed pages. A choice of two different text fonts for drawing annotation is available, and the annotations may be placed either horizontally or vertically.

ROBOCAD-2: FOR DRAWINGS OF LIMITED COMPLEXITY

This package is relatively inexpensive and very straightforward and simple to use. It handles 2D drawings of limited complexity quickly and easily. However, changing drawings is an awkward process, and some features like automatic dimensioning are only partially effective

RoboCAD-2 runs on Apple II+ IIe computers. It sells for $1495, and the price includes a "controller" device with joystick, dial, and pushbuttons. It is available from Chessel-Robocom Corp., 111 Pheasant Run, Newtown, PA 18940 [(215) 968- 4422].

With this package users can keep their eyes on the computer display screen, maneuvering and creating the drawings with the help of a joystick-dial controller and making very little use of the keyboard.

Memory countdown

Drawings are created a screenful at a time. To help users keep track of the computer memory space currently available for drawing, RoboCAD displays a countdown counter. The correct procedure is to avoid reaching the memory limit (10K) by storing drawings on disk as they begin to grow too large.

Disk-stored drawings can be retrieved as needed to be incorporated in larger, overall drawings. These retrieved drawings can be rotated, reduced, flipped about vertical or horizontal axes, stretched or squeezed, but their details cannot be altered.

To modify a drawing, it can be put through an editing process. This is inconvenient since the user has to step through the lines of the drawing, one at a time, to find the one that is to be altered. For $600 an accelerator card can be plugged into the computer which will speed up, but not short-cut, this process.

To find their way through partial or component stored drawings that will be used to make up a larger overall drawing, users create a skeleton or base drawing that shows how key reference points on the partial drawings relate to the overall picture. If a drawing is created in the package's scale drawing mode, it will be automatically rescaled to the correct size when incorporated into a scaled work drawing.

Screen-displayed features

Displayed around the edges of the screen are symbols and codes representing various choices available to the user. These are invoked by pointing to them via the controller joystick. Choices include straight-line or several curved drawing elements, selectable pitch cross hatching, six line colors, four line types, and a number of other drawing choices.

The package makes symbol libraries available. These are displayed on the screen, and symbols are selected from the screen rather than by entering a code on the keyboard.

RoboCAD will calculate line lengths and measure angles, arcs, and radii. It uses decimal quantities for all dimensions and will automatically annotate lines and other features with their dimensions. English and metric dimensions can be used on the same drawing and will be correctly scaled. Dimension lines, arrows, and reference marks have to be drawn by the user. Blocks of text can be rotated as needed but are limited to 40 characters each.

VERSACAD: IMPRESSIVE DRAFTING FEATURES

This package has an impressive array of useful features and options. It provides for a huge number of drawing layers, and it makes up, to some extent for speed limitations by offsetting features. In support, ease of learning and of use, VersaCAD is very much oriented to user needs.

VersaCAD runs on IBM/PCs and HP Series 200 computers; it sells for $1995. An Apple computer version called CADAPPLE is also $1995. ENTRY-LEVEL versions with more limited capabilities are available for $495. The vendor is T&W Systems, 7372 Prince Dr. #106, Huntington Beach, CA 92647 [(714) 847 9960].

Available with VersaCAD as drawing primitives are lines, arcs, circles, rectangles, fillets, and regular polygons. These can be placed on the screen at any location, in any desired size. The package also has a Bezier curve-fitting feature that allows drawing segments to be connected by smooth curves, and the ability to create ellipses by specifying their major and minor axes. There is a hatch function that works automatically to fill closed areas.

Users set up their own overall coordinate system for each drawing. Polar coordinates can be used. Drawings may be larger than the display screen. A screen readout informs the user of the location of the current display on the overall drawing.

Two monitors are used for display. One shows the drawing itself; the other is a command screen used to select drawing procedures and features. For simultaneous work on different sections of a drawing, the package allows up to five drawing "windows" to be set up and used. These can be used to provide the equivalent of zooming in and out.

Input may be by means of a graphics tablet or a joystick, or by entering coordinates, angles, etc., through the computer keyboard.

Each drawing may include up to 250 layers of material, and each layer can be shown in a different background color, provided a color display is used, to help keep track of layer location.

Many convenient features

The user controls the size, proportion, and rotation of text used with a drawing. Drawings can be conveniently modified by spotting the object to be changed on the screen and giving an appropriate change command.

Drawing primitives may be used to make up parts which can, in turn, be stored in pages containing up to 100 parts each. These stored parts can be called up from a screen display of the page that contains them and placed where desired in the currently active drawing. The user simply points to the desired symbol with a graphics tablet stylus and presses the Enter key. Once on the drawing screen, the symbol can be rotated, scaled, and moved. Until finally placed in the drawing, the symbol blinks as it is moved, making it easy to follow. The vendor makes about 5000 such symbols available. Others can be drawn and stored by users.

Dimension lines, with arrowheads, leader lines, and dimension text are automatically created; the user specifies the units of measure.

A Repeat function allows objects to be duplicated along a line, around an object, or to fill an area. Whole drawing sections can be replicated using a Copy function. And portions of drawings as well as entire drawings can be deleted. The mirror-imaging feature is a useful one. Text in mirrored objects will be displayed as if read in a mirror, but in plotter output the mirrored text can be correctly reproduced.

To aid in aligning drawing elements, an optional background grid can be displayed, and the user can define the spacing of this grid. A "snap" function allows objects placed nearby to be snapped into precise grid locations.

Attributes such as line-type, color, and plot-pen number are assigned to symbols and objects rather than to drawings or layers of drawings. This means that when these symbols and objects are moved, the attributes move with them.

An Inquiry feature allows the user to summon up stored and calculated information about specific objects in a drawing. This may include such items as lengths and areas, and the package is able to do some fairly complex area calculations.

An optional program allows the user to display sequences of drawings for presentation purposes. There is also an optional 3D program that includes a 3D "box" as a primitive element.

A bill of materials feature searches drawings for the objects they contain and creates a report. If told to search for something that does not appear in the drawings, the package will report finding no such object. Use of this feature, like similar features in other packages, is rather complicated and slow.

Speed of operation

In fact, these often excellent features tend to be offset by the fact that, like other personal computer based drafting packages, VersaCAD runs rather slowly, even with the use of a special 8087 math coprocessor chip in the IBM/PC.

However, there are some built-in features designed to speed up operation. Unused drawing layers can be switched off so that the package doesn't waste time scanning and redrawing material on the unused layers. Since recreating text after panning or zooming can be time consuming, the package allows the user to temporarily convert text lines into simple straight lines while doing a lot of moving around.

When problems arise

The "Help" feature of the package provides advice on the use of selected program options. If material is accidentally deleted, it can be restored—not just the last item but all the objects deleted from the drawing during the current session. When the user enters a program option by mistake, pressing the Esc key will provide a quick means to back out.

If an equipment or system failure should occur, VersaCAD allows the user to recover the work files completely so that valuable design effort will not be lost. Protection of work files involves frequent storage of current activity on disks, so the package is best used with hard, rather than slower, floppy disk storage.

VersaCAD is well-maintained and is frequently updated to add new features. After the first 90 days of free support, an extended warranty service is available. Revisions and new software additions are sent to users as part of this service.

Chapter 9
Symbol/Object Manipulation
Graphics Packages

The graphics packages described in this chapter allow users to construct drawings by positioning prepared symbols or objects on the screen. These packages generally incorporate the ability to do some drawing of lines as well as figures like polygons, circles, and ellipses, and they also allow users to annotate the drawings with text.

However, the packages fall short of providing drafting capability in that they are not equipped to produce standard engineering drawings efficiently. For this, the ability to automatically, or at least conveniently, handle drafting necessities like dimensioning, and to construct highly complex drawings with rapid manipulation of drawing processes, would be needed. The packages described here do not meet those requirements.

However, even with their limited capabilities, symbol and object manipulation packages have a wide range of possible applications. They can be used to draw layouts useful in conceptual and planning activities and to produce the many types of diagrams and charts that help engineers to put their projects into operation.

If they are to be more than mere toys, the implicit question that packages of this type must answer is: can they produce results that are better, or more useful, or are less expensive to achieve than what can be done by manual drawing methods?

Store and draw

The basic idea of these packages is to use the storage capabilities of the personal computer to eliminate the need to constantly redraw often-used objects or symbols. To allow creation of useful drawings, there must also be some means to connect these objects together. And, like other symbols, images of alphabetic letters and numerals should be able to be drawn from storage to form text entries on the drawings.

PC-Draw is a package that provides those basic capabilities in pretty much the expected way, and that is about all it does provide. For most of the other packages, the vendors apparently felt they had to offer something extra.

Benchmark, for example, tries to be as universal as possible. This package includes, along with its graphics capabilities, a data manager, word processor, spelling checker, and spreadsheet. Benchmark is integrated in that the graphics can be used together with the data manager and spreadsheet. However, there seems to be no useful interaction between graphics and the word processor.

Multiple text fonts are offered by the QUICK-DRAFT package. Twenty different character fonts come with the package, and these include many symbols useful in making drawings as well as different types of numerals and alphabet letters. There is a Japanese Katakana font, a Greek font, and an Esperanto font. Most of the other packages provide only a few fonts. For example, PC-Draw gives a choice of only two different text fonts for drawing annotation.

The extra feature of the TGS package is its ability to animate. TGS can put display frames containing simple shapes composed of lines and circles, along with text, into apparent motion. However, the drawings are simple and somewhat crude, unsuitable for most engineering animation needs.

MGI/Schematic Drafter has a unique approach. It divides the drawing area up into cells. There is no overall ability to draw connecting lines, but symbols in the cells can be prepared and placed so that lines that are part of one symbol match up with those in an adjacent cell.

Symbol creation and use

Current versions of PC-Draw come with symbols for software flow-charting, logic diagrams, and electrical drawings. Users can create their own stored symbols as desired, and this can be done while a drawing is in progress. Stored symbols are selected from displays, using cursor or light pen pointing, then placed on the current drawing. An excellent feature of this package is the split-screen display, with the symbol selection menu on the right and the drawing shown on the left as it takes shape.

Most of the other packages use similar approaches, providing stored libraries of symbols and allowing users to add their own symbolcreations to those libraries.

The MGI/Schematic Drafter is again unique, in that it devotes most of the computer keyboard to symbol selection. The user refers to a printed template guide for the particular symbol library in use. There the available symbols are shown in positions corresponding to those of the keyboard. The user moves the cursor to a cell in the displayed drawing space, then presses the appropriate key to call a copy of the associated symbol into that cell. The user can move the cursor from cell to cell, inserting symbols in each. An undesired symbol can be erased from a cell by moving the cursor to it, then pressing the space bar. Or it can be replaced by another symbol by a similar key action. If desired, two symbols can be placed within one cell.

Some packages provide only limited symbol or object storage. Thus QUICK-DRAFT is able to store and repeat just 20 sequences of keystrokes and cursor motions. In other words, it can automatically redraw up to 20 user-created objects on command. The object definition process is simply the sequence of keyboard actions used to draw the object. The package automatically numbers the objects as they are created, and they have to be recalled by number. So it is left up to the user to keep some record of which stored object is which.

Complexity of drawings

For engineering applications, drawings often have to show considerable detail, and this is an area where these packages tend to be deficient.

The complexity of an MGI/Schematic Drafter drawing is set at the outset by the user. To start a drawing, the user must select a mesh size for the background grid of the drawing. The grid may contain up to 50 cells across its width or may have as few as 6 cells across. A large number of cells may be needed, in order to portray complex drawings, since only one or two symbols can be placed in any cell.

The quality of the displays and printed output produced by the QUICK-DRAFT package is limited by the coordinate matrix on which the package is based. This has a width of 280 positions and a height of 192 positions. Lines and figures are always made up of straight orthogonal segments from one coordinate position to another. The result is that vertical and horizontal lines are smooth in appearance, while all lines and curves that deviate from these two directions have a discomfortingly jagged appearance.

A similar effect is seen in the drawings produced by the PC-Draw package. All lines that are not horizontal or vertical suffer visibly from the "jaggies." While these jagged angled lines are quite easy to draw, they are difficult to erase and may make the drawings unacceptable for some uses.

Manipulation of symbols

To properly place and orient symbols taken from storage, users need considerable flexibility in manipulating them. Most packages provide several different symbol manipulation modes. For example, EnerGraphics symbols can be rotated, reduced, and enlarged, as well as translated to any position.

With the MGI/Schematic Drafter, the manipulation is more discrete. Symbols can be rotated into 8 possible orientations: four 90-degree rotations, plus four more 90-degree rotations of a mirrored image of the symbol. All these are obtained from one of the function keys. Each time it is pressed, the symbol moves to the next in the sequence of eight orientations. If the user desires, these orientation changes can be imposed simultaneously on all the symbols in the current drawing. A symbol can be shifted in position within a cell—up, down, or sideways—but only in increments of 1/4 of the cell dimension.

Because the MGI package treats line segments only as symbols and has no separate line drawing ability, it gives users an extra symbol manipulation feature. Any given symbol can be rapidly copied into a series of cells. The user types the number of cells that are to receive copies, then presses the desired symbol key, and cells are filled, following the direction of the last movement of the cursor. This feature can be used to create long continuous lines from individual cell line segments.

In most of the packages, text characters and chunks of text can be manipulated in much the same way as any other symbols. However, text positioning is sometimes restricted. In the PC-Draw package, for instance, text annotations must be either horizontal or vertical.

Manipulation of drawings

Not only symbols but entire drawings must be freely manipulated in order to produce the variety of results that these packages promise. These capabilities vary from package to package.

The user can define a rectangular block of cells with the MGI/Schematic Drafter package, then copy, move, or delete that block. And the block can also be placed in, and recalled from, disk storage. However, MGI scrolling is a rather clumsy operation. The user has to key an entry to the scroll mode, then the scroll direction, and then the number of cells that are to be scrolled, before the actual scrolling can take place. Zooming is controlled by defining the block that is to be zoomed, then specifying the width of the zoomed view in number of cells. Other zoom choices include a return to the last previous view, to the original grid view, or to a view that will display all the cells in the drawing.

A QUICK-DRAFT drawing can occupy a space equivalent to four display-screen areas. The package has no zooming or panning features. But it does have a scrolling capability to allow the user to move the display about, over this four-screen area, in half-screen increments. QUICK-DRAFT also allows full-screen drawings to be stored in the computer memory. The number of such storage positions, up to 33 with a main memory of 256K, depends on the available memory space. The current contents of the drawing screen can be stored in one of these memory positions at any time, and stored drawings can be summoned to the display for viewing or alteration.

Printing and plotting the results

For most of the packages, a printout is simply a hard copy version of what is displayed on the computer screen. PC-Draw adds a bit to that capability. It allows drawings to be divided up into pages, so that each screen display can be a component page of a larger drawing. Printouts allow two screens to be shown on a single printed page; with condensed printing, four pages can be shown.

The only package reviewed here that makes use of plotting equipment is the MGI/Schematic Drafter. Drawings created with this package can be reproduced using a Houston Instruments DMP series plotter. To use the Hewlett-Packard 7580 plotter, special added software is needed. To get plotted output, the user specifies the desired paper size (A-E) and the package automatically scales the output to place the drawing on that size of paper. The drawings can also be reproduced, as displayed, using a dot matrix printer.

Special features

Something close to a bill of materials, but not quite, can be produced by the MGI/Schematic Drafter package. The user can call for a symbol listing that will show all the symbols used in a drawing and the number of times each symbol appears, and these listings can be edited to remove unwanted items.

Some of the packages offer color to users. Thus with QUICK- DRAFT, any region of the drawing that is surrounded by lines or arcs can be quickly filled with color. The user moves the cursor into the selected region, then calls for any of 22 available colors. This package can also operate in a "Wash" mode that allows the user to fill in the entire background of a drawing with a choice of eight colors. This same mode can be used to draw rays from a fixed point.

BENCHMARK: GRAPHICS INTEGRATED WITH OTHER FUNCTIONS

Reviewed by Shen C. Lee, University of Missouri-Rolla

This integrated software package includes some graphics capabilities along with a data manager, word processor, spelling checker, and spreadsheet. The strength of the package is that the graphics can be used together with the data manager and spreadsheet. However, the word processor is not able to combine graphs with text. No operational problems were encountered with the package during this review.

Benchmark runs on IBM/PC and compatible computers with minimum 256K main memory. Use of color display, with high resolution color adapter, and of color-supported printer is optional. The package sells for $795 from Metasoft Corp., 6905 W. Frye Rd. #12, Chandler, AZ 85224 [(800) 621-1908, (602) 961-0003].

This reviewer found the graphics capability of the Benchmark package most interesting. It has the ability to move and rotate the images, to zoom, and also to add text to the graphics. Since no high resolution color display or color-supported printer was available, the output was viewed on a monochrome monitor, and the reviewer was favorably impressed with the results.

The package can generate simple engineering design drawings using 18 primitive commands, such as circle, arc, ellipse, line, and rectangle. Drawings can be stored for future use, revision, or modification.

Using data from the package's spreadsheet or data manager, presentation charts and graphs can be produced. These include pie charts, clustered bar charts, horizontal bar charts, line graphs, and x,y plots. These displays are controlled by 11 presentation graphics commands.

Handling multiple functions

An overall directory program called the Benchmark Administrator provides access to the various functions the package provides. It also performs some disk housekeeping functions.

The data manager is similar to many conventional database packages for personal computers. It allows the user to design formats for data retrieval and storage. A very useful feature is the ability to transfer stored data (through a "DIF" file format) for use with the package's graphics capabilities.

The spreadsheet feature includes a three-dimensional capability. This allows the user to store, retrieve, and manage data in the columns and rows of one or of several spreadsheet pages at the same time. Spreadsheet data can also be transferred for use with graphics display.

The word processor presents the user with more operational procedures than most simple similar packages. This reviewer expected that it would provide a choice of fonts and allow graphs to be included in the text. However, the word processor seems poorly integrated with the other features of this package. The vendor has stated that an advanced word processor feature, able to work in an integrated manner with the rest of the package, was being completed at the time of this review.

For use with the word processor, there is a spelling checker with an authority file of words that will be compared to those in text. The user can add to or subtract from this authority list as desired.

Limited help for the user

The vendor has a toll-free phone number through which users can seek answers to a limited number of questions they may have about the package. For the rest, they must rely on the documentation supplied with the package.

This written material seems to be directed mainly to experienced users. There are clear instructions for configuration of the package so it can be used with the many different computers and printers for which it is designed. However, the documentation does not provide clearly illustrated procedures for tutoring an inexperienced user to become proficient with the package. During the review process, it became clear that the user manual should be expanded to include more examples so as to minimize the amount of guesswork on the part of the user in figuring out necessary procedures. The manual also needs an index for quick reference.

MGI/SCHEMATIC DRAFTER

MGI/Schematic Drafter allows the user to place and interconnect prepared symbols on a grid and to annotate drawings produced in this way with text. Symbol libraries are available for a number of engineering applications.

This package runs on IBM/PC/XT and compatibles and on Tandy 2000 computers. Use of the 8087 math chip is recommended to increase the speed *of package operation. It sells for $2495, and that price includes a choice of three of the symbol libraries offered by the vendor, Microcomputer Graphics, 13468 Washington Blvd., P.O. Box 10819, Marina del Rey, CA 90295 [(213) 822-5258].*

To start a drawing, the user must select a mesh size for the background grid of the drawing. The grid may contain up to 50 cells across its width or may have as few as 6 cells across. A large number of cells may be needed, in order to portray complex drawings, since only one or two symbols can be placed in any cell. During the subsequent drawing process, it is possible to insert blank rows and columns of cells into the drawing. And rows or columns may also be deleted.

The package uses keyboard function keys to control cursor movement rather than the customary arrow keys provided on the keyboard. Users are advised to paste arrow labels over the appropriate function keys to remind them of each key's function.

Placing symbols

Other keys are used to transfer stored symbols to the drawing cells. To do this, the user refers to a printed template guide for the particular symbol library in use. There the available symbols are shown in positions corresponding to those of the keyboard. The user moves the cursor to a cell, then presses a symbol key to call a copy of the associated symbol into that cell. The user can move the cursor from cell to cell, inserting symbols in each. An undesired symbol can be erased from a cell by moving the cursor to it, then pressing the space bar. Or it can be replaced by another symbol by a similar key action. If the user desires, two symbols can be placed within one cell.

Manipulating symbols and drawings

Symbols can be rotated into 8 possible orientations: four 90-degree rotations, plus four more 90-degree rotations of a mirrored image of the symbol. All these are obtained from one of the function keys. Each time it is pressed, the symbol moves to the next in the sequence of eight orientations. If the user desires, these orientation changes can be imposed simultaneously on all the symbols in the current drawing. A symbol can be shifted in position within a cell—up, down, or sideways—but only in increments of 1/4 of the cell dimension.

A given symbol can also be rapidly copied into a series of cells. The user types the number of cells that are to receive copies, then presses the desired symbol key and cells are filled, following the direction of the last movement of the cursor. This feature is used to create long continuous lines from individual cell line segments.

Block operations are also provided. The user can define a rectangular block of cells, then copy, move, or delete that block. And the block can also be placed in, and recalled from, disk storage.

Scrolling is a rather clumsy operation. The user has to key an entry to the scroll mode, then the scroll direction, and then the number of cells that are to be scrolled, before the actual scrolling can take place. Zooming is controlled by defining the block that is to be zoomed, then specifying the width of the zoomed view in number of cells. Other zoom choices include a return to the last previous view, to the original grid view, or to a view that will display all the cells in the drawing.

Text insertion

Text can be added to the drawing by locating the cursor at the desired start of text, going into the text mode, then keyboarding the text characters using the normal keyboard numeral and letter keys. Like symbols, text entries can be rotated in 90-degree increments. The entries can also be dragged using the cursor arrow keys, erased, and replaced.

Using and creating symbols

Library files of stored drawing symbols are provided by the vendor. Among the available libraries are those with symbols for project scheduling, space planning, pneumatic and hydraulic drawings, P & ID designs, electrical and electronic circuits.

Users may also create their own symbols and add them to existing symbol files, or to newly-created symbol library files. Like the overall drawings, the symbols are created on grids, but the procedures are somewhat different from those previously described. Straight lines, circles, and arcs can be drawn and erased. Text can also be included as an integral part of a symbol. Existing symbols can be recalled and modified. And they can also be selected and rearranged into new symbol library files. Printed guides, for use when calling up the symbols from the keyboard, can be produced.

Plots, printouts, and listings

Drawings created with this package can be reproduced using a Houston Instruments DMP series plotter. To use the Hewlett-Packard 7580 plotter, special added software is needed. To get plotted output, the user specifies the desired paper size (A-E) and the package automatically scales the output to place the drawing on that size of paper. The drawing can also be reproduced, as displayed, using a dot matrix printer.

Something close to a bill of materials, but not quite, can be produced by this package. The user can call for a symbol listing, that will show all the symbols used in a drawing and the number of times each symbol appears. These listings can be edited to remove unwanted items.

PC-DRAW

This package supplies a number of tools for drawing but not a full-fledged drafting capability. Shapes can be created, stored, and placed as desired in the drawing area.

The package runs on IBM/PC and some compatible computers. Use of a light pen is optional. Price of the package is $395. It is available from Micrographx, 8526 Vista View Dr., Dallas, TX 75243 [(214) 343-4338].

PC-Draw provides for using stored sets of prepared symbols and drawing elements. Current versions come with symbols for software flowcharting, logic diagrams, and electrical drawings. Users can create their own stored symbols as desired, and this can be done while a drawing is in progress. When selected from the symbol display, with cursor or light pen pointing, a symbol can be placed at any location on a drawing, expanded or compressed, and rotated using keyboard commands.

For most of the manipulations a single-key command is used, but there are also a number of multiple key commands that have to be remembered. A reference card, supplied with the package, lists these keyboard commands. It will take most users considerable practice to get them down pat.

Users work from menu displays to create new symbols, or update old ones, and to create, edit, and printout drawings. The keyboard commands are used in carrying out menu-selected procedures. The optional light pen can be used to make selections from any PC-Draw displayed menu, to control cursor movement, to produce freehand line drawings, to locate circles, and to perform many combination-key functions.

An excellent feature of the package is the split-screen display, with the symbol selection menu on the right and the drawing shown on the left as it takes shape.

Jagged lines

Resolution of the drawings is poor, and all lines that are not horizontal or vertical suffer visibly from the "jaggies." While these jagged angled lines are quite easy to draw, they are difficult to erase.

Drawings can be divided up into pages, where several screen displays can be component pages of a larger drawing. Printouts allow two screens to be shown on a single printed page; with condensed printing, four pages can be squeezed onto one printed page. Larger drawings must be made up by pasting together several printed pages. A choice of two different text fonts for drawing annotation is available, and the annotations may be placed either horizontally or vertically.

The user manual explains how to use the package, but it lacks an index and is therefore not useful as a reference source. There is some indexing in the online HELP material, but no facility for calling up the specific instructions pertinent to the current package operations being used.

PC-Draw can be used with a variety of dot matrix printers, or with Hewlett-Packard 7470A, 7475A, 7550A, Houston Instruments, DMP, or Roland plotters.

QUICK-DRAFT

This is a versatile symbol manipulation and drawing package. Twenty different character fonts come with the package. Up to 20 objects may be drawn, defined, and stored, then recalled and positioned on a display. A variety of drawing modes are provided. However, the quality of drawing displays and printouts is limited, producing jagged lines, and is unsuitable for showing accurate detail.

QUICK-DRAFT runs on Apple II computers. It sells for $50 from Interactive Microware, P.O. Box 139, State College, PA 16804 [(814) 238-8294].

Line segments are drawn by defining their beginning and endpoints while the package is in its LINE mode of operation. When a line is drawn, the cursor automatically moves to the endpoint, allowing a series of connected segments to be easily constructed. Arrowheads can be added to the ends of lines by simply pressing the A key.

Circles are drawn by defining a center point, then moving the cursor away to define another point through which the circle should pass. Ellipses are similarly started by locating a center point, then moving the cursor to define the width and height of the figure. Arcs of circles and ellipses are defined by angles from the centers of these figures.

To draw rectangles, squares, and diamonds, the user moves the cursor to define two opposite vertices, then keys a command for a rectangle or diamond shape. Equilateral triangles and polygons are drawn by defining the locations of a center point and one vertice, then specifying the desired number of sides (3 to 9).

Movement of the display cursor can be controlled by key actions, game paddles, a joystick, or a Koala pad. The distance the cursor will move at each keystroke is adjustable. To aid in keeping track of the cursor position, its x,y coordinates can be shown at the bottom of the display. It can be made to jump, on command, to any x,y position on the drawing.

To locate items more accurately in a drawing, a background grid of dots can be called for. There is a slight problem here. Items drawn after the grid is put in place will have grid-dot holes in them if the grid is removed, and if the user wishes to fill these holes, this will have to be done one at a time.

Objects can be defined and used

QUICK-DRAFT is able to store and repeat up to 20 sequences of keystrokes and cursor motions; in other words, to automatically redraw up to 20 user-created objects on command. The object definition process is simply the sequence of keyboard actions used to draw the object, but that sequence must be preceded by pressing the O key and immediately followed by pressing the $ key, to define it as a stored-object sequence.

The package automatically numbers the objects as they are created, and they have to be recalled by number. So, it is left up to the user to keep some record of which stored object is which.

This feature has a procrustean peculiarity. If the user tries to place an object recalled from memory in a position where it would run over the boundaries of the screen, the object will be drawn in a distorted manner so it will fit within those boundaries.

Drawings in memory

A QUICK-DRAFT drawing can occupy a space equivalent to four display screen areas. The package has no zoom or panning features. But it does have a scrolling capability to allow the user to move the display about, over this four-screen area, in half-screen increments. QUICK-DRAFT also allows full-screen drawings to be stored in the computer memory. The number of such storage positions, up to 33 with a main memory of 256K, depends on the available memory space. The current contents of the drawing screen can be stored in one of these memory positions at any time, and stored drawings can be summoned to the display for viewing or alteration.

To help users keep track of where they are in the four-screen drawing space, "row" and "column" numbers can be displayed at the bottom of the screen. These indicate a division of the drawing space into three horizontal and three vertical regions. However, this notation is hard to grasp and has to be rehearsed before it can be helpful.

Color filling

Any region of the drawing that is surrounded by lines or arcs can be quickly filled with color. The user moves the cursor into the selected region, then calls for any of 22 available colors to be used.

The package can also operate in a "Wash" mode that allows the user to fill in the entire background of a drawing with a choice of eight colors. This same mode can be used to draw rays from a fixed point. These are constructed much like line segments, except that the cursor returns to the same beginning point each time the user defines another endpoint. With the help of a joystick or Koala pad, this feature can be used to fill areas of the screen with rays.

Selectable cursor symbol

Text for this package is made up of dot characters, and the standard symbol set contains 122 characters, including about two dozen squares, circles, crosses, and such, that may be useful for drawing figures. Nineteen additional text fonts, including a Katakana Japanese and a Greek font, can be called up from storage. And tables of other symbols can be stored as well.

Many of these characters can be chosen as the cursor symbol. In the PAINT mode of the package, the chosen symbol can then be continuously replicated along the path over which the cursor is moved. Further freedom in this mode is offered by the ability to rotate the position of the cursor character, to scale it in one of nine different sizes, and to have different colors as well.

To remind the user of how cursor use is currently arranged, there can be a display of the last-chosen scale factor and rotation angle at the bottom of the screen.

There is a TEXT mode of operation for entering text onto a drawing from the keyboard. When in this mode the available symbols are split into three fonts, and the user must be aware of which symbols are in each font, which font is currently in use, and also be able to manipulate a few special keyboard text commands.

Output on a dot matrix printer can be obtained at any desired point. The printout simply replicates what is shown on the screen. No plotting equipment is supported.

Limited graphics quality

The quality of the displays and printed output is limited by the coordinate matrix on which the package is based. This has a width of 280 positions and a height of 192 positions. Lines and figures are always made up of straight orthogonal segments from one coordinate position to another. The result is that vertical and horizontal lines are smooth in appearance while all lines and curves that deviate from these two directions have a discomfortingly jagged appearance.

The QUICK-DRAFT manual includes explanations of each of the package's commands, and there is a HELP facility that calls up a menu of 26 chunks of explanation text which the user can choose to display.

TGS: ANIMATED GRAPHICS

Simple shapes composed of lines and circles, along with text, can be created and put into apparent motion with this package. It is not designed for animation of engineering drawings.

TGS runs on Apple II computers. It sells for $149.95 from Accent Software, 3750 Wright Place, Palo Alto, CA 94306 [(415) 856-6505].

Drawing is done by pointing the display cursor in the desired direction. It can then move off in that direction until the user stops it, or changes its direction, or until it reaches the edge of the drawing area on the screen. The movement can be used to relocate the cursor or, at the user's command, to leave a drawing trace behind it. To remove what has been drawn, the cursor can be run over existing traces in an erase mode. Alternatively, an entire screenful of drawings can be erased at a keystroke.

In addition to lines, circles and text can be created and located on the displays.

Drawing can take place at two levels. At the LO level a drawing can be composed on the screen. Drawings made in this way can then be dropped into small rectangles on the HI level display. To alter the LO level drawings, they can be elongated or compressed on command, scrolled to move them about, and mirror-imaged.

These windows can then be moved about to place them as desired on the HI level display area, and they can be replicated. For example, a square can be replicated and moved to form a cube. New images, formed on the HI display, can then be transferred back to the LO display to make changes, such as removing the hidden lines in the cube.

A sequence of operations allowed by the package can be easily combined into a single "macro" instruction. The user simply gives a keyboard command that means "I'm starting the macro," then keyboards the sequence itself, followed by instructions that say, "I'm ending the macro." Thereafter, pressing R will automatically reexecute the whole sequence.

Animation technique

HI level displays can be quickly stored and retrieved. To make a square move across the screen, the user would create and store a series of HI level display frames, placing an image of a square at successive positions in each frame. Then, when the frames are rapidly displayed one after another, a moving square will be seen.

The package gives the user control over the speed at which such frames will be displayed. It also gives the user control over the sequence in which frames will be shown, allowing a sequence to be created, then frames to be removed from that sequence and other frames inserted in any desired position.

To see what is in a sequence, the user can step through it, frame by frame. Objects in the frames can be colored, backgrounds for the images created and changed.

Chapter 10
Curve and Chart Graphics Packages

Charts that display data points, curves, bars, and pie-sections are familiar tools to engineers who use them in reports, conference papers, and other presentations. In the past, preparation of such curves and charts, beyond those for personal recordkeeping, have usually required application of some drafting skills.

The packages discussed in this chapter provide a way to prepare curves and charts in acceptable presentation form with the help of a personal computer. The idea is that, with the help of these packages, such charts can be quickly set up, then displayed, printed, or output on a computer-connected plotter.

Plotting data points

Some of the packages are devoted entirely to producing plots of data points. For example, the SCIENTIFIC PLOTTER package produces point plots, with the option of having the points interconnected by straight-line segments.

Despite its title, there is no actual use of plotters with PCPLOT. This little bargain-priced package will display or print plots of x,y data points. Up to four data sets can be shown on one plot. But it can be fully used only by those with some knowledge of programming. The PLOTPRO package produces similar plots, operates from displayed menus, and sells for even less than PCPLOT.

For those who program, the ASYST package provides a set of computer commands specifically designed to produce charts of data points.

Most of the point-curve packages have few user conveniences built in. Apparently they were put together with the idea that engineers are so handy with computers that they can afford to spend a good deal of time doing little programming tricks. In actuality, these packages are in competition with manual methods of drawing data plots. An engineer cannot be expected to turn to a software package if it will be easier and faster to turn out the same graph on a drafting board.

It is by no means clear that, for the occasional user, point-charting packages represent an improvement in the state of the art of graphmaking. In terms of convenience for the occasional user, SCIENTIFIC PLOTTER is probably the best of those discussed in this chapter.

Bars, pies, text, and more

A large number of graphics packages capable of producing presentable line, bar, pie, and other charts, using personal computers, have recently become available. Most of these packages arc sold for use in business applications, but they can be very helpful in preparing materials for engineering presentations as well. Vendors of these packages seem to have given careful attention to making them easy to learn and easy to use in preparing a wide variety of professional-looking charts.

For example, users of the Graphwriter package have a choice of 23 different graph and chart formats. Ten of these are variations on the bar chart, with bars vertical or horizontal, solid or segmented, single, clustered, paired, or ornamented. Then there are pie charts, line, surface-line, and scatter charts, text display formats including tables, Gantt charts and range-bar charts, flow charts and pie-bar, bar-line combinations.

The KeyChart package produces a similar variety of charts by cleverly combining common characteristics of the different formats. And the CURVE II CRT package gives the user the option of employing standard line, bar, and pie formats, or of custom designing their own charts.

In addition to these more or less general purpose curve and chart packages, there are some with much more specific applications. Thus, for those who need contour plots, the GEOCONTOUR is available. Specifically designed for this purpose, this is truly a bare-bones package, put together with little thought for convenience of the user, and with very few options of which the user can take advantage.

Giving graphics instructions

To give an idea of the difference between packages that cater to user needs and those that ignore the user, let us take a brief look at some of the ways these packages help users to express what they want.

Perhaps the best arrangement is the one provided by the KeyChart package. Users input information for setting up their charts directly onto data displays. For example, there is a screen for naming, sizing, and labeling charts. Altogether it has spaces for 24 user-supplied inputs. Pressing the

Return key moves the screen cursor from one data entry item to another, and the keyboard arrow keys can be used to move back and forth between items. When entry items are keyboarded, they show up in bright or inverse-video characters. Users can also move easily from this input screen to others, back and forth if necessary, by pressing the PgUp and PgDn keys.

To attain this high level of operational simplicity, yet still provide for complex options, the designers of this package found they had to combine keyboarded commands with display entry. Altogether, the user has to remember about 22 special key actions to master full control of the data entry process. The manual includes a handy reference sheet listing these actions, but it will still take some practice to become familiar enough with them to make convenient use possible.

Graphwriter uses a menu display approach to present the many choices users can make. To navigate from one item and one menu to another, the user presses appropriate keys. And this package has an alternative approach that should be well suited to experienced users. It is not necessary actually to wait to see a menu before making selections. If users are familiar enough with what is on the menus, they can "type ahead," entering their choices in advance. The package will then move immediately through one typed option after another to bring the user to the desired point in the package's operations.

If these are the best of the lot, from the point of view of ease of learning and use, what do the others look like?

The regular procedures offered by the SCIENTIFIC PLOTTER package are spelled out by a lengthy and fixed sequence of screen-displayed prompts followed by user answers. The sequence includes setting up a graph format, inputting and scaling the data, plotting the data, labeling the graph, and storing the results of these steps. There is, however, some flexibility. At any point in the sequence, the user can call for a current view of the graph, manipulate the files, go into a BASIC language programming mode, or return to the display of prompts. And if users are dissatisfied with one of the steps, they can return directly to it through a redraw menu. The package will then erase the graph, automatically redraw it to the indicated step, and the user can proceed from there.

The CURVE II CRT package also uses long sequences of prompts-and-replies. Thus, a sequence of more than 60 prompts leads the user through construction of bar charts and includes the options of horizontal or vertical bars. Another 28 prompts provide for placing text on the chart. The procedures for putting pie charts together are similar.

The prompt sequences are rather rigid. If errors are made, and not caught immediately, a whole sequence must be replayed to make a correction. And it is not easy for users to keep track of the choices they have made. Experienced, constant users of this package will find little difficulty in visualizing their results as their instructions are entered, but novices and occasional users may find they have to cycle again and again through the procedures to get the results they want.

The ASYST package assumes that the user is ready to do programming. Although, from a programming standpoint, ASYST commands are very powerful (that is, one command will cause a lot to happen), all that power does little good for those who are not programmers.

Data entry

Point-plotting can often involve entering a lot of point data. That creates a special problem, in terms of presenting the data in a form that the software package can accept while imposing minimum work on the user. Some packages handle this problem well, while others seem to give it little consideration.

With KeyChart, the input data are assumed to be arranged in a row and column manner, and the package receives one column of data at a time. The entry action is arranged so the cursor skips from position to position as the user methodically enters a column title, row name, and value for each item of data in the first column. When the screen for that column is completed, it is entered and the package presents another column entry screen, and so forth until all the input data have been entered.

In lieu of keyboard entry, row and column data can be fed directly into KeyChart from packages like Lotus 1-2-3, Symphony, Supercalc, Multiplan, and several other popular spreadsheet programs.

CURVE II CRT will accept data from the keyboard or from stored files in the DIF format used by VisiCalc spreadsheets and similar packages. In either case, the data to be used can be reviewed, 10 points at a time, and edited to correct errors or make desired changes.

PCPLOT draws upon data files to trace out its plots. However, users have to rely on their own programming skills to provide and enter those files. If that sounds inconvenient, consider the GEOCONTOUR package where the input information is required to be formatted as if it were being read into the computer by a data-processing card reader. Thus, the first line of element data gives, in positions 1-5, the total number of elements involved. The second line shows, in positions 1-5, a number identifying an element. Then in positions 6-10, 11-15, and 16-20 it shows the three node numbers for that element. Other input must be keyboarded in similar rigidly-prescribed formats.

Graph Construction

Packages that handle formats for a number of different types of graphs need to have a way to make those formats available to users. For instance, Graphwriter comes with a total of ten different floppy disks. Two of these are concerned with the main program and with setting up for specific kinds of plotters and printers. The other eight contain the software needed to set up particular chart and graph formats. To get a desired format the user has to insert the correct disk into the computer's disk drive.

The KeyChart package takes a different approach. In this nicely integrated package, once the user creates an input description file for a set of data, that same file can be used to create bar, line, and pie charts with minimum added effort. To adopt the stored chart data for presentation of other types of display, such as x,y graphs, stacked bars, or exploded pies, added input has to be entered. For this, the user works through an Options Screen. Here, with surprisingly few entries, the necessary added instructions are given.

See and do

One of the main problems in using this kind of package is to form a clear picture of what effect various choices will have on the actual appearance of the graph that is to be produced. Most of the packages make the user wait until virtually all instructions and data have been entered before allowing any view of an actual graphics display.

CURVE II CRT has the advantage of letting the user see a displayed version of the partially completed plot. This works particularly well in the line chart procedures, since the display can be viewed quite early in the chart construction process. For bar and pie charts, there is a lot more input before a displayed chart can be seen.

SCIENTIFIC PLOTTER is something of an exception. At any point in the input sequence, this package allows the user to call for a current view of the plot. But other packages are much less generous. With Graphwriter, it is only after all the entry material is completed that the user gets a look at what the visual results will be. That is done by calling for a "Preview on Screen" from the plot menu. If that display seems acceptable, the user can go on and produce plotted or printed output.

Keychart also requires users to complete the input process before getting any screen display of graphs. But then this package relents and actually allows editing of the graph while it is being displayed. At this time the size of the chart can be expanded or reduced, and it can be moved about within the plotting space. While observing the chart display, users can also edit titles to change their size and location. Charted variables may be edited to show them in alternative formats. For example, a variable shown in bar form can be changed so it will be displayed in line format. Types of cross-hatching can also be changed.

The ideal method of constructing charts and curves would be to give instructions and enter data while using a split or windowed screen to simultaneously watch the desired display take shape. None of the packages reviewed in this chapter provide this capability.

Editing procedures

No user, even the most experienced, can expect to flawlessly enter exactly the right instructions and specifications to produce a perfect graph. That is one reason why editing procedures, that provide for changes in what has been entered, are needed. Another is that a new chart is often very similar to one that may have been previously constructed and stored. In this situation, a lot of effort can be saved by simply recalling the previous chart and editing it to meet the new requirements.

With the completion of the last data entry screen, the KeyChart package stores the whole set of chart data. The package includes a cataloging arrangement in which stored charts are listed by name for later recall and use. When a chart is to be updated, or another chart very similar to one already stored is to be created, the user can call up a copy of the stored chart. The displayed input screens will then appear with all the previously entered data in place, and the user need only change items that need updating. To aid in keeping track of the stored data, the package provides for printing out the contents of any selected file of chart data.

SCIENTIFIC PLOTTER uses three files for each graph. Format, Data, and Picture information are each stored in their own named file. These files can be recalled to speed the construction of similar future graphs, since the user is allowed to quickly skip through the entire graph construction sequence, accepting previously installed values and altering only those that need changing.

Graphwriter has a similar arrangement. Users can go through the entire sequence of prompts, keyboarding the answers that are requested. Or they can call up a previous chart from a storage file and make changes only in selected segments, to alter that chart to meet current needs.

ASYST: GRAPHICS LANGUAGE

ASYST is a computer language, in the same sense that BASIC and FOR-TRAN are computer languages. It was designed with engineering and sci-

entific problem solving in mind and has a variety of capabilities, including those in the areas of equation solving and instrumentation. Here we will discuss only the graphics abilities of this language.

ASYST runs on IBM/PC and compatible computers. The Systems module, which sells for $795, includes graphics and statistics. The vendor is Macmillan Software Co., 866 Third Ave., New York, NY 10022 [(212) 702-3241].

ASYST is not a package designed to do curves or charts conveniently. It provides the user with no menus of available functions, nor does it have predesigned formats to organize its use. Instead, like the BASIC language, it simply presents the user with an OK prompt and waits for commands to be keyboarded. As with any other language, these commands must reside primarily in the user's head, which means that the ASYST language must be learned before it can be used.

As with any other computer language, regardless of its intrinsic merits, the success or failure of ASYST will rest on the extent to which it is adopted and used by programming-minded engineers and scientists. If and when these users write programs that can, in turn, be put to use by the vast majority of engineers who have little or no interest in doing programming, then ASYST will indeed become a significant engineering tool.

The graphics capabilities of ASYST are directed specifically to making plots of mathematical functions and of sets of data. Some of the commands are very powerful. For example, plotting can be called into action by a single command, Y.AUTO.PLOT, that scales the x and y axes, sets up tick marks, and provides a background grid of dots. The same command goes on to plot a data set which the user has previously put into place.

Of course, a command that does so much leaves the user with little power to control the details of the graphs it produces. However, other commands give the user more detailed control of the appearance, scaling, and labeling of plots of functions and data points. There are also commands for controlling Hewlett-Packard 7470 and 7475 plotters.

CURVE II CRT

This package is used to create, print, and plot line, bar, and pie charts. Users able to do BASIC programming can produce custom-designed graphs from programming subroutines provided with the package. Other users can *work from standard chart formats that do not require any programming. An added feature is the ability to produce plots of three types of equations. CURVE II CRT runs on IBM/PC, Victor 9000, and Apple II,IIe computers. The package sells for $325 from West Coast Consultants, 4049 First St., #234, Livermore, CA 94550 [(415) 449-0900].*

Operation of this package proceeds from a main menu choice like LINE CHART to a sequence of prompts and user replies. For a line chart the user first replies to 12 such prompts to specify the scaling, placement, and appearance of the chart. Then the data to be charted are entered.

CURVE II CRT will accept data from the keyboard or from stored files in the DIF format used by VisiCalc spreadsheets and similar packages. In either case, the data to be used can be reviewed, 10 points at a time, and edited to correct errors or make desired changes.

Sequences of prompts

Following data entry and editing, the user responds to another set of nine prompts that provide for fitting a plotted curve to the data points and establish further details of the appearance of the plot.

At this point, the user can take a first look at a display of the plot itself. While viewing this display, the user gives further instructions, again in response to prompts from the package. These concern the makeup and position of labels on the chart. The labels and title appear on the display as the user creates them. When they have been completed, the package permits the user to order plotted output.

A sequence of file storage and data editing prompts follows. The file storage provisions for the chart data are flexible. Users can save *x*- and *y*-data in separate files. All the data or only selected portions can be saved, and data points can be edited. Then new plots can be constructed.

A similar sequence of more than 60 prompts leads the user through construction of bar charts and includes the options of horizontal or vertical bars. Another 28 prompts provide for placing text on the chart. The procedures for putting pie charts together are similar.

Still another sequence of prompts controls the creation and placement of plotted text and numbers. These can be added to already completed charts with a choice of 15 character sizes, pen color, and standard or bold characters. Block characters can also be produced.

CURVE II CRT supports the use of several plotters, including the HP 7470A and the HIPLOT DMP-3, -4, -6, -7, and -29.

Equation plotting

Aside from the fact that users have to enter their equations in BASIC language format, the equation plotting features of this package operate on much the same basis as chart construction. Three types of equations can be plotted: Cartesian equations of the form $y=f(x)$; parametric equations $y=f(t)$, $x=g(t)$; and polar equations $r=f(s)$.

Limits on usefulness

There are drawbacks to the incessant use of prompts in this package. The prompt sequences are rather rigid; if errors are made and not immediately caught, a whole sequence must be replayed to make a correction. And it is not easy for users to keep track of the choices they have made. Users might be better served if full screen displays were used, on which entries could be made, compared and edited before being processed.

One of the main problems in using this kind of package is to form a clear picture of what the effects of the various choices are on the actual plot that is to be produced. CURVE II CRT has the advantage of letting the user see a displayed version of the partially completed plot. This works particularly well in the line-chart procedures, since the display can be viewed quite early in the chart construction process. For bar and pie charts, there is a lot more input before a displayed chart can be seen.

Experienced, constant users of this package will find little difficulty in visualizing their results as their instructions are entered, but novices and occasional users will probably find they have to cycle again and again through the procedures to get the results they want.

In the end, the usefulness of this kind of package rests on its ability to provide an improvement over manual composition and drafting of charts. To succeed fully, it must be fast and convenient for an engineer, even one who only occasionally uses the package, to turn out the needed results.

GEOCONTOUR

This package is specifically designed to make contour plots. It is truly a bare bones package, designed with little thought for convenience of the user and with very few options of which the user can take advantage.

GEOCONTOUR runs on IBM/PCs. It sells for $500 from GEOCOMP Corp., 342 Sudbury Rd., Concord, MA 01742 [(617) 369-8304].

To produce results with this package, three sets of input information are needed: the first describes the data points (elevation, or temperature, or whatever is being contour plotted) involved, the second contains x,y node coordinates for each data point, and the third (optional information which will speed the plotting process if supplied) describes how the plot can be made up from triangular elements, each containing three node points.

Data processing input formats

This input information is required to be formatted as if it were being read into the computer by a data processing card reader. Thus, the first line of element data gives, in positions 1-5, the total number of elements involved. The second line shows, in positions 1-5, a number identifying an element. Then in positions 6-10, 11-15, and 16-20, it shows the three node numbers for that element. Other input must be given in similar rigidly pre-scribed formats.

The information for controlling the appearance of the plotted output is input in a similarly rigid format. Included here are such items as the number of contours to draw, scale factor, height of letters in the legend, location of legend, specification of any circles or rectangles that are to appear.

When the actual run is made, the package will prompt the user for the file names in which node coordinates, contouring information, and data are stored. The user is asked if node locations are to be plotted, if contours are to be plotted, and if element information is being supplied. Users are also given the choice of plotting on the display screen or on the plotter.

Plotters supported by this package include the HP 7470A, 7475A, IBM XY/749, 750, DMP 4,5,6,7,29,40,41, and Calcomp M84.

GRAPHWRITER

This package is for putting together display charts and graphs. It allows a person with little or no knowledge of typeface specification to produce a wide variety of lettered graphics, suitable for use at professional meetings and presentations.

Graphwriter runs on IBM/PC/XT computers. It sells for $595 from Graphic Communications, 200 Fifth Ave, Waltham, MA 02254 [(617) 890-8778].

Users of this package have a choice of 23 different graph and chart formats. Ten of these are variations on the bar-chart, with bars vertical or horizontal, solid or segmented, single, clustered, paired, or ornamented. Then there are pie charts, line, surface-line, and scatter charts, text display formats including tables, Gantt charts and range-bar charts, flow charts, and pie-bar, bar-line combinations.

The first step in using the package is to select which of these choices is appropriate for the use at hand. Once that choice is made, the user is led, through a series of menu choices, to set up the desired graphic display and can produce printed or plotted output.

Along the way there are lots of choices to be made. The displays have to be scaled, colors and fill patterns have to be chosen. Headings and titles have to be composed. These choices are made through menu displays. To navigate from one item to another, the user presses appropriate keys. Experienced users do not have to actually wait to see a menu before making their selection. If they are familiar enough with what is on the menu, they can "type ahead," entering their choices in advance. The package will then move immediately through one typed option to another to bring the user to the desired point in the package's operations.

A total of ten floppy disks comes with the package. Two of these are concerned with the main program and with setting up for specific kinds of plotters and printers. The other eight contain the software needed to use particular types of charts and graphs, and to do so the correct disk must be inserted into the computer's disk drive.

Entering the graph description

The prompts that ask for answers from the user are arranged in a number of series or segments: chart headings, with up to three 48-character lines of text usually allowed; notes; axis titles and scales; text for legends; color and fill; and, finally, the data that are to be represented.

To allow data to be fed in from existing files, prepared with other software, the package can read the DIF files used by some spreadsheet packages.

Once a block of text has been added to a graph, it can be moved (up, down, left, right). The user follows prompts that ask for the movement distances in millimeters.

Users can go through the entire sequence of prompts, keyboarding the answers that are requested. Or they can call up a previous chart from a storage file and make changes only in selected segments, to alter that chart to meet current needs.

Within the limitations of the available graph and chart formats, the package offers considerable freedom in selecting line types, colors, and bar widths, as well as fonts, character sizes, color and placement of legends, and comments, and other stylistic treatments, such as rotating the pie chart orientations.

These choices can be quite detailed, bringing the user into design territory usually occupied by graphic artists. For example, one page of the user manual spells out the relationship between length of text lines and number of characters used, for various choices of font size. The bulk of the user manual is actually devoted to explaining the various available text and graphics alternatives.

Choice of plotters

Some menu-choice controls are also provided for the plotted output. The size of the plot area can be chosen from a list of seven possibilities. There is a choice of output for plain paper, transparencies or coated paper; paper sizes A or B can be selected. Slides, sized for 35mm projectors, can also be produced with the help of Polaroid Palette Computer Image Recorder equipment.

It is only after all this entry material is completed that the user gets a look at what the visual results will be. That is done by calling for a ''Preview on Screen'' from the plot menu. If that display seems acceptable, the user can go on and produce plotted or printed output.

An impressive list of plotting devices is supported by the package. These include the HP 7220C, HP 7470A, HP 7475A, HP 7550A, IBM XY/749,750, Mannesman Tally PIXY3, and Calcomp M84.

KEYCHART

This package is designed to easily and conveniently produce charts in such formats as line, bar, pie, x,y, and scatter, as well as text for display and presentation. Single charts or several at a time, can be plotted on a single sheet. The package will work with a variety of different types of plotting equipment.

KeyChart runs on IBM/PC and compatible computers and also on Kaypro and Epson personal computers. It sells for $375 from SoftKey Inc., 2727 Walsh Ave, Santa Clara, CA 95051 [(408) 986-8148].

One of the key features of this nicely integrated package is that once the user creates an input description file for a set of data, that same file can be used to create bar, line and pie charts with minimum added effort.

Data input screens

Users input information, for designing a chart, onto data displays. For example, there is a screen for naming, sizing, and labeling charts. Altogether it has spaces for 24 user-supplied inputs. When these are keyboarded they show up in bright or inverse-video characters. Pressing the Return key moves the screen cursor from one data entry item to another. The PC arrow keys can be used to move back and forth between items. Users can also move easily from one input screen to another, back and forth if needed, by pressing the PgUp and PgDn keys.

Altogether, the user has to remember about 22 special key actions to master full control of the data entry process. The manual includes a handy reference sheet listing these actions, but it will still take some practice to become familiar enough with them to make convenient use possible.

The input data are assumed to be arranged in a row and column manner, and the package receives one column of data at a time. On the naming screen, the user enters the number of columns that are to be charted. When that screen has been completed and entered, the package will next show the user a screen for the first column of data. Here the way that column is to be graphically handled is spelled out by filling in several input items.

The user then fills in the column data. The entry action is arranged so the cursor skips from position to position as the user methodically enters a column title, row name, and value for each item of data in the first column. When the screen for that column is completed, it is entered and the package presents another column entry screen, and so forth until all the input data have been entered.

In lieu of keyboard entry, row and column data can be fed directly into KeyChart from packages like Lotus 1-2-3, Symphony, Supercalc, Multiplan, and several other popular spreadsheet programs.

The final data entry screen is concerned with the scaling of the chart. Using the already-received data, the package calculates and inserts provisional scaling values on this screen. The user can either accept these or change them.

Chart storage and retrieval

With the entry of the last data entry screen, the package stores the completed set of chart data. The package includes a cataloging arrangement in which stored charts are listed by name for later recall and use.

When a chart is to be updated, or another chart similar to one already stored is to be created, it may pay for the user to call up a copy of the stored chart. The displayed input screens will then appear with all the previously entered data in place, and the user need only change items that need updating.

To aid in keeping track of the stored data, the package provides for printing out the contents of any selected file of chart data.

Shaping specific chart types

Selection of the desired type of display is ordinarily made from the main menu, where the choices are pie, bar/line, or text charts.

To adopt stored chart data for presentation of other types of display, such as x,y graphs, stacked bars, or exploded pies, added input has to be entered. To do this, the user retrieves the desired chart data and then calls for the Options Screen. Here, with surprisingly few entries, the necessary added instructions are given.

Choice of each specific type of chart also involves giving plotter instructions for pen speeds, use, and changes. Text charts require the use of an added input screen to define and locate the lines of text that are to be used.

Editing what is displayed

Before actually plotting, the user can call for a displayed version of completed charts. These can be viewed one at a time, or several can be viewed on the same display.

At this time the appearance of the charts can be edited. The size of the chart can be expanded or reduced, and it can be moved about within the plotting space. The same thing can be done when several charts are to be plotted on one sheet.

While observing the chart display, users can also edit titles to change their size and location. Charted variables may be edited to show them in alternative formats. For example, a variable shown in bar form can be changed so it will be displayed in line format. Type of crosshatching can also be changed.

The package supports: HP 7074A, 7475A; Calcomp M84; DMP 29,40; Zeta 8; MP 1000; 6-Shooter; Sweet P; Strobe 200, M260; and Roland DG DXY 800 plotters.

PCPLOT

Despite the title, there is no actual use of plotters here. This little package will display or print plots of x,y data points. Up to four data sets can be shown on one plot. It can be fully used only by those with some knowledge of BASIC and FORTRAN programming.

PCPLOT runs on IBM/PC, Compaq, and Columbia personal computers. It sells for $62.95 from BV Engineering, 2200 Business Way #207, Riverside, CA [(714) 781-0252].

The user replies to a few screen-displayed prompts and questions, and this package produces a plot. The procedure is very simple because the choices available are very limited. Nevertheless, the plots can be linear, log-log, or semilog (x or y).

The locations of the title and labels for the vertical and horizontal axes are fixed, but the user can decide what characters to use in these labels and what the axis scaling should be. Once a chart of a given type has been formatted, that format can be stored and reused.

The trick, with this package, is to make up the data files that are to be drawn upon to trace out the plot. The only clue the manual gives to the needed file format is to list for the user a short, 17-line BASIC program that can be run to set up the needed data file from a given function with specified increments of the variable. The equation used in the example is $y = (\sin x)/x$. It will be helpful to those familiar with programming to know that the variables are to be stored in string variable format, with data points each entered as separate lines. But this explanation can hardly be of interest to the non-programming user.

PLOTPRO

PLOTPRO produces point plots from data which may be entered through the keyboard or from a previously prepared data file. The plots can be displayed or printed on a dot matrix printer. The package can also produce continuous plots limited in length only by the length of available printing paper. The package works from menu displays. There is no provision for output to plotting equipment.

The price is a bargain. What the user gets is a package with some obvious, though correctable, faults and a manual that could stand considerable improvement.

PLOTPRO runs on IBM/PC, Apple II+, TRS-80 Models I,III,IV, and Victor 9000 computers. It sells for $52.95 from BV Engineering, 2200 Business Way #207, Riverside, CA 92501 [(714) 781-0252].

This package operates from two menus. The main one allows the user to choose whether to make a normal or a "quick" graph, enter data, create a graph template, ask for HELP, or exit the package.

If no graph templates (formats) exist, the user must start putting one together by calling up the second menu display. Here a set of format parameters is shown, including titles, type style and scaling (automatic or manual), along with choice options for changing these parameters. Each menu choice brings on a series of screen-displayed prompts that call for keyboarded answers from the user. As these responses are completed, the display returns to the second menu, until the "Done with changes" option is selected. Then the first menu display reappears.

Once created in this way, a graph template is automatically stored for further use. The storage file will have the name assigned by the user to the template. This name must conform to the rules for file naming required by the particular computer system on which the package is being run. The manual assumes that users are familiar with these requirements.

Data files for programmers

For the user who does no programming, the only realistic way to get data into this package is through the keyboard. The manual sketchily describes the file formats needed for input and shows some sample lines in BASIC and FORTRAN for generating such files, but these will be meaningless to nonprogrammers.

There are some cautionary rules to be observed when keyboarding data. For example, the user who enters the point 0,0 in the middle of a data set will find that entry is abruptly terminated. The "solution" to this defect in the package is to substitute a very small number for one of the zeros.

Curve creation and cautions

With data in place and a plotting template ready, the user is ready to call for a graph to be produced. When one of the appropriate menu choices is made, the series of prompts that follow will ask whether grid lines are desired, and what character is to be used to trace out the curve. If several curves are called for, this last question is repeated for each one.

There are a number of package peculiarities that require caution on the part of the user at this point.

Grid lines, made up of strings of the period character, can be invoked by the user. But there is a defect here. Because the period character is used, these lines show up about a half character space below their true position. As a result, curves that should pass through grid intersections will miss.

As many curves as desired can be plotted on one set of axes. However, the automatic scaling of the axes will be controlled by the first curve that is plotted. If the option of two sets of axes is used, automatic scaling of the second set will be controlled by the first curve entered after that set is introduced.

When a quick graph is drawn, up to ten curves can be plotted on it. However, the user must open a special buffer file for each such curve. This requires a knowledge of the particular version of the BASIC language in use on the computer on which the package is being run.

The package has an automatic phase plotting feature that is invoked by properly name-labeling a file of input data. The manual assumes that users have the minimum programming skills needed to create such a file.

The PLOTPRO manual is a sketchy affair. Its 25 pages do not include any complete and detailed explanation of the various keyboard commands and menu choices available to the user, so it cannot be employed as a reference guide. And it fails to meet the information needs of those who have no programming background. The vendor might find it worthwhile to clear up some of the package's foibles and provide an improved manual, thus justifying an increase in the current bargain price of this package.

SCIENTIFIC PLOTTER

Construction of point and line charts follows a rigid, compulsory prompt-and-reply sequence in this bargain-priced package. Users can store their data and charts, and modify an existing chart by rapidly skipping through the sequence. Output can be displayed, printed, or plotted.

SCIENTIFIC PLOTTER Version II runs on Apple II computers. It sells for $25. There is also a version, called Scientific Plotter-PC for the IBM/PC. Adaptation software packages for use of Hewlett-Packard, Houston Instruments, or Apple pen plotting equipment sell for $25 each. The vendor is Interactive Microware, PO Box 139, State College, PA 16804 [(814) 238-8294].

Users are led into operation of this package through a series of screen displayed prompts. In addition, about 12 special keyboard commands have to be kept in mind, since these control viewing of graphs, use of a cursor, and other package activities.

Fixed procedures

The regular procedures offered by the package are spelled out by a lengthy and fixed sequence of screen displayed prompts followed by user answers. The sequence includes setting up a graph format, inputting and scaling the data, plotting the data, labeling the graph, and storing the results of these steps. If users are dissatisfied with one of the steps, they can return directly to it through a redraw menu. The package will then erase the graph, automatically redraw it to the indicated step, and the user can proceed from there.

At any point in the sequence, the user can call for a current view of the graph, manipulate the files, go into a BASIC language programming mode, or return to the display of prompts.

Formatting and data procedures

After defining the graph name, the first step in the sequence is to set up the way a graph will appear. This is done by answering a series of questions that define a format for the graph. Thus, for the x-axis, the user is asked to set the coordinates of the ends of the axis, assign numeric values to the endpoints, specify if logarithmic scaling is to be used, what the interval between numeric labels will be, how many digits will appear to the right of their decimal points, and at what interval tick marks should appear. A similar series of prompts and answers sets up the y-axis. Users can select to have a background grid of dots over the graph, at tick mark intervals, and a rectangular frame that surrounds the graph.

The next step is to provide data for the graphs. This can be done by keyboarding the data, by reading previously prepared data from disk storage, or by a user-composed short program that calculates the desired data from a formula or equation. The SCIENTIFIC PLOTTER manual shows a five-line BASIC language program for storing data points on disk and assumes that users are able to do programming. If the data are keyboarded, they can be stored on disk by a keyboard command.

Scaling and labeling

To display a set of data properly on an existing set of graph axes, it may be necessary to scale the data, and this is the next step in the graph construction procedure. The package allows users to multiply x and y values by scale factors, and to add offset values to them as well.

When whatever scaling is desired has been completed, the next step is actually to plot the data. Several different sets of data can be plotted using the same set of axes. SCIENTIFIC PLOTTER also allows the use of a second set of axes on a graph. If there is room on the display, it even allows users to show several different graphs simultaneously.

Points on the graphs can be shown with a choice of five plotting symbols, each available in four different sizes. In addition, the larger sizes can be filled if desired. The points can be interconnected with straight-line segments in a choice of seven colors.

Graphs can be labeled with text. Upper and lower case letters plus 32 plotting and mathematical symbols can be used. With the graph displayed on the screen, the user moves a cursor to the desired position and types the label.

Storing the graphs

The final step in the SCIENTIFIC PLOTTER procedures is to store Format, Data, and Picture information, each in its own named file. These files can be recalled to speed the construction of similar future graphs, since the user is allowed to quickly skip through the entire graph construction sequence, accepting previously installed values and altering only those that need changing.

Chapter 11
Cost Estimation
and Tracking Packages

Micro/personal computer packages are available to aid cost evaluation in many aspects of engineering work. Some packages are concerned with the problem of estimating project costs in advance, producing the kind of detailed reports that are needed for passing through bidding, financing, and other approval procedures.

CES-II from Contract Micros is an example of a package set up to deal with construction bids. Users enter bid information for each job on a separate record that can include the results of bidding, showing which contractors made the three lowest bids and who won the bidding. Displayed (or printed) reports on the bid records can be produced, showing one-line partial descriptions of the bid records in bid-number order, or sorted by date of the bid or by the estimator.

The estimation functions of this package operate from stored files. These may be used to hold cost/unit information and line items that may be repeatedly used in many estimates. Other files can be used to hold complete estimates. The package allows the user to readily select and transfer any of these items to estimates in preparation.

As with any package of this type, the first estimate made with the "help" of the computer will normally take far more time and effort than would the more familiar manual preparation process. But once the stored files begin to build, items from storage can be used directly with no need to key in their descriptions. To further simplify the whole process, complete stored estimates can be retrieved under new names to serve as the basis for new, similar estimates.

When the user has to key in all the items stored in the files, the keyboarding process can become a whole project in itself and may stretch out for months. If you have ever tried to enter an item description correctly into a computer, you can imagine how long it might take to fill up the slots in files containing thousands of items.

With this in mind, vendors of packages like the Design Estimator, from Cost Information Systems, offer the user files with items already recorded in them. Design Estimator, for example, provides an on-disk version of the Dodge Cost Information Data Base which contains over 6000 construction materials and their costs.

Estimates can be useful as internal documents and also for customers and others outside the company. Such packages should, therefore, provide for estimate reports to be printed either with cost or with selling price amounts shown.

Job cost tracking

The basic idea in a job cost tracking package is to compile ongoing information on costs as they are met, keeping a running record. The computer produces to-date summaries and projects future costs to the completion of the project. For example, in the Job Costing package from Rambow Enterprises, there are two kinds of item entries. One is the line item, much like the line items used in estimating packages. The other is the "daily entry," which describe such things as invoices, bids, and purchase orders that are to be entered as they are received and added to the line-item cost totals in the reports this package produces.

Percent Complete

When job costs are being tracked, there is a need to compare the current cost totals to those expected at the completion of the job. For example, the MBA Job Cost package compares actual compiled cost figures to the estimates users make. In one job review display, actual figures are compared to the percentage of the estimated figures that should have been reached. The difference between the two is displayed as the current "variance," and this difference is projected to the end of the job to give a projected variance. Finally, the user is shown what is projected to be needed, in each cost category, to complete the job. Other displays compare original and revised cost estimates and project expected profit on the job. Similar displays are available for each individual phase of the job.

In most job cost packages, it is the user who assigns a percent-complete estimate at any given time, based on observation of actual job conditions. But some packages also provide a calculated percent complete, based on the extent to which budgeted funds for the project have been used. This is not likely to be as accurate as a user-assigned estimate, but it can be helpful when there are no better estimates at hand.

Integration foibles

Job cost tracking packages are often designed to work together in an "integrated" way with standard accounting packages. This is a good idea where both types of packages are operated by the same people. However, combining these two kinds of functions can lead to problems. For instance, to mesh smoothly with related accounting packages ABS Job Cost from Amalgamated Business Systems operates on a month-by-month basis, like the standard accounting functions. Despite the fact that a project may run for several months, with this package the recordkeeping process and the reports are broken into month-by-month segments.

The MBA Job Cost package from Micro Business Applications can work together with a general ledger package from the same vendor, assigning overhead and actual costs as general ledger accounts, but users are cautioned that the company accountant might "prefer not to use this feature" since the cost categories are assigned by the project designer.

Cost packages, even when operating on their own, may still be capable of informing users about bottom line by calculating estimated profit and profit margin, for each project, and sometimes for phases within projects. And some, like the MICA Job Cost package, can also generate invoices for all active jobs.

Time-sheet costs

Packages like COSAC from ECOM West do job costing based mainly on employee time sheets. Such packages are useful in organizations whose main output is information, like engineering drawings and specifications. Such packages can maintain records of costs related to employee time plus other expenses and produce reports which include measures of job and employee progress.

A longer view of costs may be useful to some organizations. The CostPLAN package from DacorMFG addresses this need by maintaining data on 60 months of expenses for each cost account, providing history reports on them, and generating forecasts. The package is not suitable for project tracking, since it stores only one dollar figure per month stored for each cost account.

File handling features

In addition to providing line items for estimates and reports, stored files can also be used to ease the problem of keyboarding notations that will appear in the printed reports. Thus the ABS Job Cost package allows users to make entries in a list-of-phrases file. Frequently used comments are stored here by number, and can be retrieved and inserted in reports by entering their number at the proper point in the Input routine.

The Rambow Job Cost package has a helpful copying feature that allows the user to create new job cost files from existing, similar ones. All line items from one project file can be copied to another with the old daily entries eliminated. It also has a summarizing feature that allows several job cost files to be combined into one overall file.

A nice feature offered by some packages is the option to specify in advance the maximum size to which users are willing to have a file grow. Floppy disks, even hard disks, have limited storage capability, and historical files tend to grow and grow. If the storage capability is exceeded, keyboarding effort can be lost and use of the package can be disrupted. It is therefore very helpful if the package warns the user when files exceed their specified size, thus allowing for orderly purging or establishment of new file space.

Password protection

As in virtually all packages that provide password protection, users can choose to employ or bypass the password features of CostPLAN. There are at least two reasons for using passwords. Sensitive data, involving company economics and employee salaries, may need protection from intrusive eyes. But there can also be the problem of disruption of important records due to clumsy use by inexperienced employees. Even the president of a company can fall into this second category. The amount of security that is desirable is the least that will give the needed protection.

CostPLAN solves the security problem neatly by offering the ability to put password protection on a specific menu item that leads to a sensitive procedure. When a user asks for that menu item, the package will not proceed until it receives the proper password.

Few packages use graphics

Few cost estimating or tracking packages offer graphical displays. One exception is the CostPLAN package which produces two bar charts. One shows the yearly dollar cost totals for an account, along with forecast totals for future years. The other chart shows seasonal cost patterns for an account.

Another exception is the MICA Job Cost package, which has time-line charts showing estimated start and completion dates for projects and their components.

Rigid operating procedures

An important characteristic to look for is the ease and flexibility with which a package can be used. With the Rambow Construction Estimating package, for example, operation is quite flexible. Users choose whatever procedures they want by making selections from displayed menus. And the procedures themselves are simple. To enter a line item for an estimate, the user fills out a screen-displayed form. The keyboard technique used will be familiar to anyone who has used one of the popular personal computer database packages. It involves moving from one item to another by hitting the Return key, making item entries from the keyboard, and erasing mistakes by using the Backspace key.

However, not all packages live up to this standard of ease. For example, the ABS Job Cost package operates mainly on an instruction and reply basis. The user presses a special function key with a label like "Input," "Reports," "Invoices," or "Receipts." Then a specified sequence of steps begins. The package displays an instruction to the user and the user responds. If the package finds the reply satisfactory, it goes on to the next step. If not, it demands a proper reply before it will proceed. The sequences are rigid, sometimes lengthy, and the user is locked in until they are completed.

Numbers game

Several estimating packages provide files of assemblies, groups of detail items that can be represented in the estimate by a single assembly item. The CES-II package, for example, allows up to 41,600 such assemblies to be created, so you can see that it may become a problem to locate the one you want when it is needed.

Almost all packages locate stored items by ID numbers. That is tidy, but the user who does not know that number will have to do a lot of searching to find the desired item. Lacking any adequate computer-based means for searching, about the only practical way to deal with this problem is to keep a printed list of these items on hand, showing their ID numbers. Printing updated versions of these lists will undoubtedly give idle users something to do with their spare time.

ABS JOB COST: MONTH BY MONTH PROCEDURES

ABS Job Cost was specifically designed for use with engineering projects. It is, however, oriented to month-by-month accounting practices rather than to tracking of whole projects. The package can be useful in tracking labor utilization, but it will be best employed when it has the attention of a dedicated clerical employee.

This package runs on Hewlett-Packard desktop computers, including the 9835, 9845, and Series 200. It sells for $335 from Amalgamated Business Systems, 7910 Memorial Parkway #H, Huntsville, AL 35802 [(205) 882-2360].

ABS Job Cost is designed to work together with several standard accounting packages from the same vendor. As a result it operates on a month by month basis, like standard accounting functions. Despite the fact that a project may run for several months, the record keeping process must be broken into month-by-month segments. Each month's worth of information is stored on a separate disk. This means that, while the current disk will hold the to-date totals, users must go back to previous disks if they want details on what has previously occurred.

This month by month orientation extends also to the reports produced by the package. These present a useful picture of the progress of a project during any given month. However, the only way to get a picture of the details for the progress of the whole project is to run such reports from several monthly disks and paste them onto one another.

Rigid operating procedures

There is a main menu from which users select use of this Job Cost package, as opposed to one of the vendor's accounting packages. But from that point on ABS Job Cost operates on an instruction and reply basis. The user presses a special function key with a label like "Input," "Reports," "Invoices," or "Receipts." Then a specified sequence of steps begins. The package displays an instruction to the user and the user responds. If the package finds the reply satisfactory, it goes on to the next step. If not, it demands a proper reply before it will proceed.

These steps do branch. That is, the user may have several alternative choices at any given step. However, the meaning of these choices, denoted by numbers or letters, is spelled out only in the user manual. So all but very frequent and experienced users will work the package from the printed lists of sequenced instructions in the manual. The overall impression on the user is one of being caught up in a rigid procedure of someone else's devising, with no clear way of bypassing unwanted steps in order to get to exactly what the user may want to do.

User aids

To ease the problem of keyboarding notations that will appear in the printed reports, the package allows users to make entries in a list-of-phrases file. Frequently used comments are stored here by number and can be retrieved and inserted in reports by entering their number at the proper point in the Input routine.

Everything else in this package seems to be identified by number. This includes projects, employees, and job classifications as well as phrases. This means that the user must have lists of these items, showing their ID numbers, on hand in order to use the package. Printing updated versions of these lists will undoubtedly give the user something to do on slow days.

CES-II: CONSTRUCTION ESTIMATING SYSTEM

CES-II is for job estimating and bidding. The package works from stored files of line and detail items. It can be used with the Construction Specifications Institute categories.

CES-II runs on IBM/PCs and compatible computers, and on CP/M systems. It sells for $950 from Contract Micros, 5455 Buford Highway #A120, Doraville, GA 30340 [(404) 452-0550].

CES-II is set up to deal with construction bids and estimates. Users enter bid information for each job on a separate record. Each is assigned a number and must be retrieved by that number. If the user can't remember the right number, it can be taken from a display of names and numbers of the bid records that have been stored, a tedious process when many bids are involved.

The record for each bid can include the results of bidding, showing which contractors made the three lowest bids and who won the bidding. Displayed (or printed) reports on the bid records can be produced, showing one-line partial descriptions of the bid records in bid-number order, or sorted by date of the bid, or by the estimator.

Estimate preparation

The main business of the package is to put together estimates for jobs. The user constructs an estimate, line item by line item. Within each item care must be taken to keep the units that are used consistent; the package has some rather complex rules for this and they must be followed.

CES-II estimate preparation is expedited with the help of two sets of auxiliary files:

Up to 16 "Historical" files can be set up. Each is normally kept on a separate floppy disk. One of these may be used to hold cost/unit information and other line items that may be repeatedly used in many estimates. Other historical files can be used to hold complete estimates. Each disk can hold 2720 line items. The package allows the user to readily select and transfer any of these items to individual estimates.

There is also a file of "Assemblies." These are groups of up to 15 detail items. They can be represented in the estimate by a single assembly item; the package will calculate its cost from the total of the costs for the detail items it represents. The package allows up to 41,600 such assemblies to be created, so you can see that it may become a problem to locate the one you want when it is needed. Assemblies are located by their ID numbers. The user who does not know that number has to search through all the assembly descriptions to find the right one, to figure out some better method to categorize and locate needed assemblies, or to use only a modest number of assemblies so they are easily found.

The package allows assemblies to contain cost/unit items. Since these and the other items must be summed up to get an assembly cost, the units used within the assembly have to be consistent, and this involves some care in choices by the user and more rules to follow.

When preparing estimates, the user must constantly keep a mental image of what the estimate looks like. As items are taken from displays of historical and assembly file records, the package makes little notations on these displays to indicate what has been done. But the user must go through a separate review procedure to see what effect these manipulations have had on the estimate itself. A split-screen display that could show the estimate on one side and historical records on the other would make this a much neater process.

Useful reports

Estimates can be useful as internal documents and also for customers and others outside the company. CES-II therefore provides for estimate reports to be printed either with cost or with selling price amounts shown. The package provides for markups, with user-selected percentages. Reports can have up to four cost-type columns such as materials, labor, subcontractors, and other. And the reports can have up to 16 sections covering categories such as General Conditions, Sitework, and Concrete. The names used for these categories can be chosen by the user, but the 16 standard categories used by the Construction Specifications Institute will normally be the ones chosen. If the items are numbered according to the scheme used by the institute, anyone familiar with that scheme should have a relatively easy time using the package.

The package offers the option of assigning a vendor name to each line item. If this is done, the information can be used to turn out a bill-of-materials report for the job.

Varying keyboard commands

Users of this package make choices from displayed menus, are presented with sequences of questions to be answered in order to set up procedures, and make entries on data screens. Movement from one menu or screen to another is controlled by keyboard commands, and most of the appropriate commands are displayed on the screen to remind the user. The exceptions are the Function key commands, which operate during the question and answer sequences as well as at the menu displays. These commands are used to move from one type of operation to another. For each operation there are somewhat different uses of the function keys. The rules for function keys are explained in the manual, and their uses are rather simple, but the novice may have difficulty remembering which key does what in which situation.

If entry mistakes are made, the entry screen can be edited by moving the cursor around, deleting fields, and inserting or deleting characters. The use of editing key commands is something to which the novice user will have to adjust. If too many mistakes have been made, users can choose not to enter the data on the entry screen and start again with an empty screen.

The users manual for this package is voluminous but is not well organized. This reviewer found it necessary to go through detailed descriptions of the various package functions before the introductory "Sample Estimate" section became meaningful.

There are a number of built-in controls in this package to help insure correct results. For example, the package will not allow a final report to be produced if any of the line item quantity takeoffs are not completed.

CONSTRUCTION ESTIMATING: A WELL-ORGANIZED PACKAGE

This package takes advantage of contemporary personal computer software techniques to provide users with a well-organized way of making up construction estimates.

The package runs on IBM/PC and compatible computers. It sells for $300 from Rambow Enterprises, 6738 Holly Lane, Anchorage, AK 99502 [(907) 243-6839].

To enter a line item for an estimate, the user fills out a screen-displayed form. The keyboard technique used will be familiar to anyone who has used one of the popular personal computer database packages. It involves moving from one item to another by hitting the Return key, making item entries from the keyboard, and erasing mistakes by using the Backspace key. On this form the user enters an item description and an item number that approximates the Construction Specifications Institute (CSI) number. Also entered are the quantity of the item and its unit of measure. The package will automatically calculate a corresponding dollar amount.

A standard numbering scheme

The package is designed around the 16 item categories set up by the CSI. When a line-item form is complete, it can be stored. Its location in the estimate willl be determined by the CSI-style numbering. The same form is used for material, labor, and subcontract items. A second, General Data display form is used to enter general information about the estimate. This includes descriptive entries and also percentages used for labor fringes and benefits, office overhead, and profit margin. Markup fees are also entered here.

Line item entry forms can be reviewed, once entered, to edit them or simply to view what is in there. This viewing can begin at any line item number the user selects, move backwards as well as forwards from item to item, and end whenever desired. The estimate itself, with line items in place, can also be reviewed as desired. And a summary of the estimate, showing only the 16 CSI category totals, can be similarly viewed. The user can scroll through these displays and get printed output on request.

Conventional file names

Estimates are stored on disk, and each has a name limited to the eight-or-less character designations usually allowed by personal computer system software. These names are fairly easy to identify from a displayed or printed list but are not so easily remembered by the user. For example, one estimate might be named CONSTRUC, another CNSTRCTN. Both can clearly be identified as labels for the word Construction, but it might be difficult to remember which one was actually used.

Power grows with use

As with any package of this type, the first estimate made with the "help" of the computer will normally take far more time and effort than would the more familiar manual preparation process. Once that first one is stored in the computer, the user will begin to realize the benefits of the software. With the very next estimate, items from the first can be used directly from storage with no need to key in new descriptions. Since there are always items that show up on one estimate after another, it is wise to keep these in a special "estimate" file where they be found can easily and drawn upon as needed. To simplify the whole process further, complete stored estimates can be retrieved under new names to serve as the basis for new, similar estimates.

Like the package, its user's manual is well organized, clear, and easy to follow.

COSAC: JOB COSTING BASED ON EMPLOYEE TIME SHEETS

This package seems to have been designed for use in organizations whose main output is engineering drawings and specifications. It provides a means of maintaining records of costs related to employee time plus other expenses, producing reports which include some rough measures of job and employee progress. The package offers nominal assistance to users in keeping these records.

COSAC runs on Hewlett-Packard 85/86/87 computers, operating from tape-based data storage. It sells for $495 from ECOM West, 1749 Wright St., Sacramento, CA 95825 [(916) 971-0750].

COSAC will track up to 144 different jobs. Each is identified by a job number and job name. The user assigns a target budget figure for each job (zero-budget jobs are acceptable). And the user can enter the estimated number of drawings involved in the job. For those used to floppy disk-based computer operations, this tape-based package is very slow.

Cost items can be entered as dollar-amount expenses, or in the form of hours worked and charged according to the job category involved. Job category is not the same as wage or salary rate. With this package, an employee who is paid at a fixed salary rate, may perform several tasks, each of which is charged, for accounting purposes, at a different job-category rate.

A good part of the user input to the package consists of keyboarding hours spent on various jobs, taken from employee time sheets. The user must enter an employee number, a job number, and a job-category code letter for each entry of hours worked. It would seem much more natural to key in names for these items, but the package designers felt use of numbers was a better choice.

Although jobs have identifying names, as far as the package is concerned they can be located only by the job number. This means that the user will almost certainly have to keep some tattered and inevitably outdated printed lists of jobs, employees, and job categories near the keyboard. These will be used to look up the needed numbers.

The package produces a job cost report with costs broken down by job and dollar expense categories. The user assigns a percent-complete estimate for the report. Based on this, and the budget amount assigned, the package calculates a projected overrun for the job. It also calculates the projected remaining time needed for each job category. The total charges are divided by the number of drawings to get a cost per drawing for the job.

A productivity report compares the salary or wages paid to each employee with the billable charges attributed to that employee.

COSTPLAN: FOR HISTORICAL COST DATA

This package is designed to compile cost histories useful to manufacturers and other businesses. CostPLAN maintains data on 60 months of expenses for each cost account and provides history reports on them. For accounts with 12 months worth of data, the package can generate straight-line forecasts, adjusted to reflect seasonal patterns.

The package is not suitable for project tracking, since it is strictly for keeping track of monthly costs, with only one dollar figure per month stored for the cost of each account.

CostPLAN runs on IBM/PC and compatible computers. It sells for $150, from DacorMFG, 13330 Bishop Road, P.O. Box 269, Bowling Green, OH 43402 [(419) 354-3981].

A nice feature of CostPLAN is the option to specify in advance the maximum size to which users are willing to have a file grow. Floppy disks, even hard disks, have limited storage capability, and historical files tend to grow and grow. If the storage capability is exceeded, keyboarding effort can be lost and use of the package can be disrupted. CostPLAN will warn the user when files exceed their specified size, thus allowing for orderly purging or establishment of new file space.

Specific security passwords

As in virtually all packages that provide password protection, users can choose to employ or bypass the password features of CostPLAN. There are at least two reasons for using passwords. Sensitive data, involving company economics and employee salaries, may need protection from intrusive eyes. But there can also be the problem of disruption of important records due to clumsy use by inexperienced employees. Even the president of a company can fall into this second category. The amount of security that is desirable is the least that will give the needed protection.

CostPLAN solves the security problem neatly by offering the ability to put password protection on a specific menu item that leads to a sensitive procedure. When a user asks for that menu item, the package will not proceed until it receives the proper password.

Simple graphs

This package produces only two bar charts. One shows the yearly dollar cost totals for an account, along with forecast totals for future years. The other chart shows seasonal cost patterns for an account.

DESIGN ESTIMATOR: ACCESS TO REGIONAL DATA

This package offers the user an on-disk version of the Dodge Cost Information Data Base which contains over 6000 construction materials and their costs. The package is available with costs for 10 different regions of the United States.

Users enter data such as square footage, materials to use, and information on such things as HVAC, plumbing, fenestration, wage rates, and markups. Line items for the estimates are drawn from the Dodge files.

The package sells for $795 with one regional data disk. Additional data disks are $300 each. It runs on IBM/PC, Apple, and compatible computers, and is available from Cost Information Systems, P.O. Box 28. Princeton, NJ 08540 [(800) 257-5295, (609) 921-6500].

JOB COSTING: FOR BUDGET AND COST TRACKING

This package is basically for cost tracking. It was developed to produce forms similar to those commonly used by builders to justify bank loans, but it is applicable to any situation where variances from a budget are to be tracked. Its main output is a monthly report that shows the budget amount, percent completed, dollar variances extrapolated to completion, and total spent on each line item.

The package runs on IBM/PC and compatible computers. It sells for $300 from Rambow Enterprises, 6738 Holly Lane, Anchorage, AL 99502 [(907) 243-6839].

There are two kinds of item entries for this package. One is the line item, which is used for categories of building costs such as those for land, lumber, design, and testing. The second kind is the "daily entry," which describe such things as invoices, bids, and purchase orders that are to be entered as they are received and posted to the line items.

The user sets up a job file through a screen-displayed form, sets up the line items for the file through another screen form, then makes daily entries through a third screen form.

Tracking ongoing costs

To keep account of ongoing costs, daily entries are made, one after another, until all entries for that day have been completed. The package then processes the entries, adding each one to the line item the user specifies on that particular daily entry form. Each daily entry is classified by the user as being one of five possible types: Bid, Draw, Invoice, PO, or Sale. These types are used in summary reports that list the daily entries, but they do not appear, as such, on the overall job cost reports that show the status of the line items. Daily entry report listings may be displayed and printed by vendor, by type, by due date, by line item, or in the order they were entered. So there are many ways to review what has been entered.

The package has a copying feature that allows the user to create new job cost files from existing, similar ones. All line items from one project file can be copied to another with the old daily entries eliminated. It also has a summarizing feature that allows several job cost files to be combined into one overall file.

The user manual for this package is inadequate. It relies on printed versions of the display screens and accompanies them with running commentary, but there is no item-by-item explanation of the entries and procedures.

MBA JOB COST: TRACKING PROJECT PHASES

This package was designed to handle costs for jobs involving custom engineering tasks. It provides for orderly bookkeeping on six (user-selected) categories of costs, for the overall job and its phases, with progress reports including the effect on the bottom line.

MBA Job Cost runs on IBM/PC, Apple, TRS-80, and many other micro/personal computers. It sells for $595 from Micro Business Applications, 12281 Nicollet Ave S, Burnsville, MN 55337 [(612) 894-3470].

The purpose of the package is to track costs and job progress. To do this, actual compiled figures are compared to the estimates users make. In one job review display, actual figures are compared to the percentage of the estimated figures that should have been reached. The difference between the two is displayed as the current "variance," and this difference is projected to the end of the job to give a projected variance. Finally, the user is shown what is projected to be needed, in each cost category, to complete the job.

Other displays compare original and revised cost estimates, costs actually billed to customers, and project expected profit on the job. Similar displays are available for each individual phase of the job.

Timeless phases

In MBA Job Cost, the overall job is divided into phases, each with its own costs. The way these phases are defined will have a drastic effect on the usefulness of the reports the package produces, so phase selection must be done carefully.

It may sound as if "phases" refer to portions of the job that follow one another. However, users are warned against defining the phases by time-intervals since, in the real world, such phases inevitably overlap in time, and the package is not equipped to handle such overlaps. Therefore, phases are to be defined by location, type of process or procedure, or some other timeless quality.

Cost categories must be carefully chosen

For each phase of the job, users start by giving estimated start and end dates, and estimated costs. Later the actual dates and costs will be added as the data become available. Users can set up their own cost categories and are allowed just six categories for a job. In other words, they can choose five cost categories and lump everything else in a miscellaneous category. The package will report percent job completion based only on the first of these categories, so it must be chosen with care, to best reflect the overall job completion status.

Like many packages, this one limits the number of characters that can be used to spell out the names of the cost categories. The limit here is 14 characters, which does not leave room for such type-names as " Unskilled Labor" (15 characters, including the space between the two words) but will accommodate most one-word names.

Cost category units may be defined in dollars. Or they may be assigned units such as hours or cubic feet; these must then be further defined in dollars per unit. Based on further experience with the job, these definitions may be revised. Records will be kept of both the original and revised units and prices. In any case, there will be separate definitions for overhead and for billing calculations, and both these calculations provide for a fixed amount in addition to the category amounts.

By initially establishing these categories and definitions, the user sets up the job for the package. Further information is entered in the form of individual "transactions." Every time new information on ongoing costs is entered, it is keyboarded onto a transaction-entry display "screen."

Review and control procedures

To safeguard the accuracy of the records, there is a separate editing procedure that can be performed on this screen before the information is actually added to what was previously posted and stored. Further control over what is entered can be exercised by a transaction review procedure which allows each item that is to be posted to be viewed and considered separately.

Two-key menus

To operate the package, users work from menus, listing available choices. On most menu formats, items of choice are numbered or have letter designations; the user hits the key corresponding to the desired item and it is chosen. Not so on these menus. There is a list of items, and the user presses the space bar to advance the cursor from one item to another. When the cursor finally reaches the desired item, the user presses the Return key to choose it.

Integration complications

MBA Job Cost is one of several packages sold by the vendor, Micro Business Applications. These are mainly for various standard accounting functions. These functions are "integrated;" that is, they are all designed to work together. This may be a fine feature from an accountant's point of view, but it does require the Job Cost user to go through a few extra steps when setting up the package, initiating new files, reindexing existing files, or establishing password protection for files. MBA Job Cost can work together with a general ledger package from the same vendor, assigning overhead and actual costs as general ledger accounts, but users are cautioned that the company accountant might "prefer not to use this feature."

Copying could be extended

A convenient feature is the ability to use copies of job-phase descriptions that have been entered previously. These can be edited, allowing users to save considerable time in entering similar phase-descriptions. In fact, some users set up several standard phase-descriptions just to be able to get a running start in describing types of phases that frequently occur.

A desirable improvement to this package would be to extend its copying features to get the ability to make trial adjustments to the various costs and to observe their effects on the overall profit figures. This would provide a means to work out alternate strategies for completing a job. It would be important, however, that these manipulations be strictly on a trial basis and not disturb the regular cost information already in the system.

MICA JOB COST: TRACKING AND ESTIMATES

This package does job cost tracking, maintaining cost records on the "components" that make up each job, as well as the overall job, and allowing detailed job cost estimates to be presented. It has time-line schedule reports and bottom-line reports that show profitability.

MICA Job Cost runs on IBM/PC and compatible computers. It sells for $995 from Micro Associates Inc., 2349 Memorial Boulevard, Port Arthur, TX 77640 [(409) 983-2051].

The method for entering data from the keyboard is straightforward and simple. The user is presented with display-screen forms containing many items. The entry space for the first item is shown in reverse video (a light strip on a dark background). The user makes an entry into this space. When completed, the reverse video strip moves to the next item. If the package has a suggested (default) entry, it is displayed. The user can either overwrite another entry or accept the suggestion. When all items to be entered have been completed, the user presses a key to send the screen information to storage.

Standard component table

In this way, an entry screen is filled out for each new job. Each job may have up to 999 "components." These are items to which costs can be assigned. These items can be entered from the keyboard; a separate entry screen is filled out for each component. Or components can be duplicated from already stored items in a standard component table that the user constructs. This table may grow to contain as many as 994 components and can present users with a problem in locating the desired component from among so many. Like other stored items in this package, the standard components are accessed by number.

If needed, an entire existing job can be duplicated to aid in entering a similar new job. Component entries can be related to one another by designating them as "master" and "sub." Subcomponents will then be shown on listings under their master heading. This feature allows detailed job cost estimates to be prepared.

Time-line displays

Among the items entered on each job and component record are the estimated start and completion dates. These are used by the package to prepare schedule reports that show time lines for each job and component.

The package calculates a percent complete for each job based on accumulated costs divided by the total of projected completion costs. Users can also enter an actual percent completion figure.

Entering transactions

Daily transactions are entered, one to a line, on a transactions screen. Each is assigned to a job and a component within that job, by number. The package can be used together with standard accounting packages from the same vendor. If this is done, each transaction must also be assigned to a general ledger code and account number. If the user can't remember them, the required numbers for these entries have to be searched out from printed lists of jobs, components, and general ledger structure.

Job records are located in the stored files by entering a job number. If this brings up the wrong job, the user can move from job screen to job-screen to find the right one.

Bottom-line report

The bottom line is displayed by a profitability report that shows estimated profit and profit margin, along with cost and billing figures, for each job in the files.

The package can also generate invoices for all active jobs and provides for posting these invoices to a related accounts receivable package, if it is used.

Chapter 12
Project Management Packages

Close to 100 project management packages for personal computers have become available during the past few years. With such riches before us, it is possible to define some desirable characteristics for any particular use, and then search for the right package with some confidence that it exists.

One of the first characteristics to look at is the number of tasks or activities a package can include in a given project. Those packages that handle fewer than about 20 tasks can be safely ignored. It would be simpler to plan such little projects with paper and pencil than to use a computer.

At the other extreme, it may be best to handle very large projects with thousands of tasks on large, mainframe computers. Among the personal computer packages surveyed for this chapter, those that promise to handle the largest number of activities are Plantrac (65,000) and Primavera Project Planner (10,000). These packages and others like PAC MICRO and PMS II can be used on a personal computer and can also communicate with project management software housed on larger computers.

As we move from packages that handle few activities to those that handle many, we might expect that prices would steadily increase. Such is not the case. The Pathfinder package from Morgan Computing, for example, handles up to 3160 activities and costs just $80, while many other packages are priced at a dollar an activity or more. However, the Morgan package produces simple Gantt charts; these show the start and end of activities, but no interrelationships between them; and that is about all it does. If users want more, they will have to turn to other packages.

Some users may want to see PERT charts or other "network" charts that illustrate the dependencies of one activity on another, or they may want the package to produce information on factors such as cost and manpower. Frequently users want packages that will do progress tracking as well as project planning.

Look for helpful data entry

In terms of actual use of a project management package, users will spend most of their time simply entering data to describe the project tasks or activities. For that reason, the data entry facilities offered by these packages are an important consideration. A package may have very wonderful calculation, reporting, and display capabilities, but if the process of data entry is too arduous, that package may see little actual use.

Some very helpful data entry techniques have been developed by software vendors who work on business packages for personal computers. A few of the available project management packages have taken full advantage of these techniques.

For example, the Project package, developed by a leading personal computer software company, has users enter data onto an Activity screen, on which a Gantt chart is shown. An entry window is used to fill in the data for each activity. Entry of items is accomplished by hitting the TAB key to move from one item to another in the entry window. As data for each task are completed, the Gantt chart is automatically updated, so the user sees the developing effect on the overall project of adding each activity. A very similar activity entry method is used by the Timeline package.

An aspect of data entry that is ignored by many of these packages is the use of internal checks to verify the validity and accuracy of what is keyboarded. Mainframe data processing software has traditionally given close attention to such input "controls," since data for large computers are often entered by clerks who sit all day at the keyboard typing material that may be meaningless to them.

Usually, personal computer project management packages will be operated by the professionals who want to use the results these packages produce. Nevertheless, internal computer checks on such things as consistent use of numerals and alphabetic letters and on duplication of activity descriptions can be very helpful when there is a lot of information to input. The Plantrac package is one that uses some traditional mainframe techniques to try to keep the input accurate. In this package there are well-designed entry screen displays with internal checks on consistency and duplication of tasks. In addition, as each activity is entered, the package automatically prints out the data and stores them on disk.

In most of the project management packages discussed in this chapter, little attention seems to have been given to the plight of the user faced with inputting masses of activity data. Thus Gantt-Pack invites users to input data for as many as 500 activities but offers a most inconvenient format. Data entry is onto a crowded screen that becomes closely packed with entries. It is arranged in rows and columns, and only the tops of the columns are labeled, so it is often hard to see which item is on which line. The detail formats required for items to be entered are not very easy to learn, and there is no audible warning when the package rejects incorrect entries. In surprising contrast, however, the data editing facilities for this package are both convenient and rapid in operation.

Another example of poorly arranged input methods is the Demi-Plan package which prompts for the needed data. But following the entry of each activity description, the user is returned to the main menu, where the data entry option must be chosen again if another task is to be entered. Data entry itself is an unforgiving process. Users enter a six-item task description. If there are any mistakes in the entry, they have to start all over again.

Adding and deleting should be simple

It is common wisdom that plans are made only to be changed, and project management plans are no exception. Even the most perceptive and careful planner will have to make many changes to get a complex project schedule to conform to the realities it must encounter. An important feature of these packages is therefore their ability to accommodate addition, deletion, and moving of activities easily.

With the Timeline package, changes are easily made. The cursor is moved to the desired chart location and a function key is pressed. This brings up the entry window for that location. Any desired changes are made through that window, and the results are immediately reflected in the chart.

The Harvard Project Manager offers an exemplary method for removing activities. On the PERT chart for this package, milestones are shown as boxes, activities as boxes in reverse video. To delete a box, the user simply moves the cursor to it and presses a couple of keys. It disappears and the chart is redrawn. When new activities are added, the package automatically adjusts the project plan.

Not all packages provide this kind of automatic adjustment. Some require completely manual readjustment with all additions and deletions; others are half-automatic. In Pertmaster, when activities are added the user gives the relationships to existing activities, and these are incorporated into the project plan. Activities can also be deleted, but the user must then manually rearrange the relationships among the remaining activities. The reverse is true for the PRO-JECT 6 package. When an activity is deleted by the user, the package automatically removes any references to it that may appear in other activities. But when users add an activity, they must edit the other activities to include such references.

Calendars and other constraints

The real world places certain limits on any project plan. These constraints commonly have to do with time, people (called "resources" in the parlance of project management), and money.

The Timeline package has a particularly flexible approach to relating the time sequencing of one activity with another. Activities can be marked with a specific start or end date, or ASAP (as soon as possible), or ALAP (as late as possible), or they can be designated as Span activities. The Span activities are flexible in time, able to shrink or expand to accommodate the other activities. Users can decide which tasks to sequence or "join" to one another. Partial joining (starting the next task when the preceding one is only partly complete) is also allowed.

The days of a project can become difficult to describe, for work often will not be done on weekends and holidays, nor during vacations, and all of these may differ from one project to another, one year to another.

Many project management packages therefore incorporate calendars. For example, the Garland Publishing Pathfinder package uses a calendar file in which each day is represented by a code. The built-in calendar runs from 1975 to 1990, and to handle other years the user must use a text editor to build a new calendar.

Some packages provide for multiple calendars. Thus the Pertmaster package allows users to set up any number of calendars with different work-day, holiday, and shift schedules, then select which calendar will be used with any given project. The package provides convenient calendar editing features.

Resource leveling is hard to find

Some project management packages take no account of people and other limited resources that may or may not be available to carry out project activities, leaving it to the planner to incorporate such considerations in activity durations and sequencing, but most of the packages track such resources in one way or another.

Ideally, a project management package should be able not only to indicate when limited resources are close to being exhausted but also to redistribute the resources to achieve "best" results. Very few of the packages described in this chapter even attempt such redistribution, called "resource leveling." One that does is the Primavera Project Planner which averages out the availability of up to six vital resources for each task. When the package finds that the available resources are not sufficient for all active tasks, it will try to reassign resources automatically without compromising the critical path or the project completion date.

A simpler type of resource leveling is performed by the Project Management package from the Institute of Industrial Engineers. The package includes a resource allocation module that takes both activity time and available resources into account in calculating the start and finish time for each activity, so that a limited resource is efficiently used. Up to 200 activities can be handled, but only one limited resource. The module does not yield optimum results, but the solution will improve with additional iterations.

Costs and cost tracking

Not all project management packages concern themselves with costs, but most make monetary considerations an integral part of package operations.

In the MicroGANTT package, resources are always related to tasks that are billable or have billable components. The user can assign hourly and fixed costs, along with availability and time attributes, to each resource. An hourly billing rate can be assigned to an entire project, and this rate can be overridden for specific tasks. This information allows the program to calculate the resource requirements for each task, by time period.

The PAC MICRO package has an optional cost module used to track budgeted vs. actual costs, resources, and durations. Very useful bar chart displays are used to compare the actual and budgeted amounts.

Project Scheduler 5000 reports include a list of resources and associated costs. Users can graph resource costs with or without labor costs. When actual costs are input to the package, users can graph planned vs. actual cost data, and they can also graph cost comparisons of planned, revised-planned, and actual costs to date.

What-if analysis

By changing the relationships between project activities and by adjusting constraints of time, cost, and resources, planners can produce scenarios of possible outcomes for their projects. Some packages make this kind of "what-if" analysis particularly easy by providing for the kind of easy addition, deletion, and changing of activities that has already been discussed.

Plantrac is a package that is specifically oriented to this what-if analysis. It has very flexible capabilities for modifying the planning parameters and observing the results. Constraints of time, manpower, and cost can be readily imposed and removed to examine their effects on the overall project.

Flexible reports

For many users, the printed reports produced by project management packages are very significant, for such reports can be a means of communication with those who will carry out the projects and with decision makers who may have ultimate control over planning decisions.

Usually the packages turn out only a few reports, and these are fixed in format. But some, like PRO-JECT 6 have a more flexible reporting facility. With this package, users can choose to select or sort many arrangements of data for a report. Formatted report definitions can be set up and reused as needed. Documents created by word processor packages can be incorporated into the reports.

The MicroGANTT package has a feature called Select that will scan a list of projects and extract the tasks that match codes previously assigned by the users. This allows reports to be organized by employee, machine, job number, client, or any category the user chooses.

For those who deal with government agencies, it may be essential that the reports they produce conform to the specifications of those agencies. Two of the packages discussed in this chapter have been designed with this in mind. The PMS II package produces reports that meet ER-1-1-11 and DOD 7000-2 specifications. Primavera Project Planner also produces reports that meet the contracting requirements of the Department of Defense and other government agencies.

THE CONFIDENCE FACTOR

This package offers a critical path module that handles up to 100 tasks with 10 resource categories. It also performs decision-making functions.

The Confidence Factor runs on IBM/PC computers. It sells for $389 from Simple Software, 2 Pinewood, Irvine, CA 92714 [(714) 857-9179].

Critical path calculations are only part of what this package offers. It has a decision tree module for organizing considerations that go into decisions. There is a risk simulation module for making predictions, and a linear programming module as well. Other modules are Best Course of Action for optimal choices and Yes/No Decisions for ranking alternatives.

The critical path module operates with "time units" and the user decides whether these will represent days, weeks, months, etc. The actual units are never displayed by the package.

Up to 10 manpower resources, with time unit costs applied to each task in a project, can be handled.

The package calculates the critical path, manpower requirements, and costs, producing a Gantt chart, project data report, job cost report, start-finish report, resource allocation and smoothing reports.

The user's manual is skimpy and not very helpful.

CPM/PERT

This package produces a Gantt chart and an activity schedule report that includes critical path length and may include a probability of on-time completion.

CPM/PERT runs on IBM/PCs and sells for $249 from Elite Software Development, P.O. Box 1194, Bryan, TX 77806.

The CPM in the name refers to the Critical Path Method. Users can use the CPM mode, then upgrade their operations to PERT by adding two additional time estimates for each activity. The PERT method allows computation of a probability for completing a project on time.

Program operation is controlled from a master menu. The package prompts the user for inputs. There is a "beginner" operational mode in which added HELP information is displayed. These displays can be suppressed by operating in the "expert" mode.

The capacity of this package depends on available computer main memory. With 128K, up to 600 variables can be handled. Only day-units of time can be used. Project models must have one, and only one, terminating node.

Holidays can be set at fixed dates or on certain days of the week within a given date range. Vacation and weekend no-work schedules are set using up to 26 "calendar" files, and each activity can reference a different calendar file.

Legible, detailed, and clear reports are generated, including a Critical Path report, Holiday and Calendar reports, and an Activity Cost report.

Gantt charts are produced on the printer; users can specify the characters to be used for the various chart features. Since previous calculation results are not stored, they are repeated when a Gantt chart is called for, and this can take minutes of computation time.

DEMI-PLAN

This low cost package will handle up to 100 tasks but is inconvenient to operate. The package will produce task-resource listings and Gantt charts.

Demi-Plan runs on IBM/PC/XT and TRS-80 I,III,4 computers and sells for $49.95 from Demi-Software, 62 Nursery Rd., Ridgefield, CT 06877 [(203) 431-0864].

Demi-Plan operates from menus. When the user selects the Add option, the package prompts for the needed data. Following the entry of each task description, the user is returned to the main menu to select Add again if another task is to be entered.

Data entry itself is an unforgiving process. Users enter a six-item task description; if there are any mistakes in the entry, they have to start all over again. And that is the way the entire data entry process is handled.

Starting times for projects and tasks are expressed as the number of days from the beginning of the project, and it is up to the user to make the necessary conversions.

Saving project data on disk with this package also means ending program operation. The package simply quits, and the user has to reset the computer.

EMPACT

Up to 250 tasks can be handled by this package with an unlimited number of resource categories.

EMPACT runs on IBM/PCs and sells for $149.95 from Applied MicroSystems, P.O. Box 832, Roswell, GA 30077 [(404) 475-0832].

This package is quite simple to operate, and the help displays quickly clear up most misunderstandings about how it works.

Data input displays prompt the user for start and end dates, but the package does not calculate work days, so users are required to do this themselves. Since this involves taking account of various month-lengths, it is an arduous procedure for mental arithmetic. However, the package does offer a stored calendar. Users can select any month and year and get an immediate calendar display.

Those working with lengthy input for a project are living dangerously since the package keeps all the data in main memory, storing it on disk only when the user moves to another project.

Reports produced by the package are variations of a format that shows descriptions, dates, and codes for each activity. An Analysis report displays the earliest and last scheduled dates, along with the number and percentage of tasks completed for the entire project. Gantt charts with graphic symbols are also available.

EX-PERT/80

This package handles up to 999 tasks but only one resource category.
EX-PERT/80 runs on IBM/PC, TRS-80 I,III, and Apple II,IIe computers. It sells for $115 from Decision Support Software, 1300 Vincent Pl., McLean, VA 22101 [(703) 442-7900].

Data entry is clumsy. After entering a task name the package prompts for a string of six comma-separated entries. If there are any mistakes, the user must reenter all six. There is an editing mode, but one reviewer found it defective.

EX-PERT/80 has no built-in calendar function. It does take optimistic and pessimistic estimates of task duration from the user. These are used to calculate probabilities for various project completion dates.

Outputs are, with the exception of the Gantt chart, directed to the screen for display. The only way to get a printout of the displayed material, on an IBM/PC, is to use the computer's PrtSc key.

The package will not tolerate nodes on Gantt charts that are "dangling," not connected in both directions, except the first and last nodes. If the diagram topology is unsatisfactory, the package will crash.

Other outputs include a graph that shows the amount of resource needed for each project day. There is also a report that shows task beginnings and endings, and a listing can be produced of tasks that must or may be active over a specified range of days.

The user manual is clearly written; however, one text serves for all computers on which the package may run. As a result, there are a few confusing instructions about use of the keyboard.

GANTT-PACK

This package produces Gantt and critical milestone charts.
Gantt-Pack runs on IBM/PC, CP/M, and TRS-80 computers. It sells for $395 from Gantt Systems, 495 Main St., Metuchen, NJ 08840 [(201) 494-4752].

Data entry is onto a crowded screen that becomes closely packed with entries. It is arranged in rows and columns, and only the tops of the columns are labeled, so it is often hard to see which item is on which line. Formats required for items to be entered are not very easy to learn. There is no audible warning when the package rejects incorrect entries. Data editing is convenient and rapid in operation.

The package allows the user to choose among many different measures of time when the data entry format is set up. It does not take holidays automatically into consideration.

When making menu selections, the user has to simultaneously enter the first letter in the name of a menu section and a letter denoting the desired menu subsection, a procedure that is difficult to learn to use.

The package assumes that the user will memorize the names of the available files, since the name of the desired file must be typed before other package procedures can begin.

Gantt-Pack produces a Gantt chart, a critical milestone chart that shows current status of tasks and listings of original and calculated data. The charts are not set up to display the names of events, only numbers. There are no resource management reports.

The user's manual includes clear directions for the use of each screen display used in the package.

HARVARD PROJECT MANAGER

This project management software is designed to make good use of a personal computer. It has an excellent tutorial. The package is limited to handling projects that will fit within the main memory of the computer. For an IBM/PC with 128K memory, that means that a project with about 200 tasks can be handled. Subprojects can be set up, within the same memory limitations, allowing users to develop a library of standard subtasks that can be used over and over again.

Harvard Project Manager runs on IBM/PC computers. It sells for $395 from Harvard Software, 521 Great Rd., Littleton, MA 01460 [(617) 486-8431].

The Harvard Project Manager makes good use of "windowing" techniques, dividing the screen display into separate areas, each of which can show different aspects of the materials that are to be used.

The main display of this package shows four windows. The first contains a PERT chart; the second, a bar-chart project schedule that highlights the project's critical path; the third a calendar; and the forth displays a function-selection menu. Users can make a menu choice and have the chosen window fill the screen. Or two windows can share the screen so that, for example, the Gantt and PERT charts can be viewed together.

When starting up a new project, the user will get little assistance from this package. It is expected that the initial planning will be done with paper and pencil, then the results used to construct an initial PERT chart with the package. But once the initial entries are made, the Harvard Project Manager provides powerful means to monitor and change the data and to compute new costs and dates as the project proceeds. For example, once the initial project data are entered, the package automatically readjusts all costs and dates as new data are added.

Adding a task to the project is eased by further use of display windows. As tasks are added to the PERT chart, a window can be called up on which the user can key items of specific information about that task that are to be stored. Shuttling back and forth between windows is a simple process, often involving only a single keystroke.

On the PERT chart, milestones are shown as boxes, activities as boxes in reverse video. To delete a box, the user simply moves the cursor to it and presses a couple of keys. It disappears and the chart is redrawn. In general, as new information is entered, the displays will automatically adjust. There are some arbitrary restrictions on the PERT charts. For example, all tasks must branch from milestones, and milestones must always have at least one task before and after them.

The project calendar is flexible, allowing the user to factor in holidays and any other out-of-the-ordinary days. Output is also flexible, allowing the user to produce printed PERT charts, calendars, and reports. Where needed, these can be printed "sideways" so that material of almost any length can be accommodated.

Resource allocation can be done as the PERT chart is being constructed or afterwards. There is no resource smoothing, and resources cannot be allocated for only a part of a task.

An expense can be assigned to each activity, but the package does not provide for separating out fixed and variable expenses. A percent-complete figure allows the package to be used for some project tracking as well as planning.

Learning through windows

As with any package designed to perform complicated functions, there is some learning the user has to go through before the Harvard Project Manager can be mastered. For example, when the main package functions are being selected, the Back Space key and spacebar control cursor movement. Once the user is operating within a given function, the cursor arrow keys are used to control selections. When it comes to editing text for descriptions, the Tab key is used to control cursor location.

To aid the user in learning these procedures, a disk-stored tutorial is provided, and this too makes use of display windows, showing explanations in one window while the user carries out the lessons in another. This excellent tutorial is coordinated with the user's manual. Unfortunately, the manual itself is brief. It depends unduly on the tutorial and does not provide sufficient material for later reference. There is a reference card that summarizes package functions.

The charts produced by the package can be printed as well as displayed, and the printout can be either in the conventional vertical manner, or horizontal (which takes more time but is often visually much more pleasing). The package also produces detail reports showing all project information and calculation results and status reports listing information on selected activities. A calendar of a project can be printed.

INTEPERT

Many tasks and projects (1200 to 1900 of each) can be related to one another as subtasks by this package. Up to 26 resource categories can be handled.

IntePert runs on IBM/PC computers. It sells for $195 from Schuchardt Software Systems, 515 Northgate Dr., San Rafael, CA 94903 [(415) 492-9330].

Each task is entered as a separate unit. The package prompts for the needed items. Calculation of time intervals is done by the package from the project and task dates the user supplies. When a task is inserted or deleted, the package automatically adjusts. As tasks are entered, they are automatically stored in disk memory, protecting the information from inadvertent loss.

Tasks can be divided into subtasks with up to 64 hierarchy levels allowed.

The press of a key produces a PERT chart with critical path tasks shown across the top. Another key produces a Gantt chart. Both charts can be printed, using ordinary print characters.

A detailed report lists tasks and all associated data. A schedule report lists all activities by date.

The manual includes a detailed and skillfully formulated tutorial. All the material is well written, and there is a reference section, error message explanations, and a detailed index.

MICROGANTT

This package does budgeting and Gantt charts but has no PERT chart displays. Up to 100 tasks can be handled, and many projects can be interrelated by treating them as subprojects. An unlimited number of resource categories can be used.

MicroGANTT runs on IBM/PC computers. It sells for $395 from Earth Data, P.O. Box 13168, Richmond, VA 23225 [(804) 231-0300].

MicroGANTT is command, rather than menu-driven, with the needed commands displayed at the bottom of the screen at all times.

Users are prompted for entry of data, first of overall project data, then of data for task records. The records may be billable or not. The package automatically saves data in disk storage almost immediately after they are entered.

A calendar serves to keep track of the length and order of the tasks. Each project can run as long as 61 units of time, and these units can be years, quarters, months, weeks, or days.

The package does not provide for such built-in delays as holidays and other nonworking days, nor for such contingencies as sick leave and vacations. These must be accounted for by the user.

If the user does not assign a task start date (or a prerequisite task that defines that start), the package will set the start date to the beginning of the project. Since the dates can be changed at will by the user, this assumption is simple to correct, should it be wrong.

Resources like manpower can easily be allocated on a percentage basis. But allocating several workers with different billing rates to a single project or task becomes complicated.

The package has good provisions for cost tracking, in that it allows users to assign an hourly billing rate to an entire project but still override this rate for specific tasks. It also allows fixed costs to be assigned to each task.

Resources are always related to tasks that are billable or have billable components. The user can assign a cost, along with availability and time attributes, to each resource. This information allows the program to calculate the resource requirements for each task, by time period. Fixed costs may be included.

Composite task feature

The package has a powerful composite task feature. It can be used to create subprojects, and each of these can contain up to 100 tasks. However, subproject information cannot be used in a fully integrated way with the main project information. For example, detailed main project resource reports may not incorporate subproject data.

Completion of a given task can be made fully or partially dependent on completion of other tasks, or on the availability of a specific resource. Tasks can be assigned fixed durations, and selected tasks can be designated as milestones.

The limit of 100 tasks is not just arbitrary, it is quite practical. As tasks and composite tasks are added, program execution gradually slows down. Data for composite tasks are taken from disk storage so, if many of these are used, disk accessing can add greatly to the time the program takes.

Helpful displays and printouts

Results of entries can be quickly observed on a Gantt chart, displayed on the screen. This provides a convenient way to test out various changes in schedule or tasks and see the results of different alternatives. The displayed chart gives a clear picture of the various tasks at hand, of the critical path of the project, and of how near it is to being completed.

The initial planning scheme can be updated as actual results are received. The Gantt chart display is used as a basis to revise the remaining schedules. Unfortunately, it is somewhat difficult to update the project calendar, since MicroGANTT treats completed and in-progress tasks in the same way at the project timeline.

In addition to the Gantt chart, the package provides a display that shows tasks by number, name, and type, along with other important features of each task. A cost report breaks out fixed costs for each task for each period of the project schedule and also summarizes costs for each period. In addition, a report generator program provides information keyed by task code or task description.

For a more detailed presentation of costs, the package produces printouts which break out resource use as well as cost. Printing of large reports is sequenced so that completed pages can be assembled easily into larger layouts.

The package produces detailed time-cost summaries and task summaries. The fixed format reports are detailed and relatively easy to read. A report generation feature called Select is available for creation of custom reports. The charts use letter codes to key different kinds of data. One reviewer found that it took 40 minutes to print out a complex Gantt chart, an inordinately long time.

Gantt charts can be created for small work segments that may be repeatedly used during a project. These can be stored, then retrieved and inserted in a project as needed.

Those who need a refresher course in project management techniques will find the manual supplied with the package helpful. What is missing are the instructions that novice computer users will need to get the package properly installed, on a floppy or hard disk, so it can be conveniently used, and there is no hand-holding tutorial for the timid user. The package runs from menus, and there is a screen-displayed entry form for data, so the package, quite aside from the manual, is relatively easy to learn and to use.

MICROPERT

This package creates Gantt and PERT charts, activity and resource lists, based on user responses to screen-displayed prompts about tasks and times. However, it does not handle any financial data. Up to 220 tasks can be handled.

MicroPERT runs on IBM/PC computers. It sells for $350 from Sheppard Software, 4750 Clough Creek Rd., Reading, CA 96002 [(916) 222-1553].

The package requires that users state how many activities and events there will be in a project. To aid in the paper and pencil preplanning needed to get these numbers, MicroPERT provides users with printed worksheets for events, activities, and project layout.

When the activity and event numbers are entered, the package prompts the user for event and activity data. There is no display that accompanies this data entry, but MicroPERT editing facilities are good. However, when an event is deleted, the user must update all the activities that used that event. The package automatically renumbers all subsequent events, and it will handle activity deletions automatically as well.

Time periods are set up in day, week, month, quarter, or yearly units. Holidays have to be handled as dummy activities.

Output printing options include horizontal as well as vertical printing, and presentation (slow) as well as draft-quality printing. In addition to the charts, MicroPERT produces a schedule report that can be sorted by the user.

The 210-page manual is intelligently written and includes a useful tutorial and a good index.

MICROTRAK

As many as 300 tasks can be handled by this package with up to 10 resource categories.

MicroTrak runs on IBM/PC computers. It sells for $595 from SofTrak Systems, P.O. Box 22156, Salt Lake City, UT 84112 [(801) 531-8550].

MicroTrak will handle about 300 tasks on one floppy disk. Only 10 resources can be used.

Before this package begins its work, the user has to divide the project manually into task sets and must also define the interactions between tasks.

As with most project management packages, most of the time the user spends is taken up with data entry. As new activities are entered, the package automatically updates its display.

Tasks can be deleted, and the package will automatically remove all interactions with other tasks and recalculate the network.

Reports generated by the package include one on schedule, on the network, on milestones, updates, activity-within-resource, and resource-within-activity.

The user manual has an introduction to critical path scheduling that prepares the user for the terminology used with this package. Unfortunately, the manual is not very helpful beyond that point. For example, the complex network charts the package produces are not explained at all.

MILESTONE

This package will handle hundreds of tasks, with the exact number depending on the size of available memory. It has unique scrolling features that allow convenient reading of very large Gantt charts.

Milestone runs on IBM/PC, CP/M, and USCD Pascal computers. It sells for $250 from Digital Marketing, 2363 Boulevard Circle, Walnut Creek, CA 94595 [(415) 947-1000].

Data input for this package has the user tab from one displayed data item to another and keyboard the correct values for each item.

The package does rapid scrolling that operates either horizontally or vertically. Users can jump-scroll over any chosen number of jobs or work periods. With this scrolling, it is easy to make practical use of a large Gantt chart.

The number of activities that can be handled depends on the available computer main memory. It takes an IBM/PC with 448K to handle 300 tasks. The package keeps the user informed how much room is left for further input.

Milestone allows the use of only 9 resources and 12 holidays. Time units can be hours, days, weeks, months, quarters, or federal fiscal quarters.

Output reports include project description and job description. The time schedule output is a conventional Gantt chart with critical path shown. There is also a columnar job report.

Financial information is presented in a histogram format, allowing users to see cash flow along with the critical path and job loading.

The user's manual is put together well, with explanations of features and reports keyed to a sample problem.

PAC MICRO

This package offers project progress tracking as well as planning. It can readily exchange information with similar mainframe-based packages from the same vendor. Up to 400 tasks can be handled, and up to 100 resource categories.

PAC MICRO runs on IBM/PCs and sells for $990 from AGS Management Systems, 880 First Ave., King of Prussia, PA 19406 [(215) 265-1550].

PAC MICRO works from easy-to-use displayed menus. There is an entry screen for each task. Unfortunately, there is no reference on one screen to any of the previous ones, so users can easily lose track of what they are doing.

Resource data are entered on separate screens. A master list of resources is created, with associated costs. In separate steps, resource assignments to project tasks are entered. This seems to involve unnecessary duplicate data entry.

Optional printing

An optional report-printing feature is available. Without it, the package offers only displays, and users are on their own in getting their computers to print what is displayed.

There are some nice display features. Reports list the project tasks in order of criticality and show predecessor and sucessor tasks. A Gantt chart is included in the output.

The portion of a project taken up by each task is displayed in the form of a pie chart. However, this kind of display is useful only when relatively few tasks are involved, since the pie-sections soon become too fine to be significant.

A column chart can be used to display the number of resource units required on each day of the project. This quickly reveals over allocation of a resource.

Users can exit the main program of the package and use another program to produce a network diagram of their project.

The cost module used to track budgeted vs. actual costs, resources, and durations is also an optional feature. Very useful bar chart displays are used to compare the actual and budgeted amounts.

The user's manual is thoughtfully constructed to walk users step by step through the procedures required by this package. There are plenty of figures showing what to expect in the way of screen displays. Unfortunately, the manual is not designed to function as a reference.

PATHFINDER

As many as 500 tasks can be handled by this package. Resource categories are limited to 30 per project and just one per task.

Pathfinder runs on IBM/PC and CP/M computers. It sells for $299 from Garland Publishing, 136 Madison Ave., New York, NY 10016 [(212) 686-7492].

Procedures for adding, deleting, and inserting tasks work efficiently. There is an interactive dialog for entering task information.

The package uses a calendar file in which each day is represented by a code. The built-in calendar runs from 1975 to 1990, and to handle other years the user must use a text editor to build a new calendar.

Pathfinder produces exceptions reports to spot activities that need attention, cash flow reports, and Gantt charts. There can also be up to four project schedule reports in which users can sort and arrange activities as desired. There is no output that analyzes the interdependence among various tasks.

PATHFINDER

This package handles up to 3160 tasks, taking simple inputs and producing Gantt charts.

Pathfinder runs on IBM/PC computers. It sells for $80 from Morgan Computing, 10400 North Central Expwy #210, Dallas, TX 75074 [(214) 739-5895].

This is a simple package that takes in only four data items for each task: beginning and end event-numbers, a time-to-perform, and a name. It is designed to produce Gantt charts quickly, and that is just what it does—no more, no less.

Its editing features work well. If subelements of a task are deleted, the entire project will be automatically rearranged.

The package does have some awkward limitations. It will not accept unterminated activities and won't run if there is more than one activity (the final one) that has no continuing connection.

The output is a Gantt chart, which can be produced on virtually any printer including daisy wheel types. Events listings can also be produced.

PERTMASTER

Depending on available computer memory, this package can handle 1000 to 2500 tasks, with 29 resource categories per task.

Pertmaster runs on IBM/PC and CP/M computers. A version that will handle 1500 tasks sells for $695; a 2500-task version sells for $895. An optional plotting package, Pertplotter, sells for $495. Westminster Software, 3000 Sand Hill RD. Bldg. 4 #242, Menlo Park, CA 94025 [(415) 845-1400].

The package uses the IBM/PC function keys, and a list of their uses is displayed at the bottom of the screen. Users can set up their own abbreviations for tasks and resouces, which will be recognized by the package.

Users can set up any number of calendars with different workday, holiday, and shift schedules, and they can select which calendar will be used with any given project. Calendar editing features are convenient.

Time periods used by the package are user selected and flexible. They can be in seconds, minutes, hours, days, shifts, weeks, months, years, or in completed work periods.

Projects can be set up based on Gantt charts or on PERT charts. Tasks can be added, the user giving the relationships to existing tasks. They can also be deleted, but the user must then manually rearrange the relationships among the remaining tasks.

There is a standard report on activities sorted by activity number, float, early start, or description. The package also produces project and period bar charts. Users can define their own reports as well.

Pertmaster can send its graphical output to plotters as well as printers using an additional program called Pertplotter.

The user manual has good tutorial and reference sections but gives little explanation of how errors are handled.

PLANTRAC

This is a very capable package that can handle up to 25 projects with a total of 65,000 tasks per project and 200 resource categories.

Plantrac runs on IBM/PC, TRS-80, and CP/M computers. It sells for $3000 plus $1000 per year for updates and support from Computerline Limited, 755 Southern Artery, Quincy, MA 02169 [(617) 773-0001].

The menus are not the usual kind found in personal computer packages. One menu leads to another, but it is difficult for users to keep track of how to return to a menu once it has been passed.

Data entry includes internal checks on consistency and duplication of tasks. There are well-designed screen displays on which the data are entered. As each task is entered, the package automatically prints out the data and stores them on disk. That is methodical, but the printing activity may be disturbing to those accustomed to using their computers in peaceful silence. The printer is actually used as a logging device to record everything entered on the keyboard. There is no option by which the user can turn it off.

Output from the package includes PERT and Gantt charts and, for those who have plotters attached to their systems, project network drawings. There are many report options. Information on specific items can be displayed in bar chart or histogram format. The data can be sorted as desired for reporting purposes. Holidays and other work-week adjustments can be added when reports are being specified.

There are very flexible capabilities for modifying the planning parameters and observing the results. Constraints of time, manpower, and cost can be imposed and removed to examine their effects on the overall project.

The user manual has a section on the basics of PERT chart use, but there is no tutorial material on package operation. There are explanations of the operation of the various package modules but no index.

PLAN/TRAX

Up to 300 tasks can be handled with 10 resource categories allowed.

PLAN/TRAX runs on IBM/PC computers. It sells for $595 from Engineering-Science, 57 Executive Park So. NE #590, Atlanta, GA 30329 [(404) 325-0124].

The user's manual gives instructions that are difficult to understand and incomplete. However, once past the learning barrier, users will find that this package is quite simple to operate. Tasks can be easily and quickly inserted or deleted.

PLAN/TRAX will not tolerate project nodes that cannot be traced back to the initial node or do not flow into the final one. It does not handle fractional time periods.

The package does not produce PERT charts, but it does turn out Gantt and manpower charts.

Users can track project progress by entering the funds spent and time taken to date. The package produces charts and graphs showing the schedule and budget status of the project. One Gantt-type chart shows current activity status and projected finish dates, assuming the present conditions continue.

PMS-II

This package is capable of handling sizeable projects, with the number of projects limited only by disk capacity. As many as 2750 tasks per project can be handled, and 96 resource categories can be used. The package does project tracking as well as planning. PMS-II is not an easy package to learn and use.

PMS-II runs on IBM/PCs; it sells for $1295. A companion resource-handling package, RMS-II, sells for $995. The vendor is Aha Inc., 147 South River St., Santa Cruz, CA 95061 [(408) 458-9119].

The main menu for this package offers users some 14 procedure choices for entering or updating project information, and producing reports.

Input data for each task are entered in response to prompts from the package. Unfortunately, the entry screen does not include any project summary or other indication that would help the user keep track of what has already been entered. For that, the user has to return to the main menu.

A variety of output reports can be produced. These include reports on activity and changes from previous activity reports, edit listings, PERT charts, funding schedules, percent-complete reports, subcontractor billing reports, and Gantt charts. Two of the reports are designed to meet government contract requirements. However, all these are printed reports and are unavailable as screen displays.

The user manual is not easy for beginners to follow. There is a sample project on the disk, but no written or displayed tutorial material accompanies it. The manual has no index that would allow it to be used as a reference source.

PRIMAVERA PROJECT PLANNER; FROM MAINFRAME TO MICRO

This is a package with powerful capacities and features, designed to meet U.S. Government reporting requirements. It can handle a total of up to 10,000 tasks, with the number of projects limited only by disk space. If that is what you need, the high price and batch-oriented operation of Primavera will not put you off.

Equipment required is an IBM/PC with 10-million-byte hard disk drive and 512K main memory. Price of the package is $2500. It is available from Primavera Systems, 29 Bala Av, Bala Cynwyd, PA 19004 [(215) 667-8600].

Originally developed for mainframe computers, this package is generous in its parameters. It will handle projects that include up to 10,000 tasks;

any task can be related to as many as 128 other tasks, whose beginning or end depends on the progress of the original task. Up to six resources, selected from an overall project total of 96 resource categories, can be associated with each task, along with six categories (and any number of subcategories) of fixed and variable costs, an events log, and constraints on the dates.

However, like many mainframe-originated programs, Primavera is essentially batch-oriented. That means that to revise a project, the user has to run a separate scheduling program, then print a revised project report to see the revisions in place. This process will take about two minutes. That is not very long, but is a far cry from the fast interaction most personal computer users expect.

Resource leveling

One of the important features of the package is its ability to do resource leveling—that is, to average out the availability of up to six vital resources for each task and, in this way, to calculate the duration of the task. When the package finds that the available resources are not sufficient for all active tasks, it will try to reassign resources automatically without compromising the critical path or the project completion date.

The Critical Path Method is used to schedule tasks into the overall project. Resources and costs can be tracked by task, and the package will compare expected to actual figures. The package can set up project schedules based on plans and on actual progress data and spell out the differences between the two.

With this package, the display screen is devoted mainly to entry of project data. As each task is initially entered, the user provides a task name and number and an estimate of the task's duration. A series of seven screen-displayed forms are then provided, on which the detailed characteristics of the task are entered. These forms cover project dates (which may be assigned by the user as well as computed by the package), time parameters, costs, resources to be used, successor tasks (which can be related by start-to-start, or end-to-end, or start-to-end succession), freeform notes, and codes to be used in connection with the task. Completed forms can be printed out on command.

Allows detailed specification

Each task may be assigned up to 20 codes. These serve as a form of indexing that allows a variety of special reports to be readily produced. For example, a code may be used to identify the geographic location of the task.

Then, in a large project a report showing the progress of all tasks in a given geographic area can be produced.

As with tasks, the specification of resources can be quite detailed. Resource availability can be spelled out in maximum and normal units that can be used each day. Up to five different availability periods can be assigned; during each of these, the maximum and normal availability of the resource can be set at different levels. In addition, the desired duration of use of each resource and it's lag-time can be specified. Given these data the package will calculate total resources needed for the task and the project. As the work proceeds, it will also compare actual data to scheduled use.

Although little is available in the way of reports that are displayed, Primavera can produce a great variety of printed reports. These are said to be adequate to meet the requirements of the Department of Defense and other government agencies. Gantt charts provide a ready view of the project's critical path, showing dates, tasks, and durations with reporting-time units set at days, weeks, or months. The relationship of a task to its predecessors and successors can be shown in a network path analysis printout. Resource reports are available to list or graph resource use, estimate resources needed for project completion, and compare resource use to project progress. Other reports spell out task and cost data.

As would be expected from a mainframe-originated package, all printouts are designed for a 132-column printer. However, the package does include a routine to use compressed printing.

PROJECT

This package can handle up to 128 tasks per project with 8 resource categories per task, 64 per project.

Project runs on IBM/PC computers. It sells for $250 from Microsoft, 10700 Northrup Way, P.O. Box 97200, Bellevue, WA 98004 [(206) 828-8080].

Project works from command choices displayed at the bottom of the screen. Users start by setting up work days and declaring holidays on a Calendar screen. Data are next entered into an Activity screen, on which a Gantt chart is shown. An entry window is used to fill in the data for each activity. Entry of items is accomplished by hitting the TAB key to move from one item to another in the entry window. Up to 128 activities can be entered on one Activity screen, and other similar screens can be linked to accommodate more activities.

Each project can be up to 10 years long and can involve up to $21 million in costs. Each activity can have up to eight predecessors and can use up to eight resources.

The package requires a lot of data. Each activity has a description, duration, predecessors, start date, and names and quantities of resources. Activities and resources can readily be added or removed, but entries often have to be completely retyped.

Resource unit costs and availability are shown in tabular format on a Resource screen. In practice, users need to move frequently from one screen to another, and each time a user moves from the Activity to the Resource screen, the package recalculates, a process that can take minutes with a fully entered large project.

The package's calendar can accommodate any 10-year period between 1900 and 2068. Holidays and weekend work can be selected as desired.

Other projects can be linked to the current one as subtasks for handling very large overall projects.

A sorting feature allows activities to be rearranged by criticality, duration, dates, or in alphabetical order.

The package produces histograms to display the daily time assigned to each resource, convenient for locating overloads and slack time.

There is a Gantt chart that prints sideways. A Project Detail report presents a page of information on each activity, including a summary of the resources assigned to that activity. There is a Table report that gives a summary for the activities, showing early and late starts and finishes and identifying critical activities. A Resource report summarizes time and costs. However, there are no PERT charts, and there is no provision for assigning fixed costs or income to tasks.

This package is very easy to learn to use. There is a half-hour tutorial and the instructions and illustrations in the manual are clear.

PRO-JECT 6

From 75 to 250 tasks can be handled by this package, depending on the available computer memory. Thirty resource categories can be used, with up to five used for any given task.

PRO-JECT 6 runs on IBM/PC computers. A 75-task version sells for $99, a 150-task version for $149, and a 250-task version for $199. SoftCorp, 2340 State Rd. 580 #244, Clearwater, FL 33575 [(813) 799-3984].

The data entry is straightforward, except that users must give an ADD command before entering data for each task instead of simply entering one task after another. The TAB key is used to advance from one entry item to another, and the ENTER key is used to end the entry for a task, a confusing arrangement for those who are accustomed to hitting the ENTER key after each item in other packages.

The package handles dates only between the years 1980 and 1989, a narrow range for some uses. If data entry is started and items are entered until the 1989 limit is exceeded, there seems to be no way to adjust to more acceptable dates without starting over.

PRO-JECT 6 accepts only integer time durations, so half-days or half-hours cannot be handled. Numbers, rather than descriptions, are used to identify tasks.

When a task is deleted by the user, the package automatically removes any references to it that may appear in other tasks. But when users add a task, they must edit other tasks to include such references.

The package has a very flexible reporting facility. Users can choose to select or sort many arrangements of data for a report. If desired, formatted report definitions can be set up and reused as needed. Documents created by word processor packages can be incorporated into the reports.

Vertical bar charts allow users to review the use of project resources.

The user manual is clear and concise. It has a command reference section and a listing of error messages, but no index.

PROJECT MANAGEMENT

Up to 500 tasks can be included in the critical path information handled by this package, and up to 300 tasks in the PERT information it produces.

Project Management runs on IBM/PC computers. It sells for $170 (or $140 to members) from the Institute of Industrial Engineers, 25 Technology Park, Norcross, GA 30092 [(404) 449-0460].

This package includes four separate modules. One determines the critical path, calculates free and total floats, and earliest and latest start times for up to 500 activities. Users have to draw their own Gantt charts, because this module doesn't do any. Once a project has been defined, activities cannot be inserted or removed, but their dates can be changed.

A PERT module calculates an estimate of the mean and variance of the time to reach each node of a project network. It will also estimate the probability of meeting scheduled completion times. The user enters three time estimates for each activity to start the calculation.

A resource allocation module takes both activity time and available resources into account in calculating the start and finish time for each activity, so that a limited resource is efficiently used. Up to 200 activities can be handled, but only one limited resource. The module does not yield optimum results, but the solution will improve with additional iterations.

A project network analysis module calculates the critical path, earliest and latest starting times, and appropriate floats for a network in which the activities (up to 300) are assumed to take place at the nodes rather than on the lines.

PROJECT SCHEDULER 5000

Project Scheduler 5000 can handle as many as 500 to 750 tasks per project, with the number of projects limited by disk storage capacity. Up to 96 resource categories can be handled.

This package runs on IBM/PC computers. It sells for $345 from Scitor Corp., 256 Gibraltar Dr. D7, Sunnyvale, CA 94089 [(408) 730-0400].

This package works from menus, with somewhat annoying delays between menu displays. The menu screens are not well organized, but the package nevertheless seems to function well.

As each task data item is entered, the cursor moves to the next item on the screen. When the data for a task are complete, there is a pause of a few seconds while the package redraws and redisplays the Gantt chart. When the user adds, inserts, or deletes tasks, the package handles the details automatically and adjusts the rest of the project as needed.

Projects can be easily modified. Each task and milestone is assigned a number on the Gantt chart. A new task can be inserted and the entire project renumbered. Tasks can also be moved about.

The package provides for detailed resource information on each task. Up to 96 different resources can be handled for each project. Users can enter both resource labor codes and fixed costs. The package will calculate the project cost on a daily basis and display it along the bottom of the Gantt chart.

As many as 30 holidays can be scheduled for a project.

Project Scheduler 5000 produces Gantt charts, a schedule of resources and costs, and several reports, but no PERT chart. The reports include a list of resources and associated costs, and a work week definition and calendar. There is a selectable report option that allows users to put together a wide variety of tailored reports.

There are similar flexible choices for the graphical output of the package. Users can graph resource allocation by time period, or resource costs with or without labor costs. When actual costs are input to the package, users can graph planned vs. actual cost data, and they can also graph cost comparisons of planned, revised-planned, and actual costs to date.

The user manual includes a tutorial exercise that takes about two hours to complete. The manual itself is well organized and has an index.

THE PROJECT MANAGER

This package calculates start and end dates as well as total entered costs; it produces Gantt charts. Projects with up to 399 tasks can be handled. It does not handle resources.

The Project Manager runs on IBM/PC computers. It sells for $495 from John Wiley and Sons, 605 Third Ave., New York, NY 10158 [(212) 850-6000].

Users have to make up their own project diagram before beginning to enter data into this package, so they can supply the required node numbers to identify the individual tasks.

Scheduling time has to be in man-days, but fractional days are allowed. Handling of dates makes no use of calendar files, and the package seems to have some difficulty handling weekends.

The package produces Gantt charts that display the entire project on a single sheet. This format gets quite cramped when lengthy projects are being shown. Five reports, none of which is headed by a title, can be produced.

Demonstration data are included on the package disk, but there are no tutorial instructions. The 95-page manual is readable, but it is not very well organized and there is no index.

PROJECT MANAGER WORKBENCH

This package does its calculations rapidly, supporting complex task interrelations and producing printed Gantt charts and reports. A network chart can be displayed. The number of projects and tasks that can be handled is limited by disk capacity, and nine resources can be used with each task.

Project Manager Workbench runs on IBM/PC computers. It sells for $1150. A version that handles up to 300 tasks sells for $750 from Applied Business Technology, 76 Laight St., New York, NY 10013 [(212) 219-8945].

Users have the option of menu operation of this package, or of using direct commands from the keyboard. The menus respond so rapidly that there seems to be little reason not to use them.

Data entry is well designed for handling large projects. Task data are entered on one display screen. Another screen is used to define relationships between the various tasks. These can be grouped into activities, which can in turn be grouped into phases of the overall project.

As these relationships are entered by the user, the package displays a growing map of the defined relationships between tasks. A detailed Gantt chart can also be displayed and scrolled through by the user.

An automatic scheduling feature adjusts for resource and dependency constraints. Activities are scheduled in increasing order of slack time. Reports are quickly produced and printed.

This is an easy-to-learn package that comes with on-disk samples and a 96-page tutorial. Unfortunately, the on-disk material has some bugs; the written tutorial is, however, well written and helpful. The user's manual has a reference section that describes all aspects of package operation in detail. It also gives the user insight into project management concepts and provides practical suggestions.

QWIKNET

The package can handle up to 250 tasks, with 100 resource categories per project, 12 per task. It can schedule backwards or forwards. Pull-down windows and a mouse device are used.

Qwiknet runs on IBM/PC computers. It sells for $800 from Project Software and Development, 14 Story St., Cambridge, MA 02138 [(617) 661-1444].

A mouse device is used to aid in moving the cursor around the display screen. By clicking the mouse button, users can move from one choice to another, when the item where the cursor is located is a multiple-choice type.

Across the top of the displays there is a line of items. With the cursor on one of these, a click of the mouse's left-button will open a pull-down menu window that allows for further choices.

In this way the user can access separate displays for entering task data, relationships between tasks, and resources for the tasks. There are also separate holiday calendars and resource lists to keyboard. This fractionated data entry is easy to use, but the process can become laborious. There seem to be difficulties in adding and deleting tasks.

Qwiknet does project tracking, following actual, estimated, and target schedules and costs. The package is capable of scheduling backwards from a given date. Several resources can be used with each task, and date constraints can be placed on tasks. Resources can be handled as distributed or lumped quantities.

Five reports are produced, including one listing task information, a task schedule, a Gantt chart, a target schedule listing, and a target schedule bar chart. A listing that includes costs for scheduled tasks and one that shows task dependencies, are displayed but not printed. There are no reports showing funding schedules or manpower loading.

Qwiknet does rapid calculations, responding almost instantaneously to user requests. Reports take only a few minutes to process. However, it cannot tolerate interruption during printing operations.

There is both a tutorial manual and a reference manual. The latter is well organized and designed to be read from beginning to end. There is an index, but without sufficient detail.

SCHEDULE-IT, GANTT-IT, UNDER-CONTROL

This group of three packages includes software for project scheduling (Schedule-It), tracking (Gantt-It), and filing (Under-Control). Up to 1300 tasks can be handled on an ordinary (320K) IBM/PC disk. The packages do not appear to be fully operational.

The packages run on IBM/PC computers. All three sell for a combined price of $180 from A + Software, 16 Academy St., Skanateles, NY 13152 [(315) 658-6918].

Schedule-It has a calendar and handles hour, day, or month time units. It calculates critical paths, slack time, and project milestones. Gantt-It is the package that does Gantt chart displays and produces standard project management reports. Under-Control manages the files and also allows users to design their own reports to supplement or replace the standard ones that Gantt-It initiates.

One reviewer reported that the packages were not satisfactorily debugged.

Data input is done with the Schedule-It package. A split-screen display shows eight previous task entries on top and the current task at the bottom.

The documentation for Under-Control is good, but the manuals for the other two packages are skimpy.

TARGET TASK

This package allows flexible schedule estimates. It generates Gantt charts and project management reports. The number of tasks that can be handled depends on the available computer main memory. With 512K memory, about 500 tasks can be handled.

TARGET TASK runs on IBM/PC computers and sells for $329 from Comshare, 5901 B Peachtree Dunwoodie Rd #275, Atlanta, GA 30328 [(404) 391-9012].

The menus from which this package operates are easy to use and are accompanied by HELP information that can be called upon to explain the options available to the user.

Data entries are checked by the package, which spots duplicate tasks. However, users cannot look back to view previously entered tasks.

Along with other input data on project tasks, users are asked to enter pessimistic, optimistic, and crash completion estimates of times needed for completion of each task. By making use of these estimates, charts and reports can be generated that reflect a variety of possible outcomes.

The package comes with a schedule of major holidays built in, and holidays can be added or deleted as needed.

TARGET TASK does not produce PERT charts, nor will it project labor resource requirements or show cost scheduling. What it concentrates on is calculating what happens when completion times change, and the package recalculates alternative scenarios rapidly. A cost estimate is given for completion of the project under each alternative schedule. A revised Gantt chart can be produced in seconds. Report generation is rather slow and can grind on for a half hour or more for a reasonably complex project.

The user's manual is clearly written, describes package operation, and also gives pointers on planning and PERT chart construction. It has a good index.

TASK MANAGER

This package is a special-purpose data manager applied to project applications. It can handle up to 999 tasks, with one person per task. Task Manager has particularly flexible reporting capabilities. However, it does no critical path calculations.

Task Manager runs on IBM/PC computers. It sells for $395 from Quala, 23026 Frisca Dr., Valencia, CA 91355 [(805) 255-2922].

Task Manager is operated from menu displays. The initial menu shows the functions that are available.

The input displays for this package a particularly well designed, making data entry an easy process. Arrow and other keyboard cursor controls are used to place data into displayed boxes, and keyboard inputs are automatically checked for length and other characteristics.

The package makes no provision for holidays or modified work schedules, so users will usually work with time durations rather than start and end dates.

Task Manager offers a choice of many different reports. In fact, users can define their own reports, then produce them one at a time or all at once in a batch. There is a list of sorting arrangements from which users can choose. When the desired sort order is chosen, users can then select a specific date range, individual, or department to be selected out and covered in the reports. Or they can include all the data that have been input. Reports cover only 4- or 12-month periods. Longer projects must be reported in segments.

The same kind of sorting and selection can be applied to Gantt charts. However, Task Manager does no critical path calculations. What it does display are dates, manpower, and percent complete for each task.

The user manual clearly explains package operation and has a good index.

TASKPLAN

Engineer C. Lamar Williams wrote this one in his spare time. It handles up to 50 tasks with one resource per task and 60 time periods, and it keeps track of project costs.

TaskPlan runs on IBM/PCs. It is a free package—no charge, but a $20

contribution is suggested. From Williams Software and Services, 1114 Pus-
ateri Way, San Jose, CA 95121 [(408) 227-4238].

The package comes with no manual, so it is very much a do-it-yourself experience to use it. Every time the package is started up, two screens of information are displayed, and users can print these themselves to get some sort of printed instructions to go by.

Data entry is done onto a display screen that has space for ten tasks. Start and end times, and cost are entered. Cost multipliers can be used, separately for each task or once for all tasks. Data can be corrected by backspacing during entry. Or corrections can be made at the end of each screen before the data are entered.

Tasks can be added as afterthoughts only by rerunning the package, with an option that preserves the previous data. A task can be deleted by setting its cost at zero and its time interval at the minimum .01 unit.

When data entry is completed, the package will report on the costs for each time period and can produce a chartlike display of incremental and cumulative costs.

One reviewer suggested that whatever TaskPlan can do might be done better with a spreadsheet or database package.

TIMELINE

Users can plan backwards from a deadline as well as forwards, with this
package. An unlimited number of resources can be used with a project.
Timeline runs on IBM/PC computers. It sells for $495 from Break-
through Software, 505 San Marin Dr., Novato, CA 94947 [(415) 898-1919].

Timeline operates from a main menu that can be recalled by pressing the / key. Commands can be invoked by typing the first letter of the command or by moving the cursor to it and pressing the Return key.

Data entry is done by filling out screen-displayed forms. First, resources are designated and option and calendar forms are checked. A task-entry window is superimposed on a Gantt chart display. As activity data are entered, the Gantt chart is drawn by the package. Activities can be marked with a specific start or end date, or ASAP (as soon as possible), or ALAP (as late as possible), or they can be designated as Span activities. The Span activities are flexible in time, able to shrink or expand to accommodate the other activities. Users can decide which tasks to sequence or "join" to one another. Partial joining (starting the next task when the preceding one is only partly complete) is also allowed.

Changes are easily made. The cursor is moved to the desired chart location and a function key is pressed. This brings up the entry window for that location. Any desired changes are made through that window, and the results are immediately reflected in the chart.

A resource-leveling facility spots overscheduled resources. Resource histograms graphically show allocation.

The package also produces a PERT chart which can be viewed as needed. On that chart, task descriptions are printed in the boxes, but the critical path is not shown. The display is not very well arranged and may be somewhat difficult to read.

A Gantt chart highlighting feature allows users, at the press of a key, to see all tasks that are joined to a specified task. A filtering function allows users to view only those tasks that match user-selected criteria.

Tasks can be sorted in various ways for reporting purposes. There is a detail report that gives full information about each task. Data from the package can be sent to various spreadsheet packages using an added program available at no cost from the vendor. Tables are used to summarize information on tasks, resources, and costs.

Timeline comes with an audio tape tutorial and manual that takes users through a sample project-planning exercise. The 126-page reference manual is easy to use, even somewhat entertaining, and it has a good index. Users are also provided with a quick reference card that shows function keys and shortcuts. On-screen HELP text displays are available for most of the situations users will face.

VISISCHEDULE

The number of tasks this package can handle depends on available computer memory. With 128K it handles 100 tasks; with 192K, 300 tasks. Nine resource categories can be used.

VisiSchedule runs on IBM/PC computers. It sells for $195 from Visi-Corp, 1953 Lindy Ave., San Jose, CA 95131 [(408) 946- 9000].

VisiSchedule works from a nicely designed set of menus that provide needed information along with selection options. As data on the various tasks that make up a project are entered, the package constructs a Gantt chart that changes with each entry.

The package allows use of different time units but not of fractional units. It is limited to eight resource categories. More than one category and one person can be assigned to each task, and the package will compute appropriate salary rates.

Color is used in the displays, and users can elect to change these colors.

The package produces four reports, all well designed. A Job Description report gives data on job length, finish dates, slack time, criticality, manpower required, and costs. There is a Gantt chart which includes added data on manpower levels and costs. A Project Description report summarizes the job schedule, resource categories, and holidays. And a Tabular Job report prints user-selected data.

VisiSchedule comes with adequate printed instruction and tutorial materials. The user manual reads easily and is convenient as a reference to the package commands and operations.

Chapter 13
Equation-solving Packages

In engineering analysis and design, a great variety of mathematical tools are used. And many computer-based solution techniques are available for dealing with polynomials, vectors and matrices, transforms, differential equations, and other types of mathematical entities that come up in engineering problems.

The ideal equation-solving package would be able to handle any mathematical problem thrown at it. It would allow the user to type the equations to be solved and define the necessary parameters. Then the package would choose an appropriate solution method from among many it had available and attempt a solution. All this would be done in a very simple manner, as far as the user was concerned, yet there would be ample means for users to intervene and control the solution process if it were to go awry.

This ideal package may not yet be perfected, but the available packages discussed in this report provide at least some of these desirable features. In the near future, we can hope, more powerful yet useful packages will become available.

Using computer languages

Familiar computer languages like BASIC and FORTRAN have very flexible mathematical capabilities. However, to use them for equation solving, the engineer has to become at least an amateur BASIC or FORTRAN programmer. Programming a solution means not only defining a solution method (algorithm) but also creating a means to input the needed information and to format and output the results.

What we can call the first generation of equation solvers assumes that users are willing to do more or less conventional programming. What these packages provide are conveniences to speed the programming process. For example, with the Calfex package, the user enters material in BASIC computer language format, using the BASIC mathematical operators and respecting all the rules of the BASIC language. The package offers input screens, output formatting, and some convenient storage and manipulation of parameters and previous work. Taking a somewhat different approach, The Scientific Desk provides a set of mathematical routines written in FORTRAN that can be tied together by programming-wise users; no standard input and output formats are provided.

BASIC and FORTRAN are not ideal tools for doing mathematics. If someone were to start out to design a special computer language for solving math problems, it would have commands and procedures not offered by these standard languages.

This is exactly what the creators of ASYST have done. ASYST is a computer language, in the same sense that BASIC and FORTRAN are computer languages. It was designed with engineering and scientific problem solving in mind. For example it's commands include those for generating a polynomial from a list of numbers, performing polynomial addition, subtraction, multiplication, division, integration, and differentiation. ASYST has capabilities not just in mathematics but also in the areas of graphics and instrumentation. As with any other computer language, regardless of its intrinsic merits, the success or failure of ASYST will rest on the extent to which it is adopted and used by programming-minded engineers and scientists.

A similar approach using a somewhat less powerful mathematical language is provided by the Equate package. With it, the user has to set up the solution method as well as the expressions to be evaluated.

Applications modules

Recognizing that most engineers do not want to be programmers, the vendors of these packages have begun to make preprogrammed applications modules available. For example, The Scientific Desk has an optional linear algebraic systems-solver module called LINGEN that manipulates matrices and vectors. Applications modules that come with the Calfex package include those for location of maxima and minima of functions, numerical integration, and solution of up to 10 simultaneous equations.

Equate comes with a potpourri of preprogrammed procedures, including production of calibration charts for thermistors, calculation of area and moments of inertia for geometric forms, vector operations, and structural column analysis.

Obviously, these available modules cover only a fraction of the math capabilities needed by engineers. The extent to which such packages can achieve wide acceptance among engineers will depend on the variety of the modules they offer.

Specialized equations only

Taking a more modest approach, some vendors provide packages with specialized math capabilities. Thus Optisolve is designed specifically to deal with nonlinear equations. This package relies on one computation method, the steepest descent minimization technique. This avoids the complication of choosing among different techniques but imposes the weaknesses, as well as the strengths, of the chosen solution method. Even when a simple pair of equations with two solutions is to be solved, the package will find only one of these solutions. To find the other, it must be prompted or steered toward the second solution. Optisolve finds the nearest local minimum, which may not be the desired solution. User intervention is called upon to steer the computation toward regions where desired answers lie.

CALCU-PLOT gives the user a choice of specific equations that can be solved. The standard equations happen to be of limited utility to engineers, since they represent only a few classical curves, such as parabolas, circles, trigonometric functions, exponentials, and damped oscillations. Users can also solve and graph single-valued equations of their own choice with this package.

Typical of a number of available small specialized solving packages is DIFFERENTIAL EQUATIONS, which solves only ordinary differential equations. The equations are limited to those that can be expressed using arithmetic operators, EXP, ATAN, SIN, and COS, and the equation solutions must be unique.

User-oriented packages

In the real world of engineering design, problems are often solved by going through supplier catalog information and doing handbook calculations. Equation solving packages like TK!Solver and Varicalc bring the computer into this situation as a practical tool. These packages are not just for making the needed calculations but also for giving the engineer opportunity to rapidly try out alternative parameters and approaches. Using these packages, engineers can try out different design approaches, different components. They can discover problem areas and modify their designs to find better solutions.

TK!Solver is by far the best example of a second-generation equation solver, oriented to meeting the practical needs of engineers. However, its mathematical capabilities are far from complete. TK!Solver can solve systems of linear and nonlinear algebraic equations, and it can deal with a variety of different functions, but the package has only limited ability for matrix algebra and numerical integration and has no capability to do nonnumeric calculus. The strength of TK!Solver lies in its ability to home in on bread-and-butter problem solving that can serve the bulk of engineering practice.

An example of the thoughtful features provided by TK!Solver is the top-of-screen available memory indicator, which keeps the user aware of how much computer main memory is being used by the current problem. TK!Solver error messages are aimed at the user, not at programmers. And there are many convenience features that speed and ease operation.

Many math packages ignore the use of units, leaving that to be solved by hand. Not so with TK!Solver. Users can solve problems with one set of units and display the results in another set of units. Units can be quite freely changed, and they can be readily converted.

Equations, particularly where engineering work is involved, are not simply solved once and forgotten. Very often solutions involving many different values of the variables need to be found. The Varicalc package is uniquely equipped to provide this kind of capability. Varicalc assumes that these values can and will change, and provides for connection of such changing inputs as those from game paddles, joysticks, keyboard arrow keys, and internally programmed "loops." It can even accommodate external process variables if an instrumentation interface is used with the computer. Variables and calculated results will be continuously updated as these inputs vary, until the user orders a stop. In a similar but less flexible way, TK!Solver allows variable values to be input from prepared lists.

Equation solver features

As personal computer packages continue to develop, users will come to expect an increasing number of useful features. The following are some of the features that have begun to emerge in the current crop of equation-solving packages.

Organized display screens. Instead of entering one line at a time, as a BASIC programmer would do, equation-solving packages can make use of screen displays. For example, there are eight different kinds of TK!Solver display screens, used in much the same way as sheets of paper would be in a manual calculation. The equations that define the problem are laid out on a Rule sheet; a Variable sheet contains variable names, values, and units; a Units sheet defines the needed unit conversions.

Most of the other packages use similar approaches. In Calfex, names corresponding to the symbols used for variables are entered on a Labels screen while input data are entered on a screen that displays all the independent variables. Working with this screen, the user can enter values and change them at will. Because many variables may be involved, this screen can be composed of several pages. Such screens can be stored and retrieved as needed.

Users key in the programs they design on an Equate worksheet display, but the worksheets are not limited in size to what the display screen can contain. With the computer's cursor and PgUp, PgDn keys, the display area can be moved around to expose all parts of the worksheet.

But not all equation-solving packages operate from screen displays. With the Optisolve package, input can be keyboarded line by line. Alternatively, prekeyboarded input prepared with the help of the user's own word processing or editing software can be used.

Handling complex numbers. Some packages are not equipped to handle complex numbers, but others, like Optisolve, have been designed with this in mind. Normally all variables in the entered equations are assumed to be real. An Optisolve command converts them all to complex variables so as to obtain complex solutions.

Calculator on the screen. While using an equation-solving package, it can be convenient to have standard hand-calculator functions available. There are separate calculator packages, like TexSolver, that can be kept in the main memory of a computer and brought into play while other software is being used. But several equation solvers have their own built-in calculator capabilities. For example, TK!Solver can operate as a calculator. If the user types an expression that contains only numbers and mathematical operators, the answer will be given as soon as the expression is entered. The Equate worksheet can also operate as a hand calculator. Users enter expressions like 2*2 and get an immediate answer.

Clear error messages. Programmer-oriented packages will display cryptic messages, often undecipherable by engineering users. But as equation-solving packages become more user-oriented, the quality of the messages they present when problems arise changes. For instance, the Equate package gives the user clear and useful error messages like "The first Calc Mark Missing," or "Input must be a valid number." And if these are not understood, the user can press a HELP function key and get further explanation. TK! Solver is another package with very clear and helpful error messages.

Constants from memory. An important computer asset, from the standpoint of user convienience and efficient operation, is the ability to store and recall items from the machine's memory. The Equate package makes particularly adept use of memory for handling constants. This package allows a "pop up" constants window to be called by pressing a function key. The package comes with about 400 physical and conversion constants in this window, and users can add their own as they wish. Other packages, like TK!Solver, have stored constants, along with functions and procedures that can be called into use, from storage, on command.

Worksheet storage and retrieval. The ability to store solution models and procedures for later use is an essential one for a well-designed package. Generally users must give material to be stored a file name. The system software conventions of the computer on which the equation-solving package is run are usually followed. The Equate package has a particularly handy approach to this kind of storage. Equate displays the file names of all existing worksheets, and it automatically creates a backup file when a revised worksheet is stored. Other packages have similar but often less convenient filing facilities.

Graphics. Some of the packages provide graphical display of the computed results. This is particularly useful in the Varicalc package, where input variables, and therefore the output results, can be so readily changed. As the inputs are varied, the display plot will take shape. The graph is automatically rescaled when the curves begin to go off screen. TK!Solver also provides graphical display of the computed functions.

Close to ideal

One package that aspires to the ideal of a universal equation solver is QuickSolver. Among the solution methods it can automatically bring to bear are substitution, Muller's iteration method, Gauss-Jordan for simultaneous linear solutions, the secant method for simultaneous nonlinear solutions, and specific intrinsic techniques such as linear programming. The lineup is potentially powerful, but it is implemented in a package that does not yet appear to have been perfected. For the user who is willing to endure incomplete documentation and somewhat puzzling operation, QuickSolver provides a window to the future of equation-solving packages.

ASYST: A Language For Equation Solving

ASYST is a computer language, in the same sense that BASIC and FOR-TRAN are computer languages. It was designed with engineering and scientific problem solving in mind and has a variety of capabilities, including those in the areas of graphics and instrumentation. Here we will discuss only the equation-solving abilities of this language.

ASYST runs on IBM/PC and compatible computers. To use its equation solving capabilities, two modules are needed. The Systems module ($795), which also includes graphics and statistics, and the Analysis module ($495). The vendor is Macmillan Software Co., 866 Third Ave., New York, NY 10022 [(212) 702-3241].

ASYST is not a package designed to solve equations conveniently. It provides the user with no menus of available functions, nor does it have predesigned formats to organize its use. Instead, like the BASIC language, it simply presents the user with an OK prompt and waits for commands to be keyboarded. As with any other language, these commands must reside primarily in the user's head, which means that the ASYST language must be learned before it can be used.

As with any other computer language, regardless of its intrinsic merits, the success or failure of ASYST will rest on the extent to which it is adopted and used by programming-minded engineers and scientists. If and when these users write programs that can, in turn, be put to use by the vast majority of engineers who have little or no interest in doing programming, then ASYST will indeed become a significant engineering tool.

Polynomial and matrix commands

The power of ASYST to perform equation-solving tasks rests in the specialized commands it makes available. For example, the POLY command generates a polynomial from a list of numbers, and the POLY[X] command evaluates a polynomial. Other commands perform polynomial addition, subtraction, multiplication, division, integration, and differentiation. The command ESTIMATE.ROOTS invokes a QR-algorithm to arrive at estimates, and the REFINE.ROOTS command uses the Laguerre algorithm.

Vectors and matrices are generated by the VECTOR and MATRIX commands from strings of supplied numbers. Among the manipulations that can be produced by related commands are vector dot product, tensor product, matrix product, matrix inversion, and determinant computation. The command SOLVE.SIM.EQS will generate a solution vector for a system of simultaneous equations, using the Gaussian elimination procedures. A number of matrix transformation commands are also available, including TRIDIAG, which transforms self adjoint matrices into tridiagonal form, TRIDIAG.DIAG, which does the tridiagonal to diagonal transformation, and HESSEN, which produces upper Hessenberg matrices. The SPEC-

TRAL.SLICE command computes the number of eigenvalues in a tridiagonal matrix.

CALCU-PLOT

This package has a repertoire of 16 Cartesian and 9 polar coordinate functions which it will tabulate and graph. Single-valued functions entered by users can also be handled.

CALCU-PLOT runs on Apple II, IIe computers. It sells for $150 from Human Systems Dynamics, 9010 Reseda Blvd #222, Northridge, CA 91324.

CALCU-PLOT gives the user a choice of specific equations that can be solved. These represent the classical curves that are part of any descriptive geometry course, including parabolas, circles, trigonometric functions, exponential, damped oscillation. By selecting menu-offered choices, the user can pick the desired equation type, then assign values to the equation constants. The package then asks for the ranges of x and y values that are desired. For the polar-coordinate equations, which include spirals, conics, and other curves, a similar procedure is followed.

With this input, the package produces tabulations of pairs of values for the defined function. And it will display a corresponding graph. If desired, two or three rectangular- coordinate functions can be tabulated and then displayed on the screen together.

Users can also enter formatted descriptions of single-valued equations of their own choice, and the package will handle these. Where second-order polynomials can be broken down into two single-valued functions, the package will solve and graph them as well.

The package is also capable of graphing arbitrary sets of data points that are provided to it. It will plot integrals and derivatives of equations and do log-log and semilog plots.

CALFEX: BASIC PLUS ORGANIZATION

This is a good package for those who practice BASIC programming. It provides a convenient way to organize the input and present the output, plus some convenient built-in features.

Calfex runs on Apple II, IIe, and III computers and on the IBM/PC. It *sells for $175 from Interlaken Technology, 6535 Cecilia Circle, Minneapolis, MN 55435 [(612) 944-2627].*

Like most engineers, the staff at Interlaken Technology were frustrated with having to write a whole new program every time they wanted to find an equation solution using their personal computers. This package is a response to those frustrations.

When inputting equations, the user enters the material in BASIC computer language format, using the BASIC mathematical operators and respecting all the rules of the BASIC language. So, to use this package, one must in the first place be familiar with BASIC.

Names corresponding to the symbols used for variables are entered on a separate Labels screen. As many as 120 independent and 120 dependent variables can be used, and these may be either simple or array variables.

Input data are entered on a screen that displays all the independent variables. Working with this screen, the user can enter values and change them at will. Because many variables may be involved, this screen can be composed of several pages. Such screens can be stored and retrieved as needed. Frequently used constants and BASIC input routines can also be saved and reused.

With input data complete, the package can be commanded, using one keystroke, to calculate. The results will appear on a display of dependent variables. They can also be readily organized into printouts formatted to the needs of the user, including comments, along with the values of the independent and dependent variables.

Trading variables

A special feature of the package is the ability to trade places between any independent variable and a dependent variable. This is convenient in situations where the same design equations are being used to find answers for different design cases. It also offers an easy way to switch and experiment.

The vendor is developing specific applications of the package for mechanical and electrical engineering. A companion package has also been developed to make plotted results available.

EQUATE: GENERAL PURPOSE CALCULATION PACKAGE

Unlike some other equation-solving packages, Equate will not simply go ahead and find a solution to a problem like a set of simultaneous equations.

The user has to set up the the solution method as well as the expressions to be evaluated. The package comes with a few prepared procedures that can be used to solve the particular problems they address. When, and if, the vendor makes a more comprehensive set of such procedures available, Equate could be a very powerful engineering tool.

Equate runs on the IBM/PC and several compatible computers. It sells for $195 from Banyan Systems, 5632 East Third St., Tucson, AZ 85711 [(602) 745-8086].

For those who, like most practicing engineers, do not wish to turn themselves into programmers and mathematicians, the only practical way to use this package is with already prepared methods. The vendor does, in fact, provide some such solution methods in the form of stored worksheets that can be readily called up and used.

A look at an Equate worksheet disk that comes with the package reveals that a scattering of useful solution techniques are provided. However, the worksheets on this disk are all "protected." This means that the user will not see the actual solution method, but only a prescribed procedure into which parameters can be plugged and which will produce whatever answers it is designed to turn out. Thus the solution techniques that have been provided cannot be incorporated easily in procedures users may want to program themselves.

Engineering problem solutions provided by these prepared worksheets include the following:

THERMX, which produces calibration charts for thermistors using three
   known temperatures and resistances. It uses the Steinhart-Hart equation
   recommended in Yellow Spring's literature.
STATS, which calculates average, standard deviation, and variance as data
   are input.
MATRIX, which solves linear equations in 2, 3, or 4 unknowns using Cramer's rule.
MOMENTXY, which calculates the area and moments of inertia for rectangles, triangles, elipses, circles, and concentric circles.
VECTOROP, which performs the vector operations of addition, cross
   product, dot product, and scalar product. It also converts between spherical and Cartesian coordinates and finds the angle between the two vectors.
COMBUCK, which finds properties of a slender compressive column, including critical bucking load, modulus of elasticity, minimum moment
   of inertia, and length of the column.

Making up worksheets

The package itself and the user's manual that comes with it are directed to those who wish to program their own solutions. Equate provides a programming language with 30 commands designed to invoke all the capabilities of the package. Users key in the programs they design on a worksheet display. Once set up, a worksheet can be used and then discarded, or it can be stored for future reuse. Worksheets are not limited in size to what the display screen can contain. Using the computer's cursor and PgUp, PgDn keys, the display area can be moved around to expose all parts of the worksheet.

What is entered on the worksheet can be edited, using convenient keyboard word processing commands. When the material has been examined and corrected, the entire worksheet is entered for use.

The worksheet can operate as a hand calculator. The user can enter calculations, like 2*2, and get an immediate answer. But this calculator use is a rather trivial application of the package.

Mathematical operators and programming commands can be entered in a similar manner. All calculations can be carried out to 24 bits of accuracy (7 digits) if single-precision is used, or to 53 bits (15 digits) with double precision calculations. The user can choose whether to put the package into single or double precision mode. The user also has a choice of the number of digits to be displayed before and after the decimal point. Another user choice is to select either fixed-point or floating-point (digits plus an exponent) style of displaying the computed results.

Along with the mathematics and commands, users can enter notes and memos on the worksheets. These will not interfere with calculations but can be helpful reminders from users to themselves or to assistants.

Mathematical operations are denoted by the usual symbols ($+$, $-$, $/$, $*$, and $\wedge$ for exponention). A variety of other operators, for trigonometric, exponential and other calculations, are provided. There is also a random number operator.

Handy constants

To assist in the proper construction of expressions, a constants window can be called up by pressing a function key. The package comes with about 400 physical and conversion constants in this window, and users can add their own as they wish. With many constants to look through, users may need searching help. Searching is eased by the fact that the constants are listed alphabetically. In addition, users can make a word-matching automatic search of the list. When first called up, the first page of the list is displayed. Users can view other portions of the list by paging up and down as needed. As the up and down arrows on the keyboard are pressed, one item after another on the list is highlighted. To enter a highlighted item into an equation on the worksheet, all the user has to do is press the Enter button.

Long calculations handled

Variables can be represented by alphabetic letters or by words interspersed with numerals, up to 60 characters per variable name. Each expression can be up to 200 characters long. Larger problems can be broken up into several expressions. Strings of expressions can be set up, and the package will use the results of each expression solution in the following expression. Calculations can be strung out at length since a worksheet can carry up to 799 lines of expressions and other information.

When a worksheet has been completed, the user presses a function key and the package does its work. If the worksheet has been prepared according to the rules, the results are calculated and displayed, and they can be printed or stored as well.

Clear error messages

Equate catches errors made in the format and content of the entries on worksheets. It gives the user clear and useful error messages like "The first Calc Mark Missing," or "Input must be a valid number." And if these are not understood, the user can press a HELP function key and get further explanation.

The package allows the user to control the number of lines printed on each page of output, and to print worksheets complete with equations or only the calculated results.

Create and store problems

Storing worksheets is a simple matter, performed with the help of a special Transfer window that can be called up onto the screen. Users must give each worksheet a file name, following the IBM/PC system software convention of limiting file names to eight characters. Using the same approach to files as that of popular word processing packages, Equate will display a directory listing the names of all existing worksheets. If the user gives a current worksheet the same name as one that is already filed, the package assumes that an updating of that file is intended. It changes the name of the old file, adding a .BAK ending to it. If a file by that name with a .BAK ending already exists, it is automatically deleted.

The similarity to word processing file procedures is not accidental. Equate worksheet files can be composed by popular word processing packages in standard (ASCII) format, then converted for use by Equate. The conversion process is a built-in and easy to operate feature of the package. Using a reverse conversion, worksheets can be put into ASCII format for editing by word processors.

Users can customize

Equate is a malleable package that allows the user to shape it to particular needs. It includes the capability to create prompting forms, allowing users to set up calculation procedures that can then be easily followed by assistants. Up to 256 such forms can be created and stored for future use. Custom table formats for output data can also be created, so that results can be easily included in reports. Automatic conversion of units and display of correct units can be incorporated as well.

OPTISOLVE: ONE SOLUTION AT A TIME

This package solves nonlinear systems of equations and finds the maxima and minima of nonlinear functions with or without constraints. It is designed with little regard for the occasional user, and its use requires familiarity with the steepest descent solution techniques the package employs.

Optisolve runs on IBM/PC and compatible computers. Use of the 8087 math chip is recommended. It sells for $195 from Optisoft, 2920 Domingo Ave. #203, Berkeley, CA 94705 [(415) 540-1224].

Equations are keyboarded, one to a line, using the usual mathematical function names and symbols. The only symbols that may seem at all unfamiliar, even to those who have never used a computer, are the * for multiplication and the ∧ for exponention. Variables are entered as alphabetic letters or names, constants as numbers. For lengthy constants a name can be defined (for example, PI = 3.141592653) and used as an abbreviation in the equations.

Along with the equations to be solved, the user enters some initialization information. Here, approximate solutions are indicated by assigning initial values to the variables.

The package is not interactive. Input can be entered from the keyboard or from prekeyboarded files prepared with the help of the user's own word processing or editing software. In any case, the input must be formatted to a set of rules prescribed by the manual.

Only one solution at a time

Optisolve produces only one solution at a time, and the solution it gives may not be a correct one.

The basic calculation technique used in Optisolve is the steepest descent minimization method. This finds the nearest local minimum, which may not be the desired solution. Most of the user intervention in the operation of this package is concerned with steering the computation away from regions where the solution diverges, or where undesired local minima exist, and toward regions where desired answers lie.

Even when a simple pair of equations with two solutions are to be solved, the package will find only one of these solutions. To find the other, it must be prompted or steered toward the second solution.

The basic Optisolve solution commands are MIN, MAX, and SOLVE. In addition, there is an ALSO command for adding constraints and a START command, which allows the user to rerun a calculation with revised initialization of the variables.

Solution times can be long

Perhaps the major limitation on the use of Optisolve is computation time. With sufficient prodding from the user, this package can find good answers, but that may take a very long time for some problems. For this reason, the vendor suggests using the 8087 math chip, which can speed up numerical solutions by a factor of about 30.

If a solution seems to be running forever, the user can hit the Esc key. Optisolve will then halt and give the best solution approximation it has to that point. The search for a better solution can then be continued by giving the CONT command. Where several distinct solutions are expected, the OTHER command can be used after each solution to find the next. There is also a GLOBAL command that initiates global search strategy

Normally, all variables in the entered equations are assumed to be real. The COMPLEX command converts them all to complex variables so as to obtain complex solutions.

In addition to the requested answers, Optisolve also provides the user with a "performance index" that indicates the extent to which the solution satisfies the input equations. However, even a perfect index of 100 does not mean that the answers given are necessarily adequate. For example, asked to find values of x between 2 and 3, Optisolve might return any value in that interval and give itself a performance index of 100.

The manual is poorly designed, with little regard for the convenience of the user. Operating instructions are intermixed with solution examples, and there is no separate, one-by-one detailed explanation of the use of the various commands. Under "Syntax Notes," buried in the middle of the manual, the user is given the needed formatting rules for entering information.

QUICKSOLVER: FOR A VARIETY OF PROBLEMS

Reviewed by Dr. Darrel G. Linton, University of Central Florida

---

QuickSolver has the potential to solve a large class of engineering-oriented problems using standard algebraic notation. Included are systems of linear or nonlinear equations; linear programming problems; multiple linear regression problems; and matrix algebra calculations.

However, incomplete documentation and program development appear to detract from its usefulness. This reviewer found that the package failed to solve a simple problem, and an example recorded on the package disk did not work. These experiences caused some loss of confidence in the package. Using a rating scale of 0 (low) to 100 (high), this reviewer's ratings of QuickSolver are: ease of use, 90; correct documentation, 70; freedom from error, 50; overall rating, 70.

QuickSolver runs on IBM/PC and compatible computers. Use of the 8087 math chip is optional. The package was designed by Conversational Computer Systems, 224 Summer St., Buffalo, NY 14222 [(716) 886-0424]. It sells for $125 from Technical Software, 3981 Lancaster Rd., Cleveland, OH 44121 [(216) 486-8535].

Virtually no knowledge of computers or of special computer languages is needed to use this package. For the novice, some practice in saving disk files and using the full-screen editing features will be needed. Since the original QuickSolver disk is copy-protected, the user cannot make backup copies to protect against damage or loss of the original.

Users enter information in an algebra-like format, one equation to a line. Special symbols are used to represent Greek letters, the constants pi and e, and the summation symbol. Keywords and other symbols are used to denote such items as maxima and minima of objective functions, and the EST for the lefthand side of multiple linear regression model equations.

Almost any problem involving mathematical equations can be solved by this package, provided only that the equations must conform to the QuickSolver format. For these problems, QuickSolver has the potential for not only solving them but also producing plotted output, saving the problem in disk storage, and allowing the problem to be edited and changed.

Included on the QuickSolver disk is a file containing supplementary documentation for using the package. This is an excellent idea for illustrating increased capability and correcting any faults in the printed documentation. However, it also carries the implication that QuickSolver is not yet a finished product and may have bugs as well as incomplete documentation. This reviewer observes that either or both of these implied characteristics may be inherent in the package.

Incomplete solutions

When two simple simultaneous algebraic equations (one containing a square root function) were entered, the package failed to obtain the solution for x. Instead, it produced a peculiar error message: 036 SINGULAR MATRIX. The message meant nothing to this reviewer since the package provides no documentation on error messages. The failure of QuickSolver to obtain a complete solution implies the possibility of an error in Quick-Solver's algorithm for solving simultaneous equations.

Another simultaneous equation test problem produced the message "Diverged," followed by a display of answers that were correct to just two significant figures. The package apparently allows the user no way to specify convergence criteria.

Missing features and peculiarities

The linear programming features of this package do not conform to standard notation. Only strict inequalities are allowed. Attempts to use greater(less)-than-or-equal-to notation resulted in error messages.

The documentation promised that a feature called ALL SLACK? could be used. Yet when this feature was tried with one of the example problems (QS.MAX) on the package disk, the response was another error message: 010 INVALID EQUATION.

The documentation implies (page 32) that there is no need to use any multiplication symbol between two (TABLE) variables when the summation operation is used. In fact, this reviewer found that the summation function would not work unless such symbols were inserted.

When the multiple linear regression capabilities were tested, this reviewer found it necessary to list the Y TABLE array last, after the independent variables, in order to get a correct result. There was no indication in the documentation that this order of things was necessary, but when it was not observed, the error message 129 MORE EQUATIONS OR VALUES ARE NEEDED appeared and the value of beta-sub-zero was unknown.

Comment by Keith Beech, Conversational Computer Systems

Our acceptance of the reviewer's criticisms of the documentation for QuickSolver is reflected in extensions we have made to our supplementary documentation, based on his review. These extensions are included on disks being shipped from today onwards and illustrate the value of the thorough and informed reviews which appear in Engineering Microsoftware Review.

However, we feel that we should draw specific attention to a new section on nonlinear systems which has been added to amplify the original information in the manual. We feel that if this had been available to the reviewer, he may not have felt a loss of confidence in the package's freedom from error and would not have felt compelled to give such a low rating on that score. The "simple" equations mentioned in the review ($2X + 4Y = 12$; $X = $ SQRT Y) are nonlinear and were solved correctly according to the revised documentation. In addition, we feel the remarks about "answers correct to two decimals" are open to misinterpretation by those unfamiliar with numerical analysis and the meaning of divergence.

We would like to stress that we are not disputing the reviewer's conclusions based on the information made available to him, and that we accept that our incomplete documentation was the principal cause of the problems encountered.

THE SCIENTIFIC DESK: LOTS OF TOOLS FOR PROGRAMMING-WISE USERS

The Scientific Desk provides a set of mathematical routines that can be tied together by programming-wise users to solve a wide variety of engineering problems. For those who do not wish to program, there are some special-

ized problem-solving modules. The package does not seem oriented toward ease of use or learning.

This package runs on IBM/PC and compatible computers. It sells for $420; problem-solving modules are extra, $110 each except the Very Small Linear Algebra Algorithms module, which sells for $50. The package requires the use of FORTRAN and comes in four versions corresponding to four popular FORTRAN compilers that are available for the IBM/PC. The vendor is C. Abaci, 208 St. Mary's St., Raleigh, NC 27605 [(919) 832-4847].

The Scientific Desk is essentially a collection of mathematical routines in areas useful to engineers, including linear algebra, optimization, nonlinear equations, and integral transforms, simulation, statistics, and probability. The most flexible way to use these routines is to incorporate them into programs written by the user. However, recognizing that most users will not want to do programming, the vendor has begun to make prepared applications modules available.

Matrix, array solver

LINGEN is an example of such a module. It is a linear algebraic systems solver that allows manipulation of and operations upon matrices and vectors. LINGEN retains up to 10 different arrays, keeping statistics on whether each array is a matrix or vector, on its dimensions, where it starts in the workspace, its length, and the remaining available space.

Factoring, solving, estimating matrix condition (and the number of correct significant digits in results), and inversion are allowed. In addition, vector and matrix arithmetic operations are provided for rectangular arrays.

Commands available to LINGEN users include those for performing array addition, subtraction, multiplication, and finding cross and dot products. A BUILD command constructs special arrays of uniform pseudo-random numbers, zeros, ones, or identity matrices, based on user prompts. Arrays can also be entered via the keyboard. Matrices can be manipulated in various ways. They can, for instance, be deleted, corrected, factored, inverted, and replicated. The matrix problem $Ax = B$ can be solved.

Other user-ready applications modules include one for Eigensystem analysis which can find the roots of polynomials and estimate eigenvalues and eigenvectors. A Statistics module takes normal or pseudo-random samples and determines the basic statistics of the sample data. An approximation and quadrature module is designed to eliminate anomalies from curve data. Another module is for evaluating definite integrals in one variable. There is also a "Very Small" linear algebra package designed to take up little storage space.

An incomplete product

To a limited extent, this package and its modules are designed with user needs in mind. The commands for the solution modules are presented in menu form to make them more readily available to the occasional user. Included are commands for printing the results. However, the user is assumed to be one who is willing to do a considerable amount of programming and experimentation with the tools provided by the package.

The documentation is whimsical, consisting of a melange of instruction, explanation, and listings of commands and other information. Apparently no one has taken the trouble to spell it all out in a form that would minimize the time taken by a novice user to understand what is available, and just how to go about solving problems. Nor is there any clear way for more experienced users to quickly find reference to command details and other needed information. Although the mathematical routines seem to have been carefully and knowledgeably constructed, the package does not fulfill what should be expected from a professionally crafted computer applications product for use by engineers.

In the basic mathematical routines of The Scientific Desk, there appears to be the potential for constructing a very useful package for solving a wide variety of engineering problems. The extent to which this potential will be fulfilled depends on how well the vendor designs and packages future problem-solving modules.

TEXSOLVER-10: HANDY CALCULATOR PACKAGE

TexSolver can be kept in the main memory of a computer and brought into play while other software is being used. Press the Alt and Ctrl keys together and a calculator screen appears. Press the Esc key and it goes away. TexSolver provides all the expected scientific calculator capabilities, with 100 storage registers and simple statistics as well.

This package runs on IBM/PCs. It sells for $44.95 from Microtex, P.O. Box 111054, Carrollton, TX 75011 [(214) 980-9837].

TexSolver can either be run from the disk or stored in the computer main memory and called up at any time by pressing the Alt and Ctrl keys simultaneously.

The screen display shows all the calculator functions performed by the package, which are those offered by a competent scientific hand calculator. Operation is not self-evident, however, and the user must study the little manual to get the idea of how to enter the numbers and math functions properly in sequence.

The screen-displayed calculator also provides 100 data registers which can be accessed as needed, and arithmetic can be performed on the contents of any storage register.

A statistical capability calculates and stores statistics of paired sets of x,y data, depositing such items as summations of squares and products in specific storage locations, where they can be examined as needed. The mean and standard deviation of the data can then be calculated at will. And a linear regression calculation will find the slope and intercept of the best fit line. A linear estimate and correlation coefficient can also be conveniently calculated.

A peculiar effect

A strange effect of this package is that while it resides in the computer main memory, the cursor used with a popular word processing package seems to be raised about a half line. This is disconcerting, but no other adverse effects were noted.

TK!SOLVER: IMPRESSIVE PROBLEM-SOLVING CAPABILITY

This package is well suited to meeting most of the practical equation-solving problems faced in everyday engineering work. User needs are kept in the forefront in the documentation and in the functional features of this package. Units are handled in as organized a manner as are the numerical parts of problem solutions.

TK!Solver is available in versions to run on most personal and microcomputers. It sells for $400 from Software Arts, 27 Mica Lane, Wellesley, MA 02181 [(617) 237-4000].

The authors of this package have given some thought to the way engineers typically solve problems involving equations and have designed procedures that are computer-based equivalents of familiar manual methods.

There are eight different kinds of TK!Solver display sheets, used in much the same way as sheets of paper would be in a manual calculation. For example, the equations that define the problem are laid out on a Rule sheet; a Variable sheet contains variable names, values, and units; a Units sheet defines the needed unit conversions.

At the user's convenience, two of these sheets, or just one, can be displayed at a time. Users type information onto these sheets, correct errors, and can store the sheets for further use. Each set of sheets is stored as a set in one file. The file names used are in the form prescribed by the operating system software of the computer on which the package is run, so users name the files in the same way as they would name files for word processors and other packages used with their computer.

Three ways to solve problems

At its simplest, TK!Solver can operate as a calculator. If the user types an expression that contains only numbers and mathematical operators, the answer will be given as soon as the expression is entered.

Two methods of equation solution are available. With the Direct method, the user must supply values for all variables except one, in one or more equations. That one unknown variable must appear once and only once in any equation. Additional equations can be solved, even if they contain more than one unknown variable, provided that the number of unknown variables can be reduced to one by solving other given equations.

To deal with the many engineering problems that require, or can best be handled with, iterative solutions, TK!Solver also has an iterative-solution mode. The user starts with an initial guess and the package will then try successive values until it converges on a solution.

The Iterative solution method is able to handle sets of linear or nonlinear simultaneous equations in which none of the variables are initially known. This solution method can also solve equations in which unknown variables appear more than once. The price of a poor guess for an initial value is likely to be slow convergence of the calculation, and this may mean an excessively long computation time for the solution. If the answer is not a real number, the Iterative-solution method will fail.

It helps if the user can do some algebra. Factoring equations before they are solved can often speed the solution. Manipulating the form of the equations, and possibly adding an extra one, can allow the Direct method to be used instead of the possibly slower and less dependable Iterative one.

Using a List sheet, the user can lay out a whole series of variable values for which a set of equations are to be solved. Portions of lists, as well as entire lists, can be processed. The answers can be displayed in tables or as plotted points on a graph.

Thoughtful features

Among the thoughtful features provided by TK!Solver is an indicator of cursor location at the top of each sheet; it is sometimes not easy to spot a cursor amidst a lot of text. More important is the available memory indicator, which keeps the user aware of how much computer main memory is being used by the current set of problem sheets. This is essential. Should available memory be inadvertently exhausted, it could take up to an hour of computer time to get the sheets stored.

Procedures are aimed at saving time for the user, and program features like error messages are aimed at the user, not at programmers. For example, for each variable in the equations typed on the Rule sheet, TK!Solver will automatically put a variable name on the Variable sheet. If the user enters values for all variables in an equation save one, the package will find the remaining value and show it on the Variable sheet. However, if too few values have been assigned, the user will be notified that the problem is underdefined. If the values assigned are inconsistent with the equations, the package will notify the user of this fact. If input values are in conflict, the package will give an "Overdefined," message.

Many engineering packages ignore the use of units, leaving that to be solved by hand. Not so with TK!Solver. Users can solve problems with one set of units, and display the results in another set of units. Units can be quite freely changed, and they can be converted, using the Unit sheet on which the user types unit names, conversion multipliers, and offset additions.

The manual is detailed and has an index for quick reference to needed information. On-screen Help messages are also provided.

Keyboard commands

The ! in the name of this package refers to the fact that the user can initiate solution of an equation or model by entering the ! symbol. To conveniently manipulate information, users have to learn some other TK!Solver commands as well. For example, by typing a colon (:) users can command the cursor to go to specific locations on a sheet. To locate a specific item on a sheet, a (") is typed, followed by the characters in the item. The package will then find those characters and move the cursor there. Items can be copied, replicated, as desired using the (/C) command.

For math operators TK!Solver uses the usual computer symbols $(+, -, *, /, \wedge)$. In addition to these operators, TK!Solver has many of the familiar scientific calculator functions built in. In addition, it has a number of other useful built-in functions, including maximum, minimum, sum, and number of elements in a list of values. The min and max functions can be used to hold solution values within defined boundaries. Dot products of the entries in two lists can also be produced. A polynomial function allows coefficients to be defined by a list for convenient evaluation.

Like mathematical functions, stored constants and procedures come with the package and can be called into use on command. And users can define their own functions, constants, and procedures using the package's User Function sheet.

Custom solutions

TK!Solver is so flexible a tool that its commands can be used to create custom solutions to engineering problems. The vendor has already addressed two areas of engineering work with special preprogrammed solution methods. A package is available to solve some mechanical engineering problems, using TK!Solver, and another similar package addresses a group of building design problems. An extensive series of TK!Solver-based solution packages, under development, will cover many aspects of engineering design.

VARICALC: FORMULA-SOLVING WITH VARIABLE INPUTS

This package is set up to do iterative solutions of formulas with variable values incrementally changed. It includes a graphical display of computed values that changes as the variables are changed, and it can take changing variable values from related formulas.

VARICALC Runs on Apple II computers. It sells for $100 from Interactive Microware, P.O. Box 139, State College, PA 16804 [(814) 238-8294].

The mathematical capabilities of this package are limited. Its basic function is to solve a formula with one independent variable, but it can also handle up to 18 dependent variables.

Users key the formulas they wish to solve onto the screen, using the usual notation for mathematical operators. Beyond $+$, $-$, $*$, $/$, and $\wedge$ operators, the formulas may also contain Ln, Exp, Cos, Sin, Tan, Arc Tan, Arc Cos, and Arc Sin. There are some rather awkward restrictions on the way the formulas have to be written, but the rules seem to be of the sort that, once learned, will be easily remembered.

When a formula is entered on the screen, it can be solved for any variable, provided values are assigned to all the others. The unique feature of this package is in the way variable values are assigned. The package assumes that these values can and will change, and provides for connection of such changing inputs as those from game paddles, joysticks, keyboard arrow keys, and internally programmed "loops." It can even accommodate external process variables if an instrumentation interface is used with the computer. The calculated result will be continuously updated as these inputs vary, until the user orders a stop.

Built-in graphics

The package also provides graphical display of changes in the variables, with the calculated variable plotted along the y-axis. The graphics display can be viewed alternatively with the VARICALC formula display. As the inputs are varied, the display plot will take shape. The graph is automatically rescaled when the curves begin to go off screen. Using the graphic display, along with the formula calculation process, the approximate minimum and maximum values of calculations can be obtained.

Once entered, formulas can be saved for future use. Up to 255 formulas can be stored on a floppy disk. In fact, the package comes with a number of frequently used engineering formulas already recorded on the disk. These formulas can be used or erased at will. Each formula is limited to two lines on the screen (79 characters). The user can enter a formula from the disk, edit and change it as needed from the keyboard, then get the solution right on the same screen display.

Injections from related formulas

The package can handle related formulas, along with the main formula that is being evaluated. When the related formulas contain some of the same variables as the main formula, the package will recognize this automatically and plug the appropriate values into all formulas.

A relatively powerful feature of the package is that values of a dependent variable in the main formula can be calculated from a related formula, then automatically "injected" into the main formula when the independent variable is calculated. This allows calculations to be chained. The example given in the package manual is calculation of the changes in mass of a rocket (as fuel is burned) by a related formula, with new values of mass injected into the main formula for the calculation of rocket thrust.

The package suffers from the limitation that it cannot deal with null quantities (zero amounts). And some fiddling with values and change intervals is sometimes required when negative values are to be handled. Outside of these anomalies, the operation seems quite straightforward.

Chapter 14
Linear Programming Packages

Linear programming has come into wider use as personal computers have become available to an increasing number of engineers. It is essentially a decision-aiding tool for use in situations where the choices are complex.

The problems it solves are often concerned with allocating available resources, such as raw materials, partly finished products, labor, capital, or time. The solution can describe how to make the allocation so that some measure of benefit, like profit or efficiency, can be optimized.

With the computation speed offered by a personal computer it is feasible to use linear programming to solve a number of problems that formerly were tackled with more approximate methods. For example, the technique is frequently used to find the most profitable mix of products to run through a production line.

Other optimization problems commonly solved with the help of linear programming include best allocation of production at several centers, so that costs of transporting raw materials and finished goods will be minimized; setting up travel routes to make preassigned stops so that total distance traveled will be minimized; specifying optimum mixtures of materials from available stocks; selecting best alternatives from cutting and trimming schedules; and even setting up investment strategies.

Linear programming concepts

To use this technique, the first task the user faces is to formulate the problem so it can be meaningfully solved by the computer. Not every decision situation can be handled by this technique, but many can.

When applying linear programming, the decision situation has to be stated so that there is an overall goal or objective that the user wants to maximize or minimize. This will be expressed in terms of a mathematical relationship, a linear equation in which desired result is set equal to a function consisting of "decision" variables, each with its own coefficient. This "objective" function may represent a cost, or any other result that is to be optimized.

Linear programming also provides for expressing the limitations or constraints under which the optimum result is to be obtained. These constraints are expressed as linear equations or inequalities in which the decision variables appear on the left with constraint coefficients, and a constant appears on the righthand side (RHS).

There are a few additional linear programming concepts, referred to in this chapter, with which the reader should be familiar.

Linear programming solutions that satisfy all the constraints are called "feasible" solutions.

Whenever a less-than-or-equal-to constraint is used, there can be slack. That is, the righthand side of the constraint can be decreased without having any effect on the solution. In a similar manner, a greater-than-or-equal-to constraint can have a surplus.

The computation method used in almost all of the packages discussed in this chapter is called the Simplex method. One requirement for its use is that inequalities be converted into equations. For this purpose, an extra or "slack" variable is added to each inequality constraint relationship, allowing it to be treated as an equation.

The shadow price of a constraint is the amount by which the objective function will change if the righthand side of the constraint is increased by 1. A large shadow price is a danger signal, warning the user that a constraint is drastically affecting the solution.

Some problems have two or more optimal solutions, called alternate solutions. The packages usually signal this situation with an alternate solutions message, alerting the user to look for additional solutions.

The job of the linear programming package is to allow users to conveniently set up the necessary equations and inequalities, to solve them as quickly as possible, and to provide a simple way to change and rerun the solutions.

Available packages

Although all linear programming packages perform virtually the same task and use the same basic mathematical method, they offer quite different features.

One major difference is the size of the problems each package will handle. Linear programming problems can become quite complex, involving many variables and constraints. Many of the packages are able to handle only smaller problems. Thus the MPS-PC package handles 70 variables and 50 constraints. Others can find solutions to considerably larger problems.

For example, the LPX88 package can handle 2510 variables and 510 constraints.

Package prices are not, however, directly related to the size of problem they can handle. The MPS-PC package, which handles 70 variables and 50 constraints, sells for $150. Eastern Software, vendor of the LPX88, sells that package for $88 and charges the very same price for each of its other packages. These include LP88 which solves problems with up to 255 constraints and 2255 variables, BLP88 which solves problems with upper or lower bounded variables, handling 255 constraints and 1255 variables, DLP88 for dual linear problems with up to 1255 constraints, and SLP88/STSA88 which solves 45 constraints and 255 variables.

In fact, taking a variety of package characteristics into account, it is fair to say that at present, prices and capabilities of these packages are not necessarily related.

The only package discussed here that does not use some version of the Simplex algorithm to produce solutions is the Dynacomp Linear Programmer. This package solves simultaneous inequalities rather than the usual linear programming problem.

Data entry can be arduous

Once the linear programming problem is set up, the next task the user faces is to input enough data to the computer so that a solution can be attempted. For problems with more than a few variables and constraints, input tasks can be formidable and users need all the help they can get to make this part of the procedure as painless and accurate as possible.

From the user's standpoint, an ideal way to enter data would be to view a display of an objective function and a set of constraints, then move a cursor through this display, entering coefficients and other values as they were reached. However, none of the packages discussed here uses this particular method.

One that comes close is LP88, where entry is done on a row-column spreadsheet format. A labeled, largely empty spreadsheet is displayed. Using row-column locations to position the cursor on this display, the user can enter desired coefficients and other values into the spreadsheet cells. The cursor can also be moved about by the arrow keys. This display can show 15 constraints and 10 variables at a time, but users can move the display to any desired area of the overall spreadsheet.

Most of the other packages cannot be given high marks on their ability to provide user-oriented data entry. The LP1 package tries, by having the user assign a unique name to each variable. The package then displays these names , one by one, and prompts the user to enter objective function coefficient values for each.

MPS-PC, data entry is on a column-by-column basis. This means that users will not be able to keep track of what they are doing merely by knowing what equations and inequalities they wish to enter. Instead, they have to make a careful handwritten layout of the entry data with all columns neatly and correctly lined up.

The Ramlp package tackles the input problem by offering users choices. They can enter or erase a single coefficient by first specifying its row and column location. Alternatively, they can enter an entire row, or column, or diagonal of data.

With the LP80 package, constraint coefficients are entered, one to a line, each accompanied by the keyboarded name of the constraint and variable to which it belongs. By the time this information has been repeated for each coefficient, a lot of typing has to be done.

LP83 makes little use of the interactive capabilities of personal computers, requiring the user to come to the package with a complete set of input data, ready to be run. This allows the package to conform readily to input procedures traditionally used with large computers, where data and instructions are frequently punched into cards, then fed to the equipment. LP83 will, in fact, accept input in the standard MPS format, used for linear programming based on large computers.

Even if they fail to take full advantage of the personal computer's ability to make things easier for the user, some of the packages do offer useful input aids. The Computer Heroes Linear Programming System package has a special sparse entry command for the situation where constraints to be entered have only a few nonzero coefficients. This command allows the user to skip around to those few positions in the constraint array where coefficients have to be entered.

LP1 has a similar method for rapid entry of scattered nonzero coefficients, and it also has a helpful data verification feature. At the completion of the objective function data, and as each set of constraint data is completed, the package prompts the user to verify that the entered data are acceptable. If not, the user can go through the appropriate set of prompts once again, skipping by those items that are OK and stopping to change any incorrect items.

Most of the packages provide editing procedures for data and allow users to store data for later use. However, some of the simpler packages lack these features. For example, neither the Computer Heroes Linear Programming System nor the Dynacomp Linear Programmer have any provision for storing data.

File entry

An alternative to keyboard data entry is to create a data file using other software, outside the package, then read the file when the package is run. About half of the packages discussed in this chapter have this capability. In most cases the formats for such files are compact and formal.

The LP88 has this outside file capability. To the probable delight of users who are large-computer programmers, this package can be run in a batch mode. To do this, a properly formatted command file, containing instructions on how the computation is to proceed, must be entered, along with a data file.

Calculation speed

Linear programming problems that involve many variables can take a while to run. The calculation time will depend not only on the number of variables and constraints, but on the computational techniques used by the various packages, and also on the equipment used to process them.

When the problems are very tiny, the run times will typically be only a few seconds, but even quite small problems can run for minutes. For example, reviewers of the LP88 package checked the run time with a 13-variable, 48-constraint problem. LP88 produced an optimized solution in 2 minutes, 15 seconds, while LPX88, which uses a revised simplex algorithm, produced an optimized solution in 54 seconds. With MPS-PC, a problem with 63 columns and 47 rows is said to have taken 68 iterations and 15 minutes to reach a solution.

Run times can be greatly reduced when packages allow the use of a math coprocessor chip. This kind of chip seems to cut the run time for most problems by about a factor of 10. Type of personal computer also had an influence. The LP83 vendor found that, using an IBM/XT with math chip, a problem with 16 rows and 33 columns ran in 6 seconds, while another with 177 rows and 548 columns ran in 41 minutes, 33 seconds. These times were decreased to 3 seconds, and to 29.5 minutes, when the same problems were run on an IBM/PC/AT with math chip.

Users of large computers are fond of pointing out that these machines run much faster than personal computers. However, a more significant measure is often how long it takes from the moment inputting of the problem starts to the moment the user gets results. Elapsed times to get answers from the IBM/PC/AT and an IBM 3081 mainframe computer were compared by the LP83 vendor. For all but the very largest problems, the ready access the user had to the PC provided the answers more rapidly, although the large machine had an advantage of almost 10 to 1 in raw computational speed.

Control over calculations

Users who are interested in how computer calculations proceed can get added satisfaction from several of these linear programming packages, since they display ongoing partial computation data. Some also give users control over the computation process.

For example, the Ramlp package displays a log of partial computation results as iterations are made towards a feasible solution. These displays indicate the number of constraints satisfied at each iteration, along with a current number of "infeasibilities" (which gives the user some idea of how close a solution may be). If the solution process should fail, this record can then be used in deciding on possible fixes.

With LP88, users can control a number of computation parameters. They can set a limit on the number of iterations (pivots) that will be performed. They can also select the number of iterations performed before the inverse is recomputed and the tolerance values below which pivot elements, inverse elements, and basis variables will be rejected.

During its calculations this package shows a display that gives current information on the state of the solution. Solutions can be interrupted while in progress, allowing users to step through the pivots, reinvert, reset tolerances and controls, save the basis, and record the current solution and pivots.

Output options

Some of the packages provide only limited output information, but others give it in considerable detail. For example, the results for the MINI-MAX package include displays of the optimal solution and of basic and nonbasic variables. (The nonbasic variables are those whose coefficient values are insignificant for a particular solution.) And the output includes an "entering value" to show at what point each coefficient value would have made that particular variable basic. A separate display shows the current values of the basic variables along with high- and low-range values, to show how much variation there can be before these become nonbasic. This output also displays slack variables, dual variables with shadow prices, and the ranges of feasibilty for the variables.

The added data are important, because getting a single optimum answer to a linear programming problem is often insufficient for practical decision making. One most important consideration is: supposing the input values do not accurately represent the actual situation, that is, what then happens if those values are changed? The answer is given by a sensitivity analysis in which inputs are varied and different results calculated. Shadow prices, slack variables, and ranges of feasibility provide measures to guide this type of analysis.

A drawback of the MINI-MAX type of output is that the user has no control over the extent of the output information. In contrast, the LP88 package organizes its output into six tables. All or any of these can be called for by the user, printed, and stored in disk files.

Roundoff and other errors

It would be nice if a user could simply run these packages and be always confident of getting a correct and useable answer. Unfortunately, there are many reasons why linear programming computations can fail to produce the desired results. Most often, such failures are due to mistakes the user makes in setting up the problem. But there are also computational errors that can occur even when the input information is logically correct.

Roundoff errors, for example, can accumulate over the numerous arithmetic computations in linear programming computations. Recognizing this situation, package designers have come up with various ameliorative approaches.

To help in identifying such problems, MINI-MAX displays a maximum error figure as part of the solution. To try to reduce this figure, users can experiment with changing or eliminating constraints. Or they can adjust the rounding of data by the package. This can be set at anywhere from 6 to 12 places after the decimal point. However, users are advised that the results of such adjustments are unpredictable.

To handle roundoff errors, LP/80 sets values less than an "epsilon" value of 0.0001, to zero. However, this does not satisfy all situations, and the package may incorrectly identify some problems as infeasible. To check whether rounding is the culprit, users can adjust the value of epsilon and try to get a better answer.

Inadequate user's manuals

Linear programming packages are generally poorly documented. Most of the manuals do not have such reference essentials as a section with detailed explanations of all command functions and menu choices, another section with explanations of all error messages, and a decent index to quickly find needed items.

In many cases, the manuals are skimpy and try to explain how to use the package only by example, without ever spelling out the options that are available to the user.

An exception is the manual for the LP83 package, which carefully explains each of the error and warning messages the user may see. The manual itself is also well organized, spelling out the information users need to know, and it has an index for reference once the package is in use.

LINEAR PROGRAMMING SYSTEM

This package is for smallish problems, with up to 50 variables, including slack and artificial variables, and 35 constraints. There is no provision for storing data once a problem has been run, and all input is from the keyboard. The package seems simple to use and, within its limitations, a terrific bargain. It has not been reviewed here for software defects.

Linear Programming System runs on Commodore 64 computers. It sells for $9.99 on tape or $12.99 on disk from Computer Heroes, P.O. Box 79, Farmington, CT 06032.

The menu screen for this package shows abbreviated names of the 14 commands that can be used. These commands initiate sequences of screen-displayed queries to which the user responds, or, like the SOLVE command, they initiate actions.

Using these commands, which are explained in the manual, the user specifies the number of decision variables, calls either for maximization or minimization of the objective function, then enters the coefficients for each term in the objective function.

Constraint relationships may be set up as equalities, or as < or > inequalities. The CON command invokes a sequence of queries that ask for entry of constraint coefficients and totals in an organized manner. What the user has to keep in mind while entering these data is the form and notation the manual shows for the objective function and constraint relationships.

When constraints have only a few nonzero coefficients, a CONSP (sparce) entry command allows the user to skip around to those few positions in the constraint array where coefficients have to be entered. The procedure seems quite simple, as long as the user is able to identify the row and column location of items in the array of constraint relationships.

Display commands allow users to view all the data that have been entered, or only selected types of data such as individual columns and rows.

A CH (change) command allows users to alter items that have been previously entered, including type ($= < >$) of constraint and type (max, min) of problem. The user can also specify "Big M," the number used to restrict the size of "artificial" variables. If not specified, M will be set to 5000. Users are warned that if M is set too high, roundoff error will be introduced.

When data entry is complete, the SOLVE command sends the package in search of a solution. If and when an optimal and feasible solution is found, a message will tell the user how many iterations have been made to reach it. Warning messages appear if there are any all-zero rows or columns, if no feasible solution is found, or if the system of relationships is unbounded. When there is a possibility of multiple solutions, the user is given the option of choosing to continue with further iterations.

The package offers displays of initial and final computed values. These are presented as short lists corresponding to the rows and columns of the array-of-constraint and objective-function relationships. The interpretation of these results is laborious the first time but much simpler thereafter.

LINEAR PROGRAMMING SYSTEM

This package has some inconveniences, but it does the essential linear programming job, and look at the bargain price. The vendor does not indicate how many variables and constraints can be handled. An example with just eight variables is given in the manual.

This package runs on Apple II+ computers. It sells for $29.95 from Microphase, P.O. Box 10461, Tallahassee, FL 32302 [(904) 877-7794].

The main menu for this package gives the user the choice to create a new data file, delete an existing file, or EDIT/PRINT/SOLVE an existing file.

New files are created from the keyboard. The package prompts for each item of data. The user specifies the number of variables (including slack variables) to be used, the number of constraints, and whether the solution is to be maximized or minimized. The package then prompts for the coefficients of the objective function, and for each constraint relationship.

Work for the user

Users have to come to this package with a clear picture in mind of the exact form of the objective-function and constraint relationships they wish to use. The prompts will call for a coefficient for every variable, including all the slack variables for every constraint and for the objective function. Any variable that should not appear has to be given a zero coefficient, so the procedure is methodical.

When this entry is complete, the user must still inform the package which (slack) variable in each constraint relationship is to be used as the "basic" variable in the computation.

At this point the package has enough information to make up a complete data file, and the user is given the option of storing the data.

Zero means trouble

To generate a solution, the user selects the EDIT/PRINT/SOLVE menu option and keys an S. The package asks for a data file name to run and, if it finds that file, goes on to a solution, displaying a list of the variables and their computed values, along with a "z" value for the objective function.

If $z = 0$, something has gone wrong. Even if z is not zero, the user manual advises that "curious results" indicate that there is some difficulty, probably with the way the problem has been set up.

In such cases, the user will want to make changes in the data and can resort to the edit command, E, to do so. The appropriate file is then called for by name, and the first display will show the number of variables, constraints, and problem type. Unfortunately, nothing on this frustrating display can be changed, except by creating an entirely new file. What can be altered are the values of coefficients, constraint righthand-side values, and "basic" variable designations.

LINEAR PROGRAMMER

This little package does not solve the conventional linear programming problem, but it does deal with simultaneous inequalities, and it is inexpensive.

LINEAR PROGRAMMER runs on IBM/PC, Apple II, TRS-80, and most other personal computers. It sells for $33.95 from DYNACOMP, 1064 Gravel Rd., Webster, NY 14580 [(800) 828-6772, (800) 828-6773].

This package does not solve linear programming problems in their conventional form. Instead it solves for the linear variables in a set of < or

> inequalities, with variables and coefficients on the left and a numerical value on the right.

LINEAR PROGRAMMER comes up with a "nearest" solution that satisfies as many of the inequalities as it can. The package also produces a partial solution that minimizes the largest difference between any variables expression and the righthand-side value. It uses a modified form of the Khachiyan technique.

Input data are entered on user-numbered lines. What is entered are the number of inequalities and of variables; the coefficient values for the inequalities; and the righthand-side values.

To run the solution, the user types RUN and is prompted to scale the problem if the coefficients are large numbers, since this can lead to an arithmetic overflow error.

The user also keys in the desired number of iterations. The manual advises that 100 iterations are usually enough, except for large problems. A sample problem with two variables and three inequalities ran through 100 iterations in about 70 seconds, according to the vendor.

LP1

This package can solve linear programming problems with as many as 100 variables and 100 constraints. It can accept input data either through menu selection, query-and-answer keyboard entry, or from files created by word processors.

LP1 runs on IBM/PC/XT computers. It sells for $99 from Micro Vision, 145 Wicks Rd., Commack, NY 11725 [(516) 499-4010].

When this package is started, an input menu appears on the screen, offering the user the alternative of entering data through the keyboard or of reading data from a previously prepared file.

During the keyboard entry procedure, names for the variables can be assigned by the user with up to seven characters per name. The package will then display the variable names, one by one, and prompt the user to enter objective function coefficient values for each.

Users can then assign a name for each constraint relationship. The package will prompt for a constraint coefficient value for each variable and a RHS (righthand-side) value for each constraint, as well as the nature of the constraint relationship ($=$, $<$, or $>$).

At the completion of the objective function data, and as each set of constraint data is completed, the package prompts the user to verify that the entered data are acceptable. If not, the user can go through the appropriate set of prompts once again, skipping by those items that are OK and stopping to change any incorrect items.

The package also provides overall editing procedures for data. These can be used to further revise just-entered data or to alter data that were previously entered and stored. The provisions here for editing constraints are particularly helpful when only a few of the variables have nonzero coefficients. The user is allowed to move directly from one such coefficient to another, skipping over variables with zero coefficients. The edited data are automatically saved, in a user-named file, when this editing procedure is completed.

Can stop at each iteration

When a problem is run, the user has the option of making the package stop at the end of each iteration to display the current results.

When the computation is complete, the package will display whether the solution is optimal, infeasible, or unbounded, or has a redundant constraint. In the last case, the user has the option of eliminating the offending constraint and rerunning the problem immediately. In all other cases, the package moves to an output menu after the computation. Through this menu, the user can display or print the results, or save the solution in a disk file. The results are shown in a row-and-column format

LP/80

This package can solve small linear programming problems, for example, with 70 decision variables and 40 constraints.

LP/80 runs on TRS-80 Model I or III computers. It sells for $70 from Decision Science Software, P.O. Box 7876, Austin, TX 78713 [(512) 926-4899].

The first choice on the LP/80 main menu is to start a New Problem. What follows this choice is a series of screen-displayed prompts. Users reply to these by typing the desired information.

After the user supplies names for each of the variables in the problem, the package prompts for objective function coefficients. As the name of each variable appears, the user keys in the corresponding coefficient value.

Constraint coefficients are then entered, one to a line, each accompanied by the name of the constraint and variable to which it belongs. By the time this information has been repeated for each coefficient, the user may be thoroughly exhausted but still will have to find enough energy to enter constraint types and righthand-side (RHS) values.

Solutions and sensitivity

The solution is started from the main menu. The display keeps the user informed of solution progress, and messages tell the user if the problem is infeasible or unbounded. Results are viewed by keying in a PRINT RE-SULTS command. These include the optimal value of the objective function, slack and surplus values for the constraint relationships, shadow prices for the constraints, and reduced costs for nonbasic variables.

The main menu choice to analyze sensitivity can then be made. This produces current RHS values and bounds to maintain the current basis. Variables that will enter and leave the basis when these bounds are exceeded are also shown.

To handle rounding errors, LP/80 sets values less than an "epsilon" value of 0.0001, to zero. However, this does not satisfy all situations, and the package may incorrectly identify some problems as infeasible. To check whether rounding is the culprit, users can adjust the value of epsilon and try to get a better answer.

Another main menu option is to change the data. This allows objective function, constraint coefficients, and RHS values to be altered. The changes can be checked on a display that shows the objective function, then, one by one, the constraints. The data can be stored in disk files. And these files can be read to provide data for a new solution.

LP83

This package can handle large linear programming problems. For example, a problem with 513 variables and 340 equality constraints was run by one reviewer. It is not, however, an interactive package. Users prepare the input for each run in advance, using their own word processor or text editor.

LP83 runs on IBM/PC/XT/AT and compatible computers. Use of a math coprocessor chip is recommended. The package sells for $795 from Sunset Software, 1613 Chelsea Rd. #153, San Marino, CA 91108 [(818) 284-4763].

LP83 makes little use of the interactive capabilities of personal computers. Instead it requires the user to come to the package with a complete set of input data, ready to be run. Users are expected to set up this input using their own word processing or text editor package, then use the input files they create to run LP83.

This allows the package to conform readily to input procedures traditionally used with large computers, where data and instructions are frequently punched into cards, then fed to the equipment. Users familiar with large-computer procedures will find the way this package is set up, even the computer terminology used in the manual, quite familiar. LP83 will, in fact, accept input in the standard MPS format used for linear programming based on large computers.

Shaped for experienced users

Learning to use this package largely consists of mastering the input file formats that are required. It amounts to learning to use a simplified computer language. The result is that the package is inherently oriented toward experienced users who employ LP83 frequently enough so they remain familiar with the many details of its input formats.

Many of the features it provides are admirable. For example, users can exert control over about 36 different characteristics of this package by typing a string of commands on the input command line. These include determining the way the output reports will be laid out on the printed page, and what reports and report information will appear. There is also a password arrangement to restrict access to use of the package.

LP83 has a number of convenient features such as use of shorthand ''symbolic'' names to represent long strings of repetitive input material and automatic conversion of numbers to percentages. Solution runs can be interrupted; the package will save the current solution so the iterative-solution process can be restarted from that point.

Diagnostics

The package produces a large number of specific error and warning messages when things go wrong, and the manual provides an explanation for each of these.

The manual itself is well organized, spelling out the information users need to know, and it has an index for reference once the package is in use.

Run times

The run times for problems with this package depend on the available size of computer main memory and on the use of the 8087 math coprocessor chip. The use of this chip seems to cut the run time for most problems by about a factor of 10. Using a larger main memory apparently affects the run time only for large problems. For example, the time for a problem with 340 rows and 513 columns was cut in half, but a larger main memory had no effect on a problem with 60 rows and 93 columns.

The vendor found that, using an IBM/XT with math chip and 640K memory, a problem with 16 rows and 33 columns ran in 6 seconds, while one with 177 rows and 548 columns ran in 41 minutes, 33 seconds. These times were decreased to 3 seconds and 29 minutes, 30 seconds when the same problems were run on an IBM/PC/AT with math chip and 512K memory.

Elapsed times to get answers from the IBM/PC/AT and an IBM 3081 mainframe computer were also compared. For all but the very largest problems, the ready access the user had to the PC provided the answers more rapidly, although the large machine had an advantage of almost ten to one in raw computational speed.

LP88 AND RELATED LINEAR PROGRAMMING PACKAGES

Reviewers: George H. Brooks, Deborah S. Fogel, University of Central Florida.

The LP88 package solves linear problems with up to 255 constraints and 2255 variables, using the revised simplex algorithm for quick and efficient solutions. The LPX88 package handles larger problems with up to 510 constraints and 2510 variables. BLP88 solves problems with upper or lower bounded variables, handling 255 constraints and 1255 variables. DLP88 is for dual linear problems with up to 1255 constraints. And there is also a student version, SLP88/STSA88, which solves simplex problems with 45 constraints and 255 variables and also handles transportation problems with 88 sources or sinks.

These packages provide users with a powerful set of linear programming tools. Operation is easy and efficient because the packages provide menu displays, function key controls, and a spreadsheet-style input editor.

All the packages run on IBM/PC, XT, or AT computers with 192K main

memory. Each package sells for $88. All but the student package are avail-
able in versions that make use of the 8087 math chip (these each cost just
$11 extra). The packages are available from Eastern Software Products,
P.O. Box 15328, Alexandria, VA 22309 [(703) 360-6942].

The reviewers checked the speed of package operation with a 13-variable, 48-constraint problem which had 198 nonzero matrix coefficients. The computer used was an IBM/XT with 256K main memory. LP88 produced an optimized solution in two minutes, 15 seconds. LPX88, which uses the revised simplex algorithm with product form inverse, produced an optimized solution in 54 seconds. The increased speed was probably due to the sparse nature of the coefficient matrix. When the DLP88 package was used, the problem was first converted to its dual. That took just 5 seconds. Then the solution itself took 9 seconds.

An unbounded problem, involving 13 variables and 9 constraints, was also run on LP88. In 15 seconds, the result "no solution" was produced.

There is a main menu to initiate the principal functions of the package, and there are also three more specialized menus. These are used to control setup of problems and data entry, execution of the solution, and the output information. The package displays all four menus on a single screen, informing the user near the bottom of the screen as to which one is currently active.

Spreadsheet input

To input a new set of data, the user calls for a New Problem on the Setup menu. On the display that follows, the user answers questions to name the problem, state whether it is to have a maximum or minimum solution, and define the number of constraints and nonslack variables in the problem. LP88 names the constraints and variables (users can later edit these, assigning six-character names) and creates a slack variable for each constraint.

Data for the coefficient matrix as well as cost and requirement vectors can be entered by selecting the Display Editor from the Setup menu. The entry is done on a spreadsheet format. The user starts the data entry process by selecting an initial row and column. A labeled, largely empty spreadsheet is then displayed. Using row-column locations to position the cursor on this display, the user can enter desired constraint and objective-function coefficients. The cursor can also be moved about by the arrow keys. Up to six characters can be entered for righthand-side values and five characters can be entered for coefficients. The package automatically computes coefficients for the slack variables.

The Display Editor cannot show all rows and columns for large problems. It is in fact set up to display 15 constraints and 10 variables at a time. Users can move the display to the desired area of the spreadsheet by identifying the constraint name and variable name of the spreadsheet cell they wish to appear in the upper lefthand corner of the screen. If desired, an array similar to the spreadsheet display can be produced in printed form.

An alternative method of entry is to create a data file using other software, outside the package, then read the file when the package is run. The format for such a file is compact and formal, with the details explained in the manual. With this input method, ten characters can be used for coefficient values.

Control over the solution

The technique used for solving linear programs involves the explicit inverse variant of the revised simplex algorithm. The algorithm can be started in four different ways: generate basis; obtain a previously computed or saved basis and optimize; restart from the most recent point of execution; and solve for a given basis without maximizing or minimizing.

Users can set a limit on the number of iterations (pivots) that will be performed. They can also select the number of iterations performed before the inverse is recomputed, the tolerance values below which pivot elements, inverse elements, and basis variables will be rejected, and the scales for display of primal and dual variables and of the objective value. If the user does not make these selections, the packages will use default values for these parameters.

During its calculations, the package shows a display that gives current information on the state of the solution. Solutions can be interrupted while in progress, allowing users to step through the pivots, reinvert, reset tolerances and controls, save the basis, and record the current solution and pivots. User control is simplified by function keys.

When operated by programming-minded users, the package can be run in a batch mode. Here a properly formatted command file, containing instructions on how the computation is to proceed, is entered, along with a data file. In the run that follows, users can exercise limited control from the keyboard.

Flexible output

Package outputs include the original problem data, primal and dual values, cost and righthand-side ranges, basis interval matrix, inverse and nonbasis column products.

Six tables are used to display this information. All or any of these can be called for by the user, printed, and stored in disk files. The solution basis can also be stored.

To rapidly solve problems that are similar but not identical, a problem can be modified using the Display Editor; then it can be rerun starting with the previous solution. If a basis inverse has been computed, and there are no changes to any of the basis columns, the modified problem can be rerun even faster by starting from the previous inverse basis.

Some cautions

When using version 3.12 of LP88, DLP88, BLP88 and version 4.07 of LPX88, users should be aware of the possibility of program crashes. When errors occur, the package may suddenly terminate its operation, forcing the user to restart from scratch in order to get a solution. During the review procedures, the printer ran out of paper and such a crash occurred. The inconvenience of such incidents can be minimized if users store their information on disk immediately after it is produced by the package, and before any printing is done. The package vendor has indicated that future versions will include error-trapping provisions to prevent such crashes.

The student version, SLP88/STSA88, already has such error trapping. This version offers most of the features of LP88. However, it is limited to six characters for coefficients, does not allow use of sequential files nor storage of results on disk, and does not support use of the 8087 math chip.

Before using the BPL88 bounded variable version, users should take care to read the documentation covering solution output. The usual printout and display will show only those variables that appear in the basis. To obtain a complete statement of the solution, users must call for a special printout. This will mark nonbasis, nonslack variables with an asterisk if they have reached their bounded value. These must then be included in the determination of the optimized objective-function value.

Documentation is comprehensive

LP88 documentation is contained in a 42-page manual. It is comprehensive and includes a sample problem. The package disk includes three sample problems that allow users to experiment before running their own problems. Explicit instructions are included in the manual on how to use the package, the meanings of the function keys, along with general information on the package. Documentation for BLP88, DLP88, and SLP88/STSA88 is recorded on the package disk and can be printed out if the user wishes.

MINI-MAX

MINI-MAX can solve linear programming problems with up to 300 variables and up to 70 constraints, but not both at the same time. For example, when 132 variables are involved, only 30 constraints can be handled.

MINI-MAX runs on IBM/PC and compatible computers. It sells for $395 from Agricultural Software Consultants, 1706 Santa Fe, Kingsville, TX 78363 [(512) 595-1937].

The package runs from a main menu and several series of screen-displayed queries to which the user keyboards responses.

Keyboarded input

One of the main menu selections is to set up a new linear programming problem. Replying to the queries that follow this selection, the user specifies how many variables and constraints will be used, and whether the problem is to be run to find a maximum or minimum result.

Names are then keyboarded to describe the problem, each of the variables, and the disk file in which the input data will be stored. Then the coefficients of the objective function are entered. At the completion of this set of entries, the user is asked to verify that they are correct; if not, the set can be reentered. The next series of input queries is designed to allow the user to enter the coefficients for the constraint relationships. This is done for one constraint at a time, with a verification step when the coefficients of each constraint have been completed.

When this problem description has been completed, the user can call for a printout of the input data. The description is automatically stored in the named disk file, and it is made ready for running the solution to the problem.

Lots of output

To run the problem, the user presses the R key with the main menu displayed. The entire problem is run, and results are displayed, a screenful at a time. The user can rerun these displays, or call for a printout of the results.

These results include displays of the optimal solution, and basic and nonbasic variables. The nonbasic variables are those whose coefficient values are insignificant for the solution, and the output includes an "entering value" to show at what point each coefficient value would have made that particular variable basic. A separate display shows the current values of the basic variables along with high- and low-range values, to show how much variation there can be before these become nonbasic.

Sensitivity analysis

The output also displays slack and surplus variables, dual variables with shadow prices, and the ranges of feasibilty for the variables.

Whenever a less-than-or-equal-to constraint is used, there can be slack; that is, the amount the righthand side of the constraint can be decreased without having any effect on the solution. In a similar manner, a greater-than-or-equal-to constraint can have a surplus variable.

The shadow price of a constraint is the amount by which the objective function will change if the righthand side of the constraint is increased by 1. A large shadow price is a danger signal, warning the user that a constraint is drastically affecting the solution.

Some problems have two or more optimal solutions, called alternate solutions. MINI-MAX will signal this situation with an ALTERNATE SOLUTIONS message. It is then up to the user to locate additional solutions by making small changes in the coefficients of the objective function.

When solutions fail

If the problem has no solution, the package will display a NO SOLUTION message and show the shadow prices. This may have happened because one or more of the constraints cannot be satisfied. In this situation it may be enlightening to examine the shadow prices, since those constraints with zero shadow prices will not be the ones preventing the solution. The user can then try altering or eliminating the remaining constraints, one at a time, until a satisfactory solution is obtained.

Another error message that may appear is UNBOUNDED SOLUTION. This usually indicates that the problem has been set up incorrectly, but it may also be due to a computational arithmetic error. To help in identifying such problems, MINI-MAX displays a maximum error figure as part of the solution. One recommended remedy is for the user to experiment with changing or eliminating constraints. Another is to adjust the rounding of data by the package. This can be set at anywhere from 6 to 12 places after the decimal point. However, users are advised that the results of such adjustments are unpredictable.

Changes and reruns

To make changes to an existing problem description, the user has to call for the file by name. If in doubt, a directory of stored files can be consulted.

A listing of the variables and coefficients in the objective function is then displayed, with variable names, and the user can choose to make changes to any individual variable or coefficient. This is done by answering a short sequence of displayed queries. In a similar manner, changes can be made to displays of any or all of the constraint relationships.

MPS-PC

This package solves linear programming problems with up to 70 variables and 50 constraints. It has procedures that could make it very easy to learn and use, but somehow falls short of achieving all it could in this area.

MPS-PC runs on IBM/PC and compatible computers. It sells for $150 from Research Corporation, 6840 E. Broadway Blvd., Tucson, AZ 85710 [(602) 296-6400].

MPS-PC is a personal computer version of the MPS-X program used on large computers. It operates from three menus and various displayed prompts that follow from menu choices.

Column by column data entry

The data entry process is an organized one, but the organization does not seem to give high priority to user convenience. In several ways, users are asked to compensate for programming peculiarities and oversights by special procedures.

Data are entered from the keyboard or read from previously prepared files. When entering data, users have to be aware of the particular rules this package uses. Thus, the number of rows the user calls for does not include the row for the objective function, and the number of columns does not include the one for the righthand-side (RHS) data. The package doesn't recognize $<$, $>$, and $=$, so users must enter L, G, and E for these relationships.

Actual data entry is on a column-by-column basis. This means that users will not be able to keep track of what they are doing by merely knowing what equations and inequalities they wish to enter. Instead, they have to make a careful handwritten layout of the entry data with all columns neatly and correctly lined up.

MPS-PC will not tolerate negative RHS values, so users must multiply all the terms in such a constraint by minus one to enter it.

Users have to be sure not to inadvertently press the F1 function key followed by Enter. That will erase whatever data entry has been done. This can be a helpful feature, but it lacks a verification step in which users are asked if they really want to take that step.

Data storage and editing

Sets of input data are stored in disk files with names that can be eight characters long, plus a three-character suffix. With enough use of the package, these files can accumulate. As with most personal computer storage arrangements, it is up to the user to keep the disks from filling up by using the PC system software to erase those files that are no longer needed.

Correcting an error is easy, if it is caught during data entry before a column is complete. All the user has to do is enter the row name and then the correct coefficient value. Once the column is entered, the user must do corrections with editing procedures that can be used after the data entry process.

To examine what has been input, the user can call for a printout of the data in row-column format. There is also an alternative printed format that first lists the row names, then shows the nonzero coefficient values for each column, with each value identified by its row name. This printout also lists righthand-side (RHS) values, each identified with a row name. Only the alternative form can be shown on the display screen. The vendor excuses this fact by stating that this is due to "limited screen space."

Data editing is done from an editing menu where the user calls for specific types of items, such as objective function values, RHS values, and constraint names. The package will not tolerate duplicate names for columns or rows. To transpose two names that have been wrongly placed, a third temporary name must be used.

How solutions run

When the data for a problem are complete, the user can start the solution portion of the package. During the solution calculation, the user is given a running account of each iteration on the display screen. Added information will be printed at each iteration.

It is not uncommon, we are told, for this package to run through 100 iterations to solve a problem with 50 rows. Users are warned by the manual that they may be "somewhat disconcerted" by how long it takes to solve problems. A problem with 63 columns and 47 rows is said to have taken 68 iterations and 15 minutes to reach a solution. However, all the constraints in this problem were equations, and $<$, $>$ constraints are said to take longer.

There are some tricks that can speed things up a bit. For example, problems with many greater-than-zero constraints can be speeded up by changing these to less-than-zero. The only affect on the solution will be changes of sign in the coefficients of the affected rows. Couldn't the package have included a built-in feature to do all this automatically?

MPS-PC notifies the user when it fails to solve problems because of infeasibility and identifies the row where the logical problem arises. It also notifies the user of unbounded conditions that prevent a solution. In this case it is entirely up to the user to find the trouble.

Occasionally solutions with this package may not diverge, but instead may fail to converge to a solution. The designers of the package decided to tolerate this situation because the procedures that could avoid it would slow down the entire solution process. The manual advises on various measures users can take if faced with this kind of solution failure. To stop the package while it is cycling through one of these infinite iteration sequences, it is necessary to terminate package operation and exit to the computer system software.

Options with cautions

The user then has the option of performing calculations that will produce an upper and lower bound for each objective function coefficient and for the righthand-side (RHS) values of the constraints. This provides a measure of how much these quantities can change, for one variable at a time, without changing the optimal solution.

Another optional calculation allows the user to make changes to objective function coefficients and RHS values, then rerun the solution. The procedures for this seem annoyingly complicated and indirect. Instead of making specified changes to selected items, the user has to manipulate a change vector, with operations that could better have been done internally by the package. Even more constricting is the requirement that the user make up these change vectors before running the problem, while what the user needs is to make the changes on the basis of the calculated results.

However, when a solution is completed, the package automatically stores the solution information on a disk file, so it is not too difficult to make a rerun with an appropriate change vector.

An existing solution file can be used as the starting basis for a solution to another problem. But here the package offers little control over the situation. There will be an automatic check to see that the number of columns and rows in the problem file and the solution file are the same. But the package will not check to see that the nature of the constraints and the values of the constraint coefficients match up. And unless they do, the calculated answers will be wrong.

OPERATION RESEARCH PACKAGE

Reviewer: Darrell G. Linton, University of Central Florida

The four programs in this package are not intended for solving very large and complex problems. Instead, they permit the user to obtain quick and inexpensive answers to problems, provided that the underlying assumptions approximate those of the model. The programs are written with user convenience in mind. The example and documentation are easy to follow. This reviewer's grade rating for this package is a 95.

Programs included are for linear programming, maximum flow analysis, inventory models, and queueing models. The package as reviewed runs on an IBM/PC. Versions for TRS-80 I, II, III, and 4 and for Apple II, II+, IIe are available, all from The Institute of Industrial Engineers, 25 Technology Park/Atlanta, Norcross, GA 30092 [(404) 449-0460]. Price of the package is $175, or $140 to IIE members.

The linear programming portion of the package optimizes a linear objective function subject to linear constraints. Problems with up to 30 constraints and 40 decision variables can be run. Typical objective functions involve total cost or profit, while the constraints impose limits on such items as raw materials and personnel.

A typical maximum flow problem would be one where a commodity is to be shipped from one point (the source) to another (the sink). There may also be several intermediate locations, called transshipment points. The problem is to maximize the flow of the commodity from source to sink, subject to the paths connecting the various points. The total flow into a transshipment point must always equal the total flow out. Although this problem can be solved by linear programming, the maximum flow algorithm is usually more efficient. The total number of points that can be handled is limited by the available amount of computer memory.

Input to the inventory models program may include the total annual demand for a product, the per-unit price, procurement cost per order, annual holding cost, shortage cost, maximum storage space, and number of price breaks. Depending on the user input, the program selects from among eight possible models, including a basic economic order quantity model, a price-break model, a shortage-cost model, and a storage-limitation model. The program outputs include the optimum order quantity, total inventory costs, number of order cycles per year, cost per unit, maximum inventory, and number of units back ordered per cycle.

The queueing models program analyzes single- and multi-server waiting line problems. It assumes a first-in first-out serving procedure and steady-state operation of the queue. Problems with exponential interarrival and service time distributions are handled. Users can choose from four models: a single-server, infinite waiting room model; a multiple-server, infinite waiting room model; a parallel-server, finite waiting room model; and a machine servicing model.

Typical outputs for the queueing models include the steady-state probability of N units in the system, the average number of units in the system and in the queue, and the average waiting time in the system and the queue. The limitations on the program are the built-in assumptions of the models, such as Poisson arrivals, exponential service, and steady-state results.

Clear documentation

Instructions and examples in the 83-page, loose-leaf manual are clear. There is a separate section for each of the four programs, and each section concludes with an IBM/PC source listing for programming-minded users. The reviewer found a few minor errors in the text of the manual. These will undoubtedly be corrected in the next edition.

As for recovery from errors, the reviewer found that the programs are designed to recover from almost every conceivable error and allow easy editing of input data.

RAMLP

This package runs fairly large problems, with the size limited by the main memory of the computer. For instance, with a 128K main memory, Ramlp can handle up to about 100 constraints and 100 variables.

Ramlp runs on IBM/PC and Colombia computers. It sells for $149 from Miniware, 205 Winchester Rd., Annapolis, MD 21401 [(301) 757-5626].

For problems involving a lot of input data, the main task the user faces is putting the data into the computer and verifying that it is correct. Ramlp offers some alternative ways to do data entry, but the basic input format is to enter rows and columns of data.

To enter data from the keyboard, the user has to be aware in advance of how these rows and columns will look, and specify how many of each will be needed.

In the rows and columns, everything must be in its place, and each has a name. The first row contains the coefficients for the objective function. Subsequent rows each contain data for a constraint function. The first column contains constraint levels and is called the RHS (righthand side) column. Subsequent columns, each assigned to one decision variable, contain constraint coefficients. Users can assign convenient names to all but the first row and column.

Shown on this data array is the user's choice of either a maximum- or minimum-value solution for the objective function. Whether a constraint function is an inequality or an equality, the appropriate symbol is shown in the RHS column. At the bottom of each of the user-named columns, lower- and upper-bound values for each decision variable can be entered.

To set up the rows and columns for their problem, users call for an Edit menu. The choices on this menu allow changing row or column names, bounds, and =, <, > designations. They also provide for editing coefficient values once they are entered.

Data entry aids

A coefficient menu provides some aids for the main data entry task, keyboarding the coefficients for the objective function and constraint expressions. Choices here allow users to enter or erase a single coefficient by first specifying its row and column location. Other choices allow entering an entire row, or column, or diagonal of data. Then, as each coefficient is entered, the package will display location numbers for the next.

But keyboard entry is not the only means for getting data in. When the package is first started up, a displayed menu allows users to choose the type of data input they want. In addition to input from the keyboard, data can be taken from previously stored disk files.

When a problem is run, the data that went into it are discarded. So, if users want to reuse those data, they have to deliberately store the information. This choice is one of several that can be made from the package main menu, from which users can also order printed listings of rows, columns, and bounds, or of the entire array of input data.

Getting a solution

The main menu also offers a "Solve" choice. This is to be selected after a complete array of input data is in place and ready to be processed. With Solve underway, the computer display shows a log of the partial results as iterations are made toward a feasible solution. Remarks shown on these displays indicate the number of constraints satisfied at each iteration, along with a current number of "infeasibilities" (which gives the user some idea of how close a solution may be). If the solution process should fail, this record can be used in deciding on possible fixes.

Based on computation results, the user may decide to change the input description of the problem by deleting or adding data array rows or columns. This can be done through the main menu.

If and when a solution is found, the package prints out a final report showing the computed value of the objective function and of each of the rows and columns in the input array.

Ramlp runs problems entirely in computer main memory, thus avoiding the need to store and retrieve data from disk storage during the computations. This eliminates slow disk accesses, giving a fast computation. However, it limits the size of problems that can be run, since main memory space is limited. In a 128 kilobyte main memory, the package can run problems of a size equivalent to about 100 constraints and 100 real variables. The package automatically checks to see if the problem size fits the allowed limits before it is run.

Chapter 15
Comprehensive Statistical Packages

Comprehensive statistical packages, those that offer the user choice of a wide variety of statistical tools, come in two basic varieties. In the first, the procedures are invoked by keyboarded commands. The second type of package operates from displayed menus.

Command-based packages are for serious users who are willing to invest the time to learn to use a new language. For those who will find frequent, consistent use for such a package, this will be a worthwhile investment. With the use of commands, there is no need to wait for menus to be shown nor to move from one menu to another to reach a desired function.

Other users, who may turn only occasionally to personal computer-based statistical tools, will probably feel that learning to use a command-based package is an overly burdensome task. With menus always there to remind the user of the available choices, there is no need to memorize commands or the syntax rules of use that inevitably surround them.

It would be ideal to have a package that made menus available to those who need them, while it offered direct commands to more practiced users. Some word processing packages have such combined facilities, but there do not seem to be any statistical packages that do.

There are some command-based packages that do have features designed to ease the process of learning and use. For example, the SYSTAT package uses about 100 commands, but the package is divided up into modules, one for handling data and others for various types of statistical procedures. Each module has a set of commands peculiar to its operations, so the SYSTAT language can be learned piecemeal, starting with those procedures the user needs first. At the end of each user session, SYSTAT prints a log of all the commands that were used, providing a convenient reference for performing similar procedures in the future.

The language of statistics

For those readers who may not be familiar with the terms used to describe statistical procedures, it seems worthwhile to put some of the terms used in the reviews into context.

Statistical analysis starts with a set of data, and the first step is to weed out errors in the data. Packages may include procedures for scanning the data to see that no inappropriate symbols are included with the numeric data. Histogram displays of individual variables can be used to spot "outlier" values. Statistics like the Mahalanobis distance can reveal unusual variation in a row of data, compared to other rows. Since not all data sets are complete, there should also be some way to handle missing data.

Descriptive statistics can include about a dozen measures such as the mean, median, maximum and minimum, variance, standard deviation, skewness (left- or right-handed tendency), and kurtosis (peakedness) of a set or "sample" of numeric data.

Often the user wants to compare one data sample to another or to a larger data "population." The so-called null hypothesis is that the sample is representative of the population. And a number of statistical tests are used to test this hypothesis.

The choice of tests depends, in the first place, on whether the population and sample are normally distributed along the bell-shaped curve that is typical of many populations. Statistical tests like the Kolmogorov-Smirnov and Wilk-Shapiro are used to test for normality.

The null hypothesis for normal distributions is ordinarily tested by "parametric" procedures such as the various types of t-tests and the F-test. However, there are also "nonparametric" tests that are appropriate for use with data sets that are not normally distributed.

In some cases, it is desirable to transform such data sets by taking the logarithm, or square root, or performing some other mathematical operation on each of their members, such that the resulting distribution is normal. The parametric tests can then be used, and these are considered more sensitive than the nonparametric in detecting departures from the null hypothesis.

Two types of errors occur in these tests. (I) The null hypothesis may be rejected, when in actuality it is true. (II) The hypothesis may be accepted when it is false. The probability of an error of type I is called the significance level of the test; values on the order of .05 to .01 are considered small.

Correlation tests measure the extent to which two data samples are linearly related to one another, so that knowledge of data points in one can be used to predict the data points in the other.

Analysis of variance (ANOVA) is used to determine to what extent different "factors" contribute to the total variance of a data sample. Thus an engineer might be interested in the extent to which maximum temperature or processing time contributes to the variance of the dimensions of the items in a production sample. One-way ANOVA tests the effects of a single factor on the sample. Two-way ANOVA can test the simultaneous effect of two factors.

Analysis often involves separating the data into common-characteristic groups. The software can provide for coding and segregation of such groups. One-way or two-way analysis of variance and other procedures can be used to check for differences and similarities between groups. Cross tabulations can be used to summarize the ways that data separate out into groups.

When two or more variables are involved, graphical displays can be used to reveal whether or not relationships exist. Regression analysis, linear and nonlinear, can shed further light on these relationships.

There can be situations where it is difficult to identify groups or sub-populations. Clustering algorithms provide a way to identify possible groupings of variables and data. Where there are complex functional relationships between variables, factor analysis can be used to study the correlations between them.

One of the key assumptions underlying ANOVA tests is that the variables involved are normally-distributed and independent of one another. The chi-square test is used to draw inferences about their dependence or independence.

For data that clearly violate normality, there are nonparametric tests, like the Kruskal-Wallis one-way analysis of variance test and the Friedman two-way analysis of variance, that can be used.

Specialized procedures are available for dealing with time-series data, and such analyses may use either frequency or time domain approaches. Survival analysis techniques can be used to study outcomes over various time intervals.

A variety of statistical procedures

At a minimum, every one of these comprehensive statistical packages offers some basic, standard procedures. There are always some descriptive statistics, a suite of tests for normally distributed variables, nonparametric tests, correlation, regression, and analysis of variance (ANOVA) procedures. Graphics such as histograms and scatter graphs are also standard. Some of the packages also include procedures such as cross tabulation, factor and cluster analysis, time-series analysis, and survival estimation.

The predominant approach is simply to present a kit of statistical tools, a kind of statistician's smorgasbord, from which the user can choose whatever seems to meet the current need. Two command-operated packages that exemplify this approach are BDMPC and SPSS/PC. Both are personal computer versions of mainframe computer packages. Both offer such a large number of procedures that it takes user manuals running over 600 pages to describe what is available. And both offer powerful procedures. Thus, while most packages provide one-way , perhaps two-way, ANOVA, the SPSS/PC ANOVA command will handle up to five dependent variables, 10 factors, and 10 covariates.

This approach is not restricted to command-based packages. For example, the NCSS menu-based package also aims to be a wholesale supplier of everything in statistics that a user might need. The NCSS manual is thinner, mainly because its descriptions are more succinct.

Working with a more restricted set of procedures, the DAISY package (command-based) is organized to meet the needs of users who want to analyze their data by first plotting to get a preliminary impression of whether there is a relationship between the variables. Product-moment, partial, and time-shifted correlations, along with four nonparametric measures, are provided as means of further measuring relationships between variables. Linear and stepwise regression procedures are provided to establish trends in the data and to set up predictions. The other statistics offered by the package are specifically selected to support these basic capabilities by testing the results.

The SYSTAT package proudly offers two unique procedures. An MLGH (Multivariate General Linear Model) procedure can estimate and test any univariate or multivariate general linear model, allowing linear contrasts on vectors of dependent as well as independent variables. And there is also a multidimensional scaling procedure for up to 5 dimensions.

Convenient data entry

Using a package for statistical manipulation is a relatively easy matter. Once having decided which procedure to use, a few buttons are pressed and the computer churns away until results are produced. Entering and checking the data that are to be analyzed can be much more arduous.

Some of these packages seem to recognize that personal computer users will often be faced with the task of keyboarding large amounts of data, then correcting and checking what has been entered. For example, the DAISY package has spreadsheet-like data entry and editing capabilities. A table for data entry is displayed, and users can make entries one after another, moving from one location to the next by hitting the appropriate arrow key. Other keyboard actions make the cursor jump to the start of the next row or column. Editing consists of typing a new number over the existing one at the cursor position. Users can even split the screen and compare nonadjacent columns side by side.

Most of the packages provide for entering data in a much more piecemeal manner, usually a row at a time. Thus the ELF package displays an entry form for the first row that shows the variable names, each followed by a space for 10 characters. As each data item is filled in, pressing the space bar will move the cursor to the next item space. When the data for that row are complete, the user can call up the display for the next row by pressing the return key. Or, if there are any typing errors, the process of entering that row can be repeated. MICROSTAT users follow a similar procedure, straightforward, but not as convenient as working with a full-screen display of a data table.

Less desirable procedures, in other packages, prompt the user for one item at a time, never giving an overall view of even one complete row of data.

StatPac users can devise their own input "screens." This capability permits either row-by-row or column-by-column input procedures. The idea appears to be that operators with little or no knowledge of statistics will do data entry and that these screens can be designed for their use.

Emulating punched cards

When punched cards are used to input data into large computers, the processes of verifying and correcting the data take place on the punching equipment, not in the computer. The authors of the SPSS/PC package have apparently assumed that the data input to the personal computer will be as pure and correct as that from punched cards. There seem to be no convenient built-in procedures in this package that would allow users to correct errors in the data they type into the keyboard.

BDMPC users will find that this package takes a similar approach. It seems, incredibly, to be set up to take data as if the information were coming from punched cards. The user first has to write a short program that reserves storage space and specifies the format in which the information is being presented, as well as describing the information itself (title, number of variables, maximum and minimum values, etc.). The procedure, appropriate for mainframe processing, is inappropriate for personal computer use. But there does not seem to be any alternative.

Manipulating files

Given the choice, any user would rather work with existing files of data than have to enter new data through the keyboard. An important part of most of these packages is their ability to store data files on disk and to retrieve and manipulate those files to present just the desired data for analysis by statistical procedures.

These data manipulation facilities can be quite flexible. For example, with the NCSS package two tables may be joined, one above the other, or side to side. Individual columns may be copied from one table to another. Portions of tables may be selected out. Tables can even be rotated so that the rows become columns and vice-versa.

Another important capability is to be able to take data from other computer packages and adjust the formats so these data can be treated by the statistical package. Most of the packages discussed here can accept files in standard ASCII format. In addition, the DIF format used by some personal computer spreadsheets can be accepted and used by packages like MICROSTAT, ELF, and DAISY. Some of the packages will also accept files in the popular dBase II database format. ABSTAT can accept files produced by such computer languages as BASIC and reformat its own files so they can be used in BASIC programs.

Transforming the data

Often statistical analysis involves transforming the data before actually carrying out statistical procedures. All of these packages provide some facilities for making such transformations. Usually this involves operating on a table of data recalled from storage.

One of the most extensive facilities is offered by the NCSS package where transformations of the data may be done by adding, subtracting, multiplying, or dividing the items in one column by those in a second column, or by a constant, to form a transformed column. Single-column transformations include taking the absolute value, cumulative totaling, forming truncated or rounded-off integers from decimal numbers, calculating modulo remainders or signature values, taking Tukey's folded log or root, natural logs, exponents, square roots, trigonometric functions. Columns of uniform-random or sequential numbers can be generated. There are also smoothing and lagging transformations, and values within a column can be sorted, or ranked.

The ABSTAT package uses a single, flexible procedure that allows users to construct transformations using algebraic functions that can include expressions in parentheses; arithmetic, trigonometric, exponential, and log functions; modular arithmetic, absolute values, truncation; and a variety of constants including the mean and standard deviation of the variable. Transformations are also provided to convert times and dates.

The ELF package takes this idea one step further, requiring users to write short programs in a special computer language in order to make data transformations. Allowed operations include arithmetic, selections based on <, >, =, and "odd" conditions, trigonometric, exponential, logarithmic, modulo 10, rounding, truncation and absolute value.

Statistical graphics

Graphics provided with these packages are generally crude, with points represented by printed characters. The SYSTAT package makes the most of such plotting capabilities by offering variety. Scatter plots, function plots, and histograms can be easily produced. With the help of some BASIC programming, crude contour plots can be made. There is also a stem-leaf plot, a histogramlike display made up of numerals, that can give users insight into the repeated appearance of certain discrete values in the data. Box plots are used to quickly identify median, hinges, and outside values in the data. SYSTAT will also produce probability plots, which show a variable plotted against corresponding percentage points of a standard normal variable.

The DAISY package is unusual, providing high-resolution plotting for those users whose computers will accommodate it. There are histograms, useful for examining the data items in a single variable, and sequence plots that can help to discover trends, repeating cycles and unusual data points in a variable. To compare one variable to another, high resolution scatter plots are available in linear, semilog or, logarithmic form. If requested, the package will draw a regression line of best fit for the scatter plot.

ABSTAT

This package provides most of the standard statistical procedures, and it also does correlation, regression and cross tabulations. Operation is based on stored files of data, and about 64 keyboarded commands are used. There are graphics, but they are primitive. ABSTAT will handle up to 64 variables and can make use of a math coprocessor chip.

ABSTAT runs on IBM/PC/XT/AT and compatible computers. It sells for $395 from AndersonBell, P.O. Box 191, Canon City, CO 81212 [(303) 275-1661].

"Since the number of commands is too large for an effective single menu" (a rather lame excuse), the authors of this package have elected to require users to remember keyboard commands rather than work from menu choices. ABSTAT is therefore a specialized computer language, oriented to statistical procedures. As with any computer language, the user has to carefully examine the functions of the commands, and remember as many as possible, as a prerequisite to serious use of this package.

Once a user knows the command names, there is a HELP facility that can call up and display explanations of any named command.

To ease the learning process, the commands are divided up into five categories: data manipulation, statistical analysis, graphic functions, report writing, and miscellanous. In the first two categories are about 50 commands, and only about 14 more in the other categories. Most of the user manual is taken up with explanations of what these commands mean and how to use them. A runthrough of how to use the package to solve a typical problem is given in a short appendix. Another appendix gives the calculation formulas used by the package. A third lists the errors which the package may trap and gives a brief explanation for each of them, a handy feature. Appropriate to a manual that is primarily a reference source, there is an index.

Serial data entry

Data entry is accomplished with the EDIT command, after the user has set up a file using the CREATE command. Entry is made using a serial query and reply procedure in which the user keys in each of the variable values for case one, then enters case two, etc. During the entry process, the user can back up to previous queries to correct typing errors. Once the data have been entered, there is a command for making changes in selected cases. A LIST command causes the whole data table, or selected variables, to be displayed or printed out for detailed examination and verification. There is also a command that allows data entry one variable at a time. The package does not seem to provide a means for entering data onto a displayed tabular form.

A flexible transformation procedure allows users to construct transformations using algebraic functions that can include expressions in parentheses; arithmetic, trigonometric, exponential, and log functions; modular arithmetic, absolute values, truncation; and a variety of constants including the mean and standard deviation of the variable. Transformations are also provided to convert times and dates.

ABSTAT can accept files produced by the BASIC computer language and reformat its own files so they can be used in BASIC programs. It can also exchange files with the dBase II and III database packages. However, one reviewer found that this capability had some undocumented defects.

Statistical procedures

Most of the statistical commands involve a specification, by the user, of the data file and the variables within that file that are to be operated upon. The DESC command will produce a standard set of descriptive statistics. There are t-tests for comparing matched and independent variables, and a t-test for comparing a sample mean to a population mean. The package also has a group of probability calculations based on user-keyboarded information. For example, the user can enter chi-square and degrees of freedom values and get a probability for the combination. Similar calculations are provided for F distribution, Student's t distribution, binomial and Poisson's distributions, and Z-scores.

Other commands perform such tests as chi-square goodness of fit, the Kolmogorov-Smirnov two-sample test, the Kruskal-Wallis one-way analysis of variance for ranked data, the Mann-Whitney U test, a one-sample runs test, the Wald-Wolfowitz two-sample runs test, and a sign test.

The SRANK command will rank data and produce a Spearman rank correlation matrix. The CORR command will produce a correlation matrix for selected variables.

There is an ANOVA command that comes up with a summary table for up to a 4-way ANOVA. The capacity of this procedure is limited. When the numbers of values for each of the factors are multiplied together, their product must be no greater than 400.

The REGR command performs multiple linear regressions on one dependent, and up to 19 independent, variables. The XTAB command produces cross tabulations of selected variable pairs, calculates chi-square, and performs Fisher's exact test where appropriate. There is no provision for stepwise regression.

Rough graphs

The package can also produce histograms and scatter plots for selected variables. These are made up of printed characters, Xs for the histograms, and numerals that indicate point locations on the scatter plots.

If printed output, or storage of the results in a disk file are desired, the user must specify these options before a statistical procedure is run.

BDMPC

This package contains just about any and all statistical procedures that one might want to use. The problem is that the user is assumed to be someone who is willing to learn an extensive special computer language and is familiar with mainframe-style procedures. BDMPC runs on IBM/PCs and compatible computers and is designed as if the personal computer were never invented. The package requires use of 640K main memory, hard disk storage, and a math coprocessor chip.

There are 21 software modules available. The price for all of them is $1500, or they can be purchased in groups or individually from BDMP Statistical Software, 1964 Westwood Blvd. #202, Los Angeles, CA 90025 [(213) 475-5700].

BDMPC is a personal computer version of the BDMP statistical package, long a standard for mainframe users. The BDMPC modules are essentially the same programs used with the mainframe version, and they require the full capabilities of the IBM/PC, including a 64,000 byte main memory, hard disk storage, and a math coprocessor chip. Still, there are certain limits to the statistical solutions that can be run with BDMPC modules. For example, the limit on number of data values is 16,000.

The 1985 BDMP Statistical Software Manual is a 734-page compendium, a lot of paper for $17.50, but it is not a guide to using the BDMPC package itself. There is also a small "Users Guide to BDMP on the IBM PC." This explains how to load the package into the computer and gives some other information as well, but it is not a user's manual in the usual sense.

Many commands

BDMP is a statistical computer language, and a large number of commands must be mastered by those who want to use it. Mainframe users of BDMP customarily entered data and commands by first producing punched cards, then feeding the cards to the computer equipment. The BDMPC version makes a concession to personal computer use by offering an "interactive" mode of input.

To carry out this interactive entry, the user has to learn 30 or so line editing commands and variations and get acquainted with the procedures for invoking these commands. With this knowledge, it is possible to begin to use the actual BDMP commands.

These are outlined in a 177-page "User's Digest." To use any particular BDMP module, one has to look it up in the table of contents of this digest and turn to the appropriate pages. There, a brief description of the procedure will be found, followed by setup instructions for keying in the general commands to get the procedure going, and then by descriptions of the particular commands that invoke the various features of that procedure.

For more details, and for examples of how that procedure has been applied, the user turns to the full size manual.

Getting the data into the computer

The first question a BDMPC user may ask is how to get the data into the computer. The answer is that there is no convenient way to do this from the keyboard. If the data are already stored in a computer file, there are commands to get and use that file. But BDMPC seems, incredibly, to be set up to take new data only as if they were coming from punched cards.

The user has to write a short program that reserves storage space and specifies the format in which the information is being presented, as well as describing the information itself (title, number of variables, maximum and minimum values, etc.). The procedure, appropriate for mainframe processing, is wildly overcomplicated for personal computer use. But there does not seem to be any appropriate alternative.

Statistical procedures

Despite their inaccessibility, a brief rundown of the statistical procedures seems in order. Assuming that the user does get the data to be analyzed into a readable file, the list of those procedures is formidable.

A simple set of descriptive data can be produced for each variable, or the user can call for detailed data description, including frequencies and estimates of location. There are one-, and two-group t-tests, single-column frequency counts, and flexible histograms, probability, frequency distribution, and scatter plots. For data groups, there are similar capabilities, and four methods are provided for doing correlations when data are missing.

Frequency tables available to users include two-way and multiway cross sections. Two methods are provided for estimating survival, and there is a method for analyzing survival data when explanatory variables are present.

Cluster analysis of variables includes a choice of four measures of similarity and three criteria for linking. And there are similar cluster analyses for observations and for blocks of observations. Factor analysis provides four methods of initial extraction and several rotation methods.

There is a canonical correlation analysis for two sets of variables, a stepwise discriminant analysis between two or more groups, a Boolean factor analysis, scoring based on preference pairs, a procedure that describes the pattern of missing values for multivariate data, and another that partitions a set of observations into clusters.

Regression procedures include multiple linear regression, forward and backward stepwise regression, nonlinear regression with six functions built in, regression on principal components, polynomial regression, partial correlation and multivariate regression, all possible subsets regression, derivative free nonlinear regression, and stepwise logistic regression.

There is a Box-Jenkins time series analysis procedure that can be used to build a parametric model, and also a univariate and bivariate spectral analysis for time series. A multipass transformation procedure provides data editing and univariate statistics along with transformations.

Nonparametric procedures include the sign test, Wilcoxon signed ranks test, Mann-Whitney rank sum test, Kruskal-Wallis one-way ANOVA, Friedman one-way ANOVA, Kendall's coefficient of concordance, and the Kendall and Spearman rank correlation coefficients.

ANOVA procedures include one for one-way analysis of variance and covariance, another that handles repeated measures models, a general mixed model analysis of variance that uses maximum and restricted maximum likelihood approaches, procedures for univariate and multivariate analysis of variance, and a mixed model for any complete design with equal cell sizes.

DAISY PROFESSIONAL

DAISY Professional uses manageable four letter commands to invoke its procedures. Data entry is onto a convenient full-screen display. Statistical procedures are organized around a sensible concept of user needs.

DAISY Professional runs on Apple II, IIe, and Apple III computers. It sells for $203.45 from Rainbow Computing, 8811 Amigo Ave., Northridge, CA 91324 [(818) 349-0300].

Like most statistics packages, DAISY handles data in tables with the variables in columns and with a row for each observation. The number of rows that can be handled depends on the available computer main memory space. For an Apple IIe with 128,000 bytes of main memory, about 830 rows can be used. As many as 20 columns can be handled.

Four-letter commands

Users give instructions to this package by typing four-letter commands. Thus the ENTE command invokes a sequence of displayed queries that ask for the data, one row at a time, and for the names of the columns. The

QUIK command gives the user a look at a column of data, identified by name or number. The FILE command calls up a menu of file-manipulation choices.

Plotting the data

The DAISY manual wisely suggests that a good first step in many computer-based statistical investigations is to plot the data to get an immediate impression of whether there is a relationship between the variables.

The package offers the user histograms, useful for examining the data items in a single variable. It also allows the user to set up sequence plots that can help to discover trends, repeating cycles and unusual data points in a variable. For those whose computers allow high-resolution plotting, either the sequence points or their logarithms can be graphed.

To compare one variable to another, high-resolution scatter plots are available in linear, semilog, or logarithmic form. On these plots the axes will go through the means of the two variables, and the tick marks for the plot will denote units of standard deviation. If requested, the package will draw a regression line of best fit for the scatter plot.

Correlation capabilities

Another way of measuring the relationship between two variables is to calculate a correlation. The CORR command produces a table of product-moment correlation coefficients for any columns that the user selects. Partial correlations can also be computed when it is desirable to look at the relationship between two variables, after the effects of other variables have been considered. The COVA command calculates covariances between columns. Finally, the AUTO command does a correlation between a variable and a time-shifted version of that same variable. The user selects the desired time shift (number of rows). For interpretation, standard errors, and Box-Pierce scores are shown with the calculated autocorrelation figures.

In addition to the parametric correlation measures just mentioned, DAISY offers four nonparametric measures: the Spearman rank correlation, and the Kendall rank correlation, partial rank correlation, and coefficient of concordance. These are all based on the ranking of data items rather than on the data themselves. So, in order to use them it is necessary to first transform the data using the RANK command. The package will display an error message if a user tries to use these correlation measures with unranked data.

Regression models

Often, users want to use their data to predict the future course of events. Regression procedures allow trend lines to be fitted to existing data. These give an indication of data trends that may extend into the future. The REGR command calls up a sequence of choices and queries that allows users to do simple linear regression on two variables and multiple regression. There is also a forward stepwise regression procedure in which independent variables are added, one by one, to the regression calculation, with results calculated at each step. A backward stepwise regression procedure reverses the order, starting with all the variables and eliminating one independent variable at each step. Statistics designed to test the regression results are in the reports generated by these procedures. These include the multiple correlation R, R-squared, and the standard error of estimate.

If the user wishes, an ANOVA table will be displayed for the regression. This will show the sums of squared deviations accounted for by the regression, and the residuals that are left unexplained, along with the F-ratio.

To check on whether or not the residuals are autocorrelated, Durbin-Watson and Von Neumann statistics can be generated. For those who are interested, the beta weights for the variables are also calculated.

The package sets up special data columns for both the fitted and residual values of the regressions. These can be subjected to runs tests or autocorrelations, and the columns can be plotted against one another.

Users are warned that regression calculations may strain the capabilities of the package and are easily misinterpreted. Several internal checks are run by the package to turn up possibly serious rounding errors. In addition, the package warns the user if very high correlations turn up as these may indicate multicollinearity.

Once a regression solution has been obtained, the package uses the resulting equation to make predictions. These procedures are organized under the PRED command. This command can also be used to carry through cross-validation procedures, where the data are divided into two subsets. One set is used to develop a regression equation; the other data subset is then used to check the predicted values produced by that equation.

Working with data

DAISY has spreadsheet-like data entry and editing capabilities. The DATA command causes the first 16 rows in the first two columns of a data table to be displayed. The cursor can be moved about to any position in these columns.

Users can make data entries one after another, moving from one location to the next by hitting the appropriate arrow key. Other keyboard actions make the cursor jump to the start of the next row or column. Editing consists of typing a new number over the existing one at the cursor position. Users can even split the screen and compare nonadjacent columns side by side.

The manual warns that this package may take considerable time to do its calculations, and that only the first three to five digits of the results can be considered "dead accurate."

To use data from other packages, like VisiCalc, Lotus 1-2-3, and Multiplan, the vendor of DAISY offers a package called File Freedom. It runs on Apple II,IIe,IIc computers and sells for $99.95.

ELF

This menu-operated package offers standard statistical procedures along with stepwise regression and discriminant analysis.

There are versions of ELF that run on Apple and CP/M computers. These sell for $250 each. An IBM/PC version sells for $350. The Winchedon Group, 3907 Lakota Rd., P.O. Box 10339, Alexandria, VA 22310 [(703) 960-2587].

Up to 750 variables can be entered and stored in an ELF data file using an IBM/PC, and there can be up to 10,000 data items in a file.

One row at a time

Once the user names the data file and the variables that are to be in it, ELF displays an entry form for the first row that shows the variable names, each followed by a space for 10 characters. As each data item is filled in, pressing the space bar will move the cursor to the next item space.

When the data for that row are complete, the user can call up the display for the next row by pressing the return key. Or, if there are any typing errors, the process of entering that row can be repeated.

After all data for a file have been entered, there is a review and editing procedure that allows the user to leaf through displays of row data or jump to any row designated by its number. Here, the user can move the cursor, using the arrow keys, to any item and type over it with a corrected value. New rows can be added as desired.

New variables can also be added, using the review and editing procedure.

However, there seems to be no way to enter a new column of data without reviewing and editing complete rows of data, one at a time.

There seem to be no built-in procedures for merging files or extracting portions of files, but complete files can be translated to and from the DIF format used by such packages as VisiCalc.

Transformations

ELF requires users to write short programs in a special computer language in order to make data transformations. Allowed operations include arithmetic, selections based on $<$, $>$, $=$, and "odd" conditions, trigonometric, exponential, logarithmic, modulo 10, rounding, truncation, and absolute value.

Statistical procedures

Users select desired statistical procedures from a menu. In each procedure there is a series of screen-displayed queries. The user replies by typing appropriate answers, entering the files and variables to be processed and selecting procedure options, if any.

The STATISTICS procedure produces a set of descriptive measures including the mean, variance, standard deviation and error, minimum, maximum, and range, sum, kurtosis, and skewness. Significance and level of a normal distribution, t, F, and chi-square statistics are calculated by a "probabilities" procedure. There is also a separate procedure for t-tests on means for variables and groups of variables.

A correlation procedure produces a matrix of correlation coefficients for normally distributed variables. There do not appear to be any rank correlation procedures in this package.

There are procedures for one-way and two-way analyses of variance. Both are simple procedures that produce tables showing sum-of-squares and mean-square values and F statistics.

A cross-tabulation procedure produces tables for up to three variables.

There is a discriminant analysis procedure for separating rows into categories using one or more of the variables to perform the classification. A factor analysis procedure performs principal-components or principal-factors analyses. There is a choice of rotations.

A multivariate linear regression procedure uses a stepwise technique to enter and remove variables at the user's choice. A crude graph of actual and predicted values (standardized) can be produced. For time series data there is a procedure that corrects a regression for autocorrelated error terms. Up to 24 independent variables can be handled.

MICROSTAT

The authors of the MICROSTAT package have chosen to make all of its operations available through menu displays. Its data files have relatively large capacity. A good variety of statistical procedures are available. Data entry is on a query-and-answer basis.

MICROSTAT runs on IBM/PC and compatible computers and on CP/M computers. It sells for $375 from Ecosoft, 6413 N. College Ave., Indianapolis, IN 46220 [(317) 255-6476].

MICROSTAT data are stored in files, then recalled from storage when statistical procedures are to be applied. Data storage is controlled from a data management menu display. This display provides options for a number of data transformations, including arithmetic, logarithms and exponents, conversion to z-values, a linear transformation, rounding, truncation, random numbers, grouping, scaling, deletion, rank-ordering, sorting, and lag transformations.

The package also allows factorials, permutations, and combinations to be calculated, and will generate data for a number of different probability distributions, based on user-selected parameters. Available distributions include binomial, hypergeometric, Poisson, exponential, normal, F distribution, student's t, and chi-square.

There is a file directory display, and files can be renamed and erased by MICROSTAT menu choices. Files from some other packages and computers can be used by MICROSTAT. It will accept certain ASCII files, DIF-format files, and dBase II files.

As for the capacity of MICROSTAT files, an IBM/PC with 128,000-byte main memory can handle about 120 variables for most of the procedures. For multiple regression, about 60 predictor variables can be handled with such a computer.

Data entry

To start a new file, the user enters a file name and descriptive label, specifies the number of variables to be used, and gives a name for each of these.

Data are then entered on a row-by-row basis; the package will prompt with the row number and variable (column) numbers and names. Adding rows to the end of an existing file follows the same procedure. There is also a procedure for inserting new rows into an existing file. Editing is also done on a row-at-a-time basis; the user calls for the desired row, gets a display of the current entries in that row, then responds to queries asking for new values. All this is straightforward, but not as flexible and convenient as full-screen entry and editing.

The package allows display and printing of any subset of rows or columns in a file. The user can elect to change the number of places to be displayed to the right of the decimal point in each entry, so as to improve the appearance of the display. There is a batch mode of operation for those so inclined.

Statistical procedures

When users ask for descriptive statistics, there are two main choices. They can call for an abbreviated output that includes only the mean, standard deviation, and minimum and maximum values for all of the variables in the chosen file. Or they can choose from a wider range of descriptive statistics and specify exactly those variables for which the statistics will be supplied. The additional choices include the mean, variance and coefficient of variance, standard error, sum and sum of squares and sum of deviations around the mean, moments about the mean, and skewness and kurtosis, and a normal curve goodness of fit.

MICROSTAT will produce frequency distributions showing grouped categories of data values or counts of coded values.

Tests for means include checking the mean against a hypothesized value, the difference between means for paired observations, and the difference between two group means with known variance or with a polled estimate of variance.

There is a one-way and a two-way ANOVA procedure, and an ANOVA for randomized cases.

MICROSTAT will produce a correlation matrix for all variables in a file or for selected variables. It will also display the raw and adjusted sums of squares and cross products, and the covariances.

The regression analysis features perform simple, multiple, and stepwise-multiple regression on selected variables and subsets of variables. This involves a two-step computation procedure that can be lengthy. Results include means and standard deviations. The package allows the user to conveniently change the dependent variable or use another set of predictor variables and then rerun the calculation.

The regression output contains the regression coefficient, standard error, F value, a partial $r2$, the constant term, standard error of estimate, R-squared or r-squared, Multiple R or r, and an analysis of variance table.

Display of residuals and Durbin-Watson test results are optional. For stepwise regression, variables entered or removed are indicated, each with a tolerance and F to enter.

Time series analysis procedures calculate a moving average, or center moving average with seasonal indexes, or will perform exponential smoothing for selected variables.

Choices of nonparametric tests include the Wald-Wolfowitz runs test, the Wilcoxin signed ranks test and rank-sum test for two groups, the Kruskal-Wallis one way ANOVA by ranks, the Kolmogorov-Smirnov goodness of fit and two group tests, an absolute normal scores test, the Friedman test and the Kendall coefficient of concordance test, a sign test, the Fisher exact test, and the Spearman rank-order correlation.

A cross-tabs procedure, limited to 20 rows and 5 columns, generates a two-way contingency table by counting selected values from two variables. It will also calculate the chi-square statistic for the table and perform a Kolmogorov-Smirnov goodness of fit test.

Finally, the package will perform hypothesis tests for two proportions from independent groups, or for a sample proportions vs. a hypothesized value, or for two proportions from one group with overlapping or with mutually-exclusive categories.

Crude graphics

MICROSTAT provides a crude histogram display in connection with its frequency count. There are also scatter plots, with the points represented by asterisks, numerals, and # signs.

With the results of the multiple regression calculation, a similar graph displays standardized residual values.

MINITAB

Minitab is a statistical computer language with about 150 commands. The Minitab Fundamental version does descriptive statistics, simple and multiple regression, analysis of variance, nonparametric statistics, and cross tabulations. It produces scatter plots and histograms, generates random data, and has macro and looping capabilities. The Standard version does all that and also has time series analysis, stepwise regressions, and does exploratory data analysis and matrix operations.

Minitab runs on IBM/PC/XT/AT and compatibles, on the Victor 9000, the Fortune 32:16, and the DEC Professional 350. The Fundamental ver-

sion sells for $250, the Standard version for $500 from Minitab, 215 Pond Laboratory, University Park, PA 16802 [(814) 865-1595].

Data are input, a row at a time, with columns defined by the user. There is, however, no display of this data entry worksheet. What the user sees are the lines of data, with spaces or commas between the items. There is also a column-by-column data entry mode. For convenience, single commands can be used to generate a column with all row entries equal to a prescribed constant or filled with selected sequences of numbers.

These data entry procedures are each initiated by specific commands. Apparently, if any data entry errors are made, they are corrected by inserting a new, correct row of data and deleting the incorrect row. There seems to be no way to go directly to an incorrect data item and just correct that item. FORTRAN-formatted data files can also be used.

Simple histograms for individual variables can be displayed, and there are special histograms with Gaussian distributions fitted on them.

Available plots include scatter plots of two and of three variables. On the three-variable plots, positions in the z-dimension are indicated by the symbols used to mark the points. This feature is ingenious but of dubious value.

Multiple two-variable plots can be displayed on the same set of axes. There are also time series plotting formats for equally spaced data and for periodic data.

Data transformations include arithmetic, exponential, logarithmic, and trigonometric functions performed on columns. Other transformations include absolute value, sign, normal scores, and scaling.

The exploratory data analysis procedures include a stem and leaf display of selected columns, as well as box plots.

Statistical procedures

Minitab has commands for calculating descriptive statistics for rows or columns: counts, sums, means, standard deviations, medians, maxima and minima, and sums of squares. The package will also calculate t-confidence intervals and do two-sided t-tests and two-sided runs tests on column data.

Wilcoxon signed-ranks tests, rank estimates, and confidence intervals can be calculated for sets of columns.

A chi-square test can be performed on data in specified columns. The CONTINGENCY command constructs a contingency table from specified data and performs a chi-square test.

The REGRESSION command fits regression polynomials to selected columns of data. There are also stepwise regression procedures

The CORRELATION command calculates the Pearson product moment correlation between two columns, and the package will perform a Kruskal-Wallis non-parametric test.

Time series operations include computation of autocorrelations and partial autocorrelations, as well as cross correlations between two time series. There is also an ARIMA procedure that uses the Box-Jenkins methodology. Smoothing can be performed by a choice of methods using running medians and Hanning averages.

Other procedures include generation of tables of binomial and Poisson probabilities, a two-sample t-test, a Mann-Whitney two-sample rank test, and one-way and two-way analyses of variance.

NCSS: NUMBER CRUNCHER STATISTICAL SYSTEM

NCSS pulls together a large number of statistical procedures, makes them relatively easy to apply, and supplements them with helpful graphical displays.

This package runs on IBM/PC, CP/M, TRS-80, and Macintosh computers. It sells for $202 from NCSS, Dr. Jerry L. Hintze, 865 E. 400 N, Kaysville, UT 84037 [(801) 546-0445].

NCSS is menu-based. Starting with a main menu, the user moves to other menus that show the statistical and data procedures the package offers.

When it come to data handling, NCSS works from stored tables of data in which the columns represent the variables and the rows are individual observations. There may be up to 250 columns in a table, and the user must choose how many are to be used. The storage space the package allots to the table will depend on that choice and on the choice of the number of rows in the table. There can be up to 32,000 rows in a table.

Flexible data tables

The tables are set up with user-selected titles and the data items filled in by making selections from displayed menus, then responding to a series of screen-displayed queries with keyboard entries. This procedure could have been improved by presenting the user with a full-screen display of the table and having entry take place in a tabular format.

Transformations of the data in the tables may be done by adding, subtracting, multiplying, or dividing the items in one column by those in a second column, or by a constant, to form a transformed column. Single-column transformations include taking the absolute value, cumulative totaling, forming truncated or rounded-off integers from decimal numbers, calculating module remainders or signature values, taking Tukey's folded log or root, natural logs, exponents, square roots, and trigonometric functions. Columns of uniform-random or sequential numbers can be generated. There are also smoothing and lagging transformations, and values within a column can be sorted or ranked.

The package can generate a number of different probability distributions including the normal, inverse normal, chi-square, Student's t, F, Weibull, binomial negative binomial, and Poisson distributions.

Users are given considerable power to manipulate the stored tables. Standard ASCII files can be easily transformed into NCSS tabular files. Two tables may be joined, one above the other, or side to side. Individual columns may be copied from one table to another. Portions of tables may be selected out. Tables can even be rotated so that the rows become columns and vice-versa.

Descriptive statistics

Any column can be chosen for summary by descriptive statistics. Included in the unusually long list of measures generated will be the mean; standard deviation; variance; coefficient of variation; standard error of the mean; number of observations; number of missing values; sum of weights; adjusted sum of squares, of cubes, and of quartics; coefficients of kurtosis and skewness; the range and inner quartile range; a percentile, and a t-value for testing whether the mean is or is not equal to zero.

In addition to these single-column statistics, the package will produce a smaller number of descriptive statistics for rows selected from a column, where the selection is based on corresponding values in a second column.

Correlation and regression

In this package correlation coefficients and information on least squares regression are generated by the same procedure. The idea is that both represent measures of the linear relationship between two variables (columns of data). In the same vein, this procedure also generates the t-statistic for testing the significance of the slope.

A multiple regression procedure is included in the package, and there is also a procedure that provides for selecting and changing the variables to be included in a multiple regression model. Since outlier points can have a profound influence on regression analysis, NCSS provides a procedure, called Robust Regression, to locate such points and minimize their influence on the results. This procedure can be used as a check on regular multiple regression analysis.

NCSS provides a discriminant analysis procedure for cases where the dependent variable in a regression analysis is discrete rather than continuous.

When a set of data is analyzed, more variables may be involved than can be readily plotted, and several variables may represent the same general factor. NCSS provides a Principal Components Analysis procedure designed to determine the underlying factors of the data and to reduce the number of variables that have to be handled.

t-Tests and ANOVA procedures

NCSS includes both paired and unpaired t-tests. In connection with a one-way analysis-of-variance procedure, Fisher's LSD test can be used to determine which of the means are significantly different from each other. After the one-way ANOVA has been completed, Duncan's New Multiple Range Test and the Newman Keuls Multiple Range Test can be used to check the differences between two means.

The package also provides a two-way ANOVA procedure and an n-way ANOVA that will handle models with three or four factors. A Repeated Measures ANOVA is provided for designs where one treatment is an error term and another is a repeated measure of an experimental unit.

Tests of independence

To check for the independence of rows and columns in a data table, NCSS has a Chi-Square procedure that produces such measures as Chi Square, Phi, Cramer's U, Pearson's contingency coefficient and product-moment correlation, Tschupro's T, Lambda A and B, Symmetric Lambda, Kendall's tau-B and C, Gamma, and Spearman's Rho.

An alternative way to check for normality of the data is to do a Z-score, or inverse-normal quartile transformation. When the resulting scores are plotted against the original data, normally distributed data will produce a straight-line plot, and the degree of departure from a straight line is a measure of the departure from normality.

Nonparametric tests

Among the nonparametric tests included in the NCSS package are the Sign or Binomial test for determining that the mean of a variable has a particular value, or that the median of the difference between two variables is zero.

The Wald-Wolfowitz test is used to check for the randomness of a sequence of numbers made up of only two distinct values. The Wilcoxon Matched Pairs test checks on the difference between two sets of paired observations. The Mann-Whitney test check on the difference between the means of two unpaired groups.The Kruskal-Wallis test does a similar check for groups with unequal sample sizes. The Friedman Block/Treatment test checks whether the means of two or more treatment groups are equal.

Nonparametric correlations can be performed using Spearman's rank correlation coefficient and Kendall's tau coefficient.

Graphic tools

NCSS allows the user to plot the values of the rows in a column in histogram form, so that the data can be easily scanned for questionable values. With a graphics board plugged into the computer, the package will produce scatter plots of the row values from a pair of columns to visually reveal relationships and outlier points.

Box plots are also available. These show the location and spread of groups of data, in relation to the 75th and 25th percentiles, and extreme points are displayed as circles. These plots are generally used with treatment groups of ANOVA or t-test data.

As for the user's manual, it provides brief and often repetitious material on the various procedures, relying on many references to published works on statistics to fill in the gaps. The overall message to the users seems to be that if they don't understand what the package can do, they should go to the library and read another book.

PC STATISTICIAN AND STATS PLUS

A variety of different statistical procedures are offered by these two packages, along with regression and cross tabulation features. Package procedures are activated by choices from menu displays, with data entered either from the keyboard or from stored files.

STATS PLUS runs on Apple II,IIe,IIc computers; it sells for $200. PC STATISTICIAN is for IBM/PCs and compatible computers; it sells for $300. Both packages are from Human Systems Dynamics, 9010 Reseda Blvd. #222, Northridge, CA 91324 [(818) 993-8536].

Both STATS PLUS and PC STATISTICIAN perform about the same statistical procedures. PC STATISTICIAN, the more recently written package, seems a bit easier to access and operate, and the database functions seem more thoroughly integrated with the statistical computation procedures. Several features have been added to PC STATISTICIAN, including the ability to use files from such popular spreadsheet packages as Lotus 1-2-3 and VisiCalc.

Statistical features

Descriptive statistics can be computed by both packages for up to eight data variables at a time, with output including sample size, sum mean, standard deviation, and minimum and maximum values. PC STATISTICIAN gives added details on the means of dependent variables.

The packages will produce a frequency distribution from a set of data values, but the values must all be whole numbers. The output can include basic descriptive statistics, frequencies or proportions, and a percentiles report, with intervals chosen by the user. The packages will also display a frequency bar or polygon graph.

Any of three types of t-tests can be performed, including those for a single sample mean against a population mean; the difference between two correlated or dependent sample means, or between two independent means.

Nonparametric test procedures include the Mann-Whitney U Test, the Signed Ranks Test, Kruskal-Wallis Test, Friedman ANOVA by ranks, Spearman Rho, and Kendall Tau. PC STATISTICIAN adds the Wald-Wolfowitz Runs Test. The input data for these tests are ranked automatically and the sorting procedures involved can be lengthy.

Correlations can be calculated for up to five sets of data at a time. If the data sets are not all of the same size, the program will truncate them to produce equal size. Results are shown on the upper right portion of a four-row, four-column table of correlation coefficients. There are some display peculiarities. Correlations of $+1$ and -1 will appear as 999 and -999. The coefficients will appear as three-digit numbers with no decimal point, and correlations smaller than .001 will appear as 000. PC STATISTICIAN also provides for multiple correlations involving three to seven variables and has a partial correlation procedure.

An analysis-of-variance procedure produces a full summary table with F-ratios, p-values and descriptive statistics. Either one or two factors with equal or unequal sample sizes may be used.

A contingency-tables procedure allows the user to perform the Fisher Exact Test (STATS PLUS only) and one- or two-variable chi-square tests. These procedures accept keyboarded data, in the form of frequency counts.

Other package features

A STATS PLUS linear regression procedure performs a least squares calculation for one independent and one dependent variable. Multiple regression can be performed for two independent and one dependent variable. The output includes correlations and first-order partial correlations, as well as an analysis-of-variance table, regression coefficients, and significance tests. PC STATISTICIAN has a unified least squares regression procedure that will handle one to five predictor variables. And that package also has a curve-fitting option that uses power polynomials. In addition, PC STATISTICIAN has an x,y plotting capability that produces either scatter or line plots.

Finally, a cross-tabulation procedure analyzes stored data files, identifying each record in a file (based on the contents of its fields) as belonging to one of a set of categories, then generating reports on category occurrence frequency or percentage, along with basic descriptive statistics.

Using the database files

The example of STATS PLUS use given in the manual is for a set of 10 measurements of the strength of a material before, and after, a stressing procedure. The before and after data are stored in two fields of a database file. They are entered as data pairs. After the last pair is entered, the user simply keys in an asterisk in response to the query for the next pair, and the package creates the desired file. This stored file can then be called upon to calculate t-test results or to be run through any other appropriate procedure that the package offers.

Keyboard data entry for the statistical procedures offered by the STATS PLUS package is through serial query and answer. When long columns of data have to be entered, this can be clumsy, time consuming, and unforgiving of keyboard errors. However, database procedures include editing as well as entry. Apparently, for all but the simplest data sets, users are expected to do their data entry into the database portion of the package. In fact, with the PC STATISTICIAN package, all data entry is done through the database route.

As might be expected from a package that gave its author a chance to update an existing product, PC STATISTICIAN extends the database capabilities of STATS PLUS. For example, it will display a listing of available data files when the user presses a function key, and it offers additional data transformations, such as percent and z-scores, beyond those in the older package.

SPSS/PC

This is a statistical language with over 175 commands and subcommands, and a 600+ page manual. It provides an extensive list of statistical procedures but poor facilities for interactive data entry and editing. Flexible report generation is provided.

SPSS/PC for IBM/PC/XT computers sells for $795. A version for DEC Professional computers sells for $595. From SPSS Inc., 444 N. Michigan Ave., Chicago, IL 60611 [(312) 329-2400].

SPSS/PC is a personal computer version of a statistics package long used with large mainframe computers. To operate the package, users give the computer commands and SPSS/PC responds. In other words, this is a specialized computer language. There is actually a total of about 175 commands and subcommands that users need to be familiar with in order to exercise the full capabilities of the package. And there are many details of syntax and usage that must be mastered as well.

Probably because of its large-computer origins, the authors of this package could not resist providing a batch processing mode of operation in which the user can enter all commands and data, then let the computer run them without further user interaction.

To document the use of this language, the package comes with a manual that is well over 600 pages long. It describes how each statistical procedure works and shows many of the equations on which the computations are based. A good part of the manual is devoted to spelling out the commands and related procedures.

SPSS/PC is a package for serious users who are willing to invest the time to learn to use a new language. For those who will find frequent, consistent use for the package, it will be a worthwhile investment. Other users, who may turn only occasionally to the statistical tools offered by SPSS/PC, will probably feel that learning to use this package is an overly budensome task.

Errorless data

The DATA LIST command is used for interactive data entry. Up to 200 variables can be defined. For "fixed format" input, the user specifies the exact row locations in which each variable will appear; this is done as if the data were being entered on a punched card, so each numeral is assigned to a specific card-column position. There is also a "freefield" format in which exact row locations of the data need not be spelled out. Freefield data items are entered with a space or comma between each item. They can be strung out to any length, on as many lines of the input display as desired. The only requirement is that they be in row-by-row order.

When punched cards are used to input data into large computers, the processes of verifying and correcting the data take place on the punching equipment, not in the computer. The authors of the SPSS/PC package seem to have assumed that the data input to the personal computer will also be pure and correct. There seem to be no convenient built-in procedures in the package that would allow users to easily correct errors in the data they type into the keyboard.

Data entered with the DATA LIST command can be displayed, using the LIST command. They can be stored and retrieved, and files of data from mainframe versions of SPSS, or files produced by other packages, can be used by SPSS/PC, provided they are in compatible formats.

Data transformations available with SPSS/PC include arithmetic, exponents, logarithms, trigonometric functions, absolute value, truncation, rounding, modulo 10, lag, and conversion of dates into day intervals. Conditional transformations can be controlled by Boolean logic operators. Pseudo-random numbers can be generated. There is also a transformation that counts occurrences of the same value across a list of variables

For those who want to turn out neat summary reports on their statistical findings, SPSS/PC provides a report generation capability. This allows result and input data to be combined, with added headings, breakouts, and comments, on printed pages formatted by the user. As with the other features of this package, a report generation program using SPSS/PC commands has to be written.

Statistical procedures

A FREQUENCIES procedure produces frequency tables and descriptive statistics, including the mean, standard error of the mean, standard deviation, median, mode, variance, skewness and standard error of skewness, kurtosis and standard error of kurtosis, range, minimum and maximum, sum, and percentiles, for selected variables. It also produces bar charts for discrete variables and histograms for continuous variables.

Means, standard deviations, and group counts are generated by the MEANS command for a dependent variable with groups defined by one or more independent variables.

A *t*-test procedure calculates Student's *t* and displays the two-tailed probability of the differences between the means. Statistics can be produced for independent or paired samples.

Nonparametric tests available in SPSS/PC include one-sample binomial, chi-square, Kolmogorov-Smirnov, and runs tests. For two related samples there are Mcnemar, sign, and Wilcoxon tests. For *k* related samples there are Cochran, Friedman, and Kendall tests. For two independent samples, there are Mann-Whitney, Kolmogorov-Smirnov, Wald-Wolfowitz, and Moses tests. For *k* independent samples, there are Kruskal-Wallis and median tests.

A CORRELATION procedure does Pearson product-moment correlations with one-, or two-tailed probabilities. It will also produce univariate statistics, covariances, and cross-product deviations.

Multiple regression equations, associated statistics, and plots can be produced by the REGRESSION procedure. Predicted values, residuals, and related statistics are calculated. The automatic variables are available for analysis by various plots.

The ONEWAY command does a one-way analysis of variance for an interlevel dependent variable, with groups defined by one numeric independent variable. The ANOVA command handles up to 5 dependent variables, 10 factors, and 10 covariates.

A CLUSTER procedure produces heirarchical clusters of items using any of six measures of similarity or distance to one or many variables. The CROSSTABS procedure does *n*-way tabulations with up to 250 rows or columns for each variable.

The FACTOR procedure does factor analyses using a choice of seven extraction methods. A HILOGLINEAR procedure fits heirarchical loglinear models to multidimensional contingency tables using iterative proportional-fitting algorithms. This procedure is for data from populations that are not normally distributed with constant variance. Up to 10 factors can be handled.

Plots and graphs

SPSS/PC can do a variety of printed plots, with plot symbols chosen by the user. These include simple bivariate scatterplots, scatterplots with a control variable, contour plots, and overlay plots.

STATPAC

This package is very well organized, sometimes tediously so. It allows users to set up their own input procedures. A reasonable selection of statistical procedures is provided, and the documentation is excellent.

StatPac runs on IBM/PC and compatible computers and on CP/M computers. It sells for $495 from Walonick Associates, 6500 Nicollet Ave So., Minneapolis, MN 55423 [(612) 866-9022].

Each of the procedures of this package is accessed through a menu display. Thus, on the Data Management menu, the user can access Enter New Data and be presented with four ways to enter data.

User-controlled input procedures

In the row-by-row keyboard entry procedure, variable names are displayed for the first row, and the user types in the data items after each name. Then the same names are displayed for entry of the values for the second row, and so on. There is also a keypunch emulation procedure in which the user types data on the screen in a rigidly prescribed format.

Data editing, after a data file has been stored, is carried out with a keypunch-like procedure. Three rows of data are displayed, and the user can scroll or page up or down to the other rows, or the package will search for a row designated by number. The cursor can be moved or tabbed along the current row and, at the cursor position, a character can be deleted or added.

Users can also devise their own input "screens." This capability permits either row-by-row or column-by-column input procedures. The order of inputting the data and the labels used for columns can be varied by the user. Data inputs can be restricted to assigned ranges of numbers or other symbols. The screens can include whatever instruction or reminder text the user wishes to add. The idea appears to be that operators with little or no knowledge of statistics will do data entry, and that these screens can be designed for their use.

There is a separate editing procedure for these screens that involves locating the desired screen, positioning the cursor, then deleting or adding characters.

Managing files and procedures

To keep stored data in order, users are required to create an overall index (called a "codebook") to all the files and variables. There is also an overall management routine for the statistical procedures. This controls the sequencing of these procedures and is also used for any needed selection and recoding of data.

What this amounts to is that if users want to run just one statistical procedure, they have to give it a title, select the procedure and the desired options for that procedure, identify by number the variables to be processed, and specify any needed data recoding or selections. All this has to be done before any actual statistical computation can begin.

It is a very formalized routine that may tend to discourage the exploratory approach to statistical analysis permitted by personal computers.

Statistical procedures

StatPac has a frequency-analysis procedure that will sort selected variables by value or by frequency of response, calculate cumulative percentages, and produce tables and bar-chart or pie-chart frequency displays.

The descriptive statistics procedure calculates all the usual measures and also gives the 95 and 99 percent confidence intervals around the mean. A chart of number of cases vs. scores can be displayed.

Cross tabulation can be done for one variable against a list of variables. A table of up to 50 rows by 50 columns can be produced, along with appropriate statistical measures.

The correlation procedure produces a coefficient and other statistics for two normally distributed variables. Spearman's rank-order coefficient will also be calculated. This procedure can also be used to display a scattergram showing the relationship between the variables. A regression line will be calculated and displayed.

The t-test procedure includes tests for matched pairs or for two independent groups.

Stepwise multiple regression can be performed for a dependent variable and a list of independent variables. This procedure will produce descriptive statistics, regression statistics and coefficients, simple and partial correlation matrices, and an analysis of the residuals.

There are one-way and two-way analysis-of-variance procedures that operate from grouped data. These produce ANOVA tables, t-tests between groups, critical F and T probabilities, and descriptive statistics for the two-way ANOVA.

Good documentation

The user's manual spells out very clearly what the user has to do. Formulas used in the computations are given and explained, and there is a list of the textbook sources for these formulas. The manual also lists the error messages that the package may produce, along with a brief explanation of each one. Finally, there is a well-organized index to the manual so it can readily be used as a reference.

SYSTAT

This package offers the user a statistical computing language with about 100 commands, plus a version of BASIC. A full-screen entry and editing procedure eases data input. Up to 200 variables can be handled.

SYSTAT runs on IBM/PCs and compatible computers, and on CP/M computers. It sells for $495 from Systat, Inc., 603 Main St., Evanston, IL 60202 [(312) 864-5670].

SYSTAT is a statistical computer language with almost 100 commands used to exercise its full capabilities. In fact, the package includes a version of the BASIC computer language that can be used to put together routines for manipulating data, sampling, and performing complex transformations. Most calculations are done in double precision with 15-digit accuracy.

The package is divided up into modules, one for handling data and others for various types of statistical procedures. Each module has a set of commands peculiar to its operations, so the SYSTAT language can be learned piecemeal, starting with those procedures the user needs first.

At the end of a procedure, SYSTAT prints a log of all the commands used during the session. This is convenient for users who expect to perform similar procedures.

Full-screen data entry

SYSTAT takes advantage of personal computer capabilities in that it uses full-screen data entry and editing. Columns for variables can be set up and filled with data by moving the display cursor to the appropriate positions on the display. When data are methodically filled in, a row at a time, the cursor will automatically jump to the next input position as each item is entered. If a change needs to be made, the cursor can be moved, using arrow keys, to the desired item, and the correct data can be typed over the existing data. Variable names can be changed in the same way.

The data display can contain as many rows as can be stored in the disk used with the package. It can accept numbers with up to 15 digits. Once entered, the data are stored and the files can be read, merged, sorted, and transposed for use with the statistical procedures of the package.

There is an alternative data entry procedure in which the user creates data files without the full-screen display. SYSTAT also has provisions for receiving similar files from packages like Lotus 1-2-3, dBase II, and WordStar and converting them to SYSTAT format. In some cases, these files will have to be pre-edited with the user's own word processor or editing package.

Transformations are handled as part of data editing procedures, using the LET command together with the name of the variable to be transformed and the mathematical operation to be used. Available operations include arithmetic, exponents, logarithms, and trigonometric functions. Ranking and standardizing are handled by separate commands.

Statistical procedures

For basic descriptive statistics, the STATISTICS command is used. This displays counts, maxima and minima, means, and standard deviations. The mean, skewness, kurtosis, range, variance, and standard error of the mean are available on request.

A correlation module calculates symmetric triangular matrices of correlation and similarity for data sets. Types of matrices that can be calculated include sum of squares and cross products, covariance, Pearson correlation, gamma coefficients, Guttman mu2 coefficients, Spearman rank correlations, Kendall tau-b coefficients, and normalized Euclidean distances.

Nonparametric statistics for groups of rows or pairs of columns include the sign test, Wilcoxon signed ranks test, the Friedman and Kruskal-Wallis one-way analyses of variance, and the Kolmogorov-Smirnov one- and two-sample tests.

A tables module produces multiway tables and can fit them with a log-linear model. Fitted models are tested with Pearson and likelihood ratio chi-square statistics.

An MLGH procedure can estimate and test any univariate or multivariate general linear model, allowing linear contrasts on vectors of dependent as well as independent variables. This procedure can perform multivariate profile analysis of repeated measures, ANOVA, multivariate ANOVA, discriminant analysis, simple regression, multiple and multivariate regression, stepwise regression, analysis of covariance, principal components analysis, and canonical correlation.

A "factor" analysis procedure produces a principal-components analysis with optional rotations and factor scores. An MDS procedure provides nonmetric multidimensional scaling of similarity or dissimilarity matrices in one to five dimensions. This procedure is said to usually be able to fit an appropriate model in fewer dimensions than can be done using principal-components or factor analysis.

There is also a cluster-analysis procedure for detecting natural groupings in data. The JOIN command produces heirarchical clustering with a tree diagram showing the relationships between columns or rows. There is also a command for *k*-means clustering.

To aid in time-series analysis, there is a SMOOTH command that can calculate moving averages and running medians and does linear filtering with Hanning weights as well as and scatterplot smoothing. There is also Fourier transform smoothing, and an ARIMA, AutoRegressive Integrated Moving Average, procedure.

Stem and leaf plots

SYSTAT can produce a variety of crude plots made up of printed characters. Scatter plots and function plots can be produced by the PLOT command. With the help of some BASIC programming, crude contour plots can also be done. The HISTOGRAM command produces plots with bars made up of asterisks.

The STEMLEAF command produces a histogram-like display made up of numerals, which can give users insight into the repeated appearance of certain discrete values in the data. The BOX command produces box plots, used to quickly identify median, hinges, and outside values in the data.

Probability plots, which show a variable plotted against corresponding percentage points of a standard normal variable, are produced by the PPLOT command. The QPLOT command compares a sample to its quartiles, or the quartiles of two samples to one another.

Chapter 16
Instrumentation Packages

Instrumentation software packages are designed to collect and interpret information from equipment outside the computer and also to exert control over that equipment. More often than not the incoming information is in the form of continuously varying analog signals.

To convert these signals into digital form acceptable to the computer, and to properly interconnect the computer to outside instrumentation, interface circuits are needed. Generally the interface takes the form of circuit boards that plug into the computer.

Many different brands and types of such circuit boards are available, some designed to accept direct connections from individual instruments, others built to feed into an instrument "bus" (wires or cable to which many instruments can be connected).

Specialized instrumentation languages

The most flexible way to exercise computer control over intrumentation is to use a set of general commands that can be sequenced to perform whatever task is at hand, in other words, to use a computer instrumentation language.

The AMPRIS package is designed for just that purpose. It provides a set of special commands that can be used as an extension of the BASIC computer language. Thus, AMPRIS analog input commands include those for taking single and serial readings and for averaging inputs from specific channels. Multiple channels, sequentially or in arbitrary sequence, can also be scanned on command.

AMPRIS also includes analog output commands that provide for sending prescribed single signals or series of signals to specific channels, and there is a command to send such signals to a set of successive channels. For digital devices, those with on-off output, there are commands to take single or multiple input readings from specific channels and to generate digital outputs on specific channels.

There are actually several versions of AMPRIS, one for each specific type (analog or digital, with 2 to 16 channels) of interface circuit supplied by the vendor.

PC-488 is a package designed for use with the IEEE-standard 488 instrumentation bus. Like AMPRIS, this package is for use by engineers who are adept at programming, but there are some striking differences. Everything PC-488 has to offer is contained on a circuit board that plugs into the computer. The software (called, in this form, firmware) is packaged along with the interface circuitry on this board.

PC-488 commands provide an instrumentation extension to BASIC, Pascal, C, and other computer languages. These commands implement the functions provided by the circuit board. On an IEEE-488, bus, all communications are centrally controlled and PC-488 equips the computer to function as such a central controller. For example, sequences of commands and data are sent using the TRANSMIT command. LISTEN and TALK designate the instrumentation device that will do the sending and those that will be receiving. SEND and ENTER establish the computer as a talker or a listener. There are SPOLL and PPOLL commands for serial and parallel polling of devices attached to the bus. In all there are about 15 of these PC-488 commands.

A more universal language

Because instrumentation software has been so closely tied to interface circuits, the software packages are usually designed to work only with one particular type of plug-in circuit. An exception to this rule is the ASYST package.

Like the packages already mentioned, ASYST provides a set of programming commands for reading and controlling instrumentation. These are actually part of a larger set of ASYST commands designed to perform data analysis, statistics, and a variety of mathematical operations useful in engineering and scientific applications.

But unlike these other packages, ASYST includes the ability to work with a number of different interfaces. At the time this report was written, ASYST included customized routines for using the Data Translation DT2801 board, and the Techmaster Lab Master, Lab Tender and DADIO boards; the Keithley DAS Series 500 instrumentation system can also be handled. ASYST is not a perfect universal instrumentation language, for there are some ifs, ands, and buts about using specific interfaces, but the basic idea is a powerful one: once a user learns to program the ASYST commands, they can be used with many different interfaces.

However, like any instrumentation package that simply provides programming commands, ASYST is not a package designed to conveniently control instruments. It offers the user no menus of available functions, nor does it have predesigned formats to organize its use. Instead, like the BASIC language, it simply presents the user with an OK prompt and waits for commands to be keyboarded.

User-oriented packages

Instrumentation software packages designed for use by engineers who are not programmers have begun to appear. Thus far, most of these packages are directed to specific types of instruments. Thus the CHROMATO-CHART package collects data from up to four chromatographs, massages the data, displays stripcharts, and stores the data. It also produces printed reports on the characteristics of integrated peaks and compares unknown to standard data.

CHROMATOCHART operates from a series of screen-displayed menus. The user makes selections by keying in the number of the desired item on the menu. When information is to be input, the user is presented with a screenful of information and choices, makes them or changes them until satisfied, then can look the screen over and enter it into active use. The keyboard arrow keys are used to maneuver around the screen while editing.

With the help of a plug-in interface board, the RTFSA package allows a personal computer to be used as a spectrum analyzer with 10-KHz bandwidth. The package accepts filtered or unfiltered data, performs fast Fourier transform analysis, and plots the magnitude of frequency spectra. Another package called SPECSYSTEM works with external acoustical spectrum analyzer equipment to implement such applications as analysis of noise, engine and machinery diagnostics, music, sound, and voice analysis.

More general instrumentation capabilities are provided by the Analog Connection package. This package logs and displays the maximum, minimum, and average values of analog signals and signal differences. Digital, on-off, inputs, and outputs are also handled. The package works with plug-in interface boards, each of which connects to up to 16 different inputs.

The Analog Connection package operates through well-designed and easy-to-use menus and display screens. There are two main menus, one for setting up the operation of the package, the other for actually using the package to monitor or manipulate instrumentation readings.

Particular attention is paid to the laborious details of setting up the individual parameters for each input. These include such items as the range that will be used, the units that will be displayed, types of thermocouples that will be used, scale and offset factors, and alarm limits. By following the menu procedures, all these parameters can be set up in an organized manner. There is virtually nothing for the user to memorize, so that neophytes and occasional users of this package should have an easy time following these procedures whenever needed.

Although use of the package is quite simple, it does take experience to most effectively use some aspects of the Analog Connection package. For example, the user can specify the resolution of input readings, the rate at which readings are taken, and the A/D conversion filtering time. But all these, in turn, affect the time required to cycle through a set of readings, so some knowledgeable juggling may be needed.

It is important to contrast the capabilities of packages intended for engineering instrumentation applications with a similar class of packages designed strictly for educational use in student laboratories. Consider, for example, the simple temperature reading package TEMPERATURE PLOTTER. It is very low cost, only a fraction of the price of the other packages discussed here, and very easy to use. However, the package has limitations that make it unuseable for most engineering applications. Thus, each reading takes a minimum of one second, only four probes can be monitored, and a total of only 512 readings can be stored. There are also limitations, which may be unacceptable, on the accuracy of the results and of the calibration procedures.

Timing considerations

As in any instrumentation situation, accuracy is a key consideration when using a computer software package. And one way the accuracy issue arises is in terms of timing accuracy.

Two main sources of timing are generally used in connection with these packages. Timing may be derived either from the computer and the software, or from separate timing circuits that are usually mounted on the instrumentation interface circuit board.

Because of the inherently unpredictable nature of computer software timing, the AMPRIS vendor recommends that all such times should be considered to have a 5 percent worst-case tolerance. Most instrumentation software package vendors do not mention the problem, but a similar tolerance should be applied for any time intervals derived in this way. If more accurate intervals are needed, separate timing circuits should be used.

Control outputs

When dealing with instrumentation, it is often as important to control the operation of external equipment as it is to collect information. With control commands, used in programs written by the user, very flexible control can be exercized. But some of the user-oriented packages, designed for nonprogrammers, also provide quite powerful control measures.

The CHROMATOCHART package, for example, is set up to produce output signals suitable for controlling gradient pumps. Two pumps can be controlled at one time to produce desired mixtures of two fluids. Gradient profiles, created by using the package, can be used to define the mixtures, and these profiles are constructed and changed with the help of a display menu.

As for more generalized control, the Analog Connection plug-in board is able to produce digital (on-off) output signals as well as accept inputs, and the package gives users very flexible control over the input conditions that will cause outputs to be generated. Not only can various logical combinations of digital inputs be used to control these outputs, but the outputs themselves can be used to define the logic of other outputs. Effects of analog inputs can be included (by specifying set points and dead bands) in determining these logical output controls.

Graphical output

Often, showing instrumentation information in graphical form is essential to interpretation and use. Some packages include their own graphical capabilities. Others ignore graphics or would have the user turn to auxiliary programs for graphical output.

Graphics are quite essential to spectrum analysis, and the SPECSYSTEM package is well provided in this area. The package assembles and stores large arrays of spectral data. These data arrays are then displayed in the form of geometrical surfaces with dimensions of time, frequency, and amplitude. Alternatively, curves representing the data for individual spectrum channels can be displayed.

The Analog Connection package has no built-in capabilities for graphics. Instead users are instructed to feed stored data to the Lotus 1.2.3 package for creating graphs, printing formatted reports, and doing spreadsheet-type analyses.

Among the packages that provide instrumentation commands for programming, ASYST includes graphical commands that can be called upon to create displays as needed.

AMPRIS: INSTRUMENTATION COMMANDS
FOR APPLE COMPUTERS

Each of the AMPRIS packages provides a set of instrumentation control commands for a specific plug-in interface board from the vendor.

The AMPRIS-02 package ($125) is for use with the AI02 8-bit, 16-channel analog input board ($299). The AMPRIS-13 package ($225) is for the AI13 12-bit, 16-channel analog input board ($550). The AMPRIS-03 package ($125) is for the AO03 analog output board with 2,4, or 8 output channels ($195, $275, $437). The AMPRIS-09 and 09 INT packages ($195, $125) are for the DI09 input-output board ($330). All packages and boards are for use with Apple II and IIe computers. The vendor is Interactive Structures, 146 Montgomery Ave, P.O. Box 404, Bala Cynwyd, PA 19004 [(215) 667-1713].

The AMPRIS commands are all written in assembly language, and they can be called in programs written in the BASIC language.

Time intervals, used in controlling the interfaces, are derived from internal computer timing. Because of the inherently unpredictable nature of this timing technique, the vendor recommends that all times should be considered to have a 5 percent worst-case tolerance. The digital interface card includes a timer implemented in circuitry to provide more accurate inter-event delays.

Analog input commands include those for taking single and serial readings, and for averaging inputs, from specific channels. Multiple channels, sequentially or in arbitrary sequence, can also be scanned on command.

Analog output commands provide for sending prescribed single signals or series of signals to specific channels, and there is a command to send such signals to a set of sucessive channels.

For digital devices, those with on-off output, there are commands to take single or multiple input readings from specific channels and to generate digital outputs on specific channels. Other commands control the operation of interval timers and of shift registers used for serial-parallel conversions of digital data. There are also commands to control interrupt signals from devices that request immediate attention.

Five binary utility commands are provided with each AMPRIS package to ease the process of doing logical, Boolean manipulation of numerical quantities.

ANALOG CONNECTION: HANDLING ANALOG
AND DIGITAL SIGNALS

This package logs and displays the maximum, minimum, and average values of analog signals and signal differences. Digital, on-off, inputs, and outputs are handled. It provides flexible user specification of both inputs and outputs.

The package runs on IBM/PC/XT/AT computers. It works with a plug-in circuit board; the price of the board and software combination is $690. A similar combination for the Apple II, II+, IIe sells for $490. The vendor is Strawberry Tree Computers, 949 Cascade Dr., Sunnyvale, CA 94087 [(408) 746-3083].

This package operates through well-designed and easy-to- use menus and parameter display screens. There are two main menus, one for setting up the operation of the package, the other (called the "display" menu) for actually using the package to monitor or manipulate instrumentation readings.

Good control over inputs

Up to 16 input signals can be handled by each plug-in circuit board. The board converts analog inputs to digital form so they can be used by the computer.

The package gives the user control over important parameters for each input, including the range that will be used, the units that will be displayed, types of thermocouples that will be used, scale and offset factors, and alarm limits. By following the menu procedures, all these parameters can be set up in an organized manner. There is virtually nothing for the user to memorize, so that neophytes and occasional users of this package should have an easy time following these procedures whenever needed.

There is one major stumbling block that can come up. The sixth choice on the setup menu list includes selecting the number of channels that will be actively used from each plug-in board. If the user makes any changes in this choice, the menu display warns "This will erase most of your setup. Make this selection first." However, for the unwary user who has already worked through dozens of screens to set up input parameters, this warning may come too late. It is not sufficiently emphasized in the manual.

If the plug-in board contains an "analog" clock, it's output can be used to control the timing of readings and outputs. If not, the digital clock set up by the computer's system software can be used for this purpose. One of the setup display screens gives the user control over this choice.

It does take some experience to most effectively use some aspects of this package. For example, the user can specify the resolution (smallest detectable change) the cicuit board will recognize in the inputs. The rate at which readings are taken can also be specified, as can the A/D conversion filtering time. These adjustments, as well as the number of active input channels, can affect the time needed to cycle through a set of readings.

For user convenience, the input channels can be assigned descriptive names, a valuable feature in readily interpreting displayed results.

Flexible digital outputs

The plug-in board is able to produce digital (on-off) output signals as well as accept inputs, and the package gives users very flexible control over the input conditions that will cause outputs to be generated. Not only can various logical combinations of digital inputs be used to control these outputs, but the outputs themselves can be used to define the logic of other outputs. Effects of analog inputs can be included (by specifying set points and dead bands) in determining these logical output controls.

The package will display and store readings, differences between readings, maximum, minimum, and average values for each input and output, under software control. It will also log these values at intervals selected by the user.

A potentially helpful feature of the package is the capability to easily feed stored data to the Lotus 1.2.3 package for creating graphs, printing formatted reports, and doing spreadsheet-type analyses. However, it would have been preferable to have some of these facilities built into the Analog Connection package itself.

An awkward manual

A potentially confusing aspect of display-screen operation is the way that multiple-choice items work. To change from one choice to another, the user has to repeatedly select the menu item containing the multiple choice. At each selection the chosen option shifts. For example, to specify when data logging is to begin, one of the menu items offers six possibilities: Immediate ON, MIN, HR, 12HR, and DAY. Initially the first of these is shown highlighted, indicating it is the current choice. If the user selects that menu item, the highlighting will shift to the MIN; a second selection of that same menu item will shift the highlighting to the HR, etc. This method of operation is not adequately explained in the documentation for the package.

To find out exactly what these various multiple choices actually mean, it is necessary to read the user's manual, and this points up futher shortcomings in the documentation. Occasional users, who can't remember that HR means logging will begin on the next even hour, may well want to look up that meaning in the manual. It is hard to find, buried on page 33, and the index to the user's manual gives little help.

ASYST ACQUISITION MODULE: AN INSTRUMENTATION LANGUAGE

ASYST is a computer language, in the same sense that BASIC or FORTRAN are computer languages. It was designed with engineering and scientific problem solving in mind and has a variety of capabilities, including those in the areas of graphics and mathematics. This Acquisition module provides about 77 commands for using the computer to control aquisition of data from instrumentation devices and to manipulate the data for use by the computer.

The package works together with the ASYST System, Graphics Statistics module; both are required to support the functions of the Aquisition module, and both run on IBM/PC/XT/AT computers. The combined price of the two modules is $1290 from Macmillan Software Co., 866 Third Ave., New York, NY 10022 [(212) 702-3428].

ASYST is not a package designed to conveniently control instruments. It provides the user with no menus of available functions, nor does it have predesigned formats to organize its use. Instead, like the BASIC language, it simply presents the user with an OK prompt and waits for commands to be keyboarded. As with any other language, these commands must reside primarily in the user's head, which means that the ASYST language must be learned before it can be used.

Will it be used?

As with any other computer language, regardless of its intrinsic merits, the success or failure of ASYST will rest on the extent to which it is adopted and used by programming-minded engineers and scientists. If and when these users write programs that can, in turn, be put to use by the vast majority of engineers who have little or no interest in doing programming, then ASYST will indeed become a significant engineering tool.

ASYST appears to be a unique language, capable of rapidly implementing procedures that more standard languages like BASIC may process at a crawl. But ASYST has its own shortcomings. It does not seem oriented toward programmers, the very people it must please if it is ever to amount to anything. For example, programs written in ASYST seem to work efficiently, but they are very difficult to understand and therefore they will be hard to debug and modify. Since a large portion of most programming projects goes into correcting and changing what has been written, it seems unlikely that ASYST will gain much popularity among those who do this work.

Customized universality

ASYST strives for universality. The acquisitions module is presented as a universal way to control an IBM/PC/XT/AT connected to instrumentation devices. What this actually involves, however, is making ASYST work with specific existing interface equipment and particularly interface boards that can be plugged into those computers.

At the time this review was written, ASYST included customized routines for using the Data Translation DT2801 board, the Techmaster Lab Master, Lab Tender and DADIO boards, and some others as well. The Keithley DAS Series 500 System can also be handled, but its use required the creation of an additional settling-time command for ASYST. There are other ifs, ands, and buts about using specific interfaces. For example, depending on how the DADIO board is set up, the operation of ASYST input-output commands may become abnormal.

CHROMATOCHART: CONTROLLING CHROMATOGRAPHS

The CHROMATOCHART package collects data from up to four chromatographs, massages the data, displays stripcharts, and stores the data. It also produces printed reports on the characteristics of integrated peaks and compares unknown to standard data.

CHROMATOCHART is used with the ADALAB plug-in board (see the review of the QUICK I/O package later in this report). The package runs on Apple II+, IIe computers and sells for $800 from Interactive Microware, P.O. Box 139, State College, PA 16804 [(814) 238-8294].

CHROMATOCHART operates from a series of screen-displayed menus. The user makes selections by keying in the number of the desired item on the menu. As users get into these menus they will discover some unusual features. For example, the symbols $, :, or # indicate that the user must key in text, integer numbers between -32767 and $+32767$, or a power of two. For a package that tries to cater to user needs, this is hardly a convenience.

A more useful feature is that the user is presented with a screenful of information and choices, makes them or changes them until satisfied, then can look the screen over and enter it into active use. The keyboard arrow keys are used to maneuver around the screen while editing.

In this manner, the user can set up needed file names and identification of chromatograph runs. For data acquisition, the user is asked to provide memory address locations for the runs, the number of points to be averaged and summed, the chart delay, width, scale, and offset. Similarly, the user specifies the reports that are to be produced on another screen.

Users can also set up a schedule of control events that are to occur in the course of monitoring the inputs and operating pumps. The package can produce output signals suitable for controlling gradient pumps. Two pumps can be controlled at one time to produce desired mixtures of two fluids. Gradient profiles, created by using the package, can be used to define the mixtures. These profiles are constructed and changed with the help of another display menu.

Integration routines, menu operated as are most of the package features, measure peak area, retention time, height, width at half-height, and skew.

PC-488: INTERFACE WITH FIRMWARE

This product is for use by engineers who are adept at programming. PC-488 is a circuit board that plugs into IBM/PC/XT computers. The software (firmware) is packaged within the circuitry on this board; it provides an instrumentation extension to BASIC, Pascal, C, and other languages used on these computers. The PC-488 commands implement the functions provided by the circuit board, and the instrumentation interface provided by the board conforms to the IEEE-488 standard.

The PC-488 board sells for $395 from Capital Equipment Corp., 10 Evergreen Ave., Burlington, MA 01803 [(617) 273-1818].

At its simplest, the PC-488 can be used to connect a printer to the IBM/PC/XT, but it is intended as a means to hook in a whole string of instruments or other bus-connected devices through a single interface to the computer.

The programs that implement PC-488 commands are written in IBM/PC assembly language and can be used by the PC-DOS system software or called from the computer language the user employs.

The commands themselves are high level, in the sense that they implement instrumentation functions. Their essential function is to control the communications between the computer and other devices attached to an IEEE-488 instrumentation bus.

On an IEEE-488 bus all communications are centrally controlled. With the PC-488 an IBM/PC/XT is equipped to function as such a central controller.

Sequences of commands and data are sent using the TRANSMIT command. LISTEN and TALK designate the instrumentation device that will do the sending and those that will be receiving. SEND and ENTER establish the IBM/PC as a talker or a listener. There are SPOLL and PPOLL commands for serial and parallel polling of devices attached to the bus. Other commands perform such functions as direct transfer of data between the IBM/PC memory and the bus. In all there are about 15 of these PC-488 commands.

QUICK I/O: INSTRUMENTATION INTERFACE SETUP AND COMMANDS

Quick I/O is a package for use by BASIC programmers. It is used with the ADALAB plug-in interface board in Apple II+, IIe computers. The software, together with the ADALAB board, sells for $495 from Interactive Microware, P.O. Box 139, State College, PA 16804. [(814) 238-8294].

Quick I/O includes a convenient means of testing the ADALAB board and its time and alarm functions. But the main feature of the package is the set of instrumentation control commands it provides.

These commands can be keyboarded to immediately control devices connected to the ADALAB board. Usually, however, they will be imbedded in programs written in the Applesoft BASIC language. From a programmer's point of view, the commands are simply and uniformly structured. They are able to handle inputs or outputs (each board has a D/A output and an A/D input) and to handle single devices or several connected in parallel to a single board.

In any case, one must be a programmer to use these commands for monitoring or controlling instrumentation devices. The vendor is, however, beginning to produce packages directed to the needs of users who do not wish to write programs in order to control instrumentation with a computer. An example is the CHROMATOCHART package discussed elsewhere in this report.

RTFSA: REAL TIME FREQUENCY SPECTRUM ANALYZER

With the help of a plug-in interface board, this package allows a personal computer to be used as a spectrum analyzer with 10-KHz bandwidth. The package accepts filtered or unfiltered data, performs fast Fourier transform analysis, and plots the magnitude of frequency spectra.

RTFSA runs on Apple II+ computers. It makes use of the AI13 interface board from Interactive Structures (see discussion of the AMPRIS package). Available as an option ($500) is a plug-in circuit card containing an anti-aliasing filter, a frequency counter/tachometer, and circuit-based multiplication to speed up the operation of the package. RTFSA sells for $400, and there are educational discounts, from Real Time Microsystems, P.O. Box 3081, Troy, NY 12181 [(518) 274-7149].

Most of the functions this package performs are displayed on a 15-choice menu that appears when it is started. Through this menu, the user specifies from which circuit board slot, and which one of 16 A/D channels in that slot, input will be taken. The user also sets up the analysis by specifying other items on the menu like A/D (voltage) range, frequency range, calibration factor, and threshold level at which data sampling of input signals will begin.

The same menu is used to shape the output plot, determining whether it will consist of discrete dots or continuous traces, what label the plot will bear, and the speed at which a synchronous marker on the frequency axis will be displayed.

The analysis itself is started when the user selects the CURRENT PARAMETERS OK menu item. With this selection, the package automatically samples and transforms input data and produces an output plot.

If the incoming signal falls out of the user-selected voltage range, the package will display an OUT OF RANGE message. The plotted data are automatically scaled to provide maximum resolution.

Normally, the display will continue to reflect changing input data. But, while in the plotting mode, the user can exercise control choices, including freezing the current display, producing a printed copy of the current display, and printing or storing on disk the currently displayed spectral data.

SPECSYSTEM: AUDIO SPECTRUM ANALYZER SOFTWARE

This package, and the software (firmware) that comes with the accompanying plug-in board, controls the operation of an Audio Spectrum analyzer and displays its output data. SPECSYSTEM can be used by nonprogrammers.

SPECSYSTEM is for use with Apple II and II+ computers together with the APX252 Audio Spectrum Analyzer plug-in board ($595). The SPEC-SYSTEM package sells for $199 from Eventide, One Alsan Way, Little Ferry, NJ 07643 [(201) 641-1200].

SPECSYSTEM and the spectrum analyzer with which it works are useful for a variety of acoustical applications, including analysis of noise, engine and machinery diagnostics, music, sound, and voice analysis.

Firmware on the board

Included on the APX252 board are software (firmware) commands that can be called by the BASIC language or invoked directly from the computer keyboard. Some of these commands perform immediately useful analysis and display functions when keyboarded. This type of use requires little or no knowledge of programming. In addition, for those who are programmers, these and other commands can be called from BASIC programs.

The RTA command displays a bar-chart representation of the frequency components produced by the spectrum analyzer from the input signals. Other commands exert more detailed control; thus SCAN performs the spectrum analysis, BARS produces the bar-chart display, AVERAGE causes the SCAN function to use averaged data. Other commands control the frequency range of the display, the amplification of input signals, and other interface and display functions.

Surface displays

The SPECSYSTEM package uses the repertoire of APX252 commands to perform more complex operations. Its basic function is to assemble and store large arrays of spectral data. These data arrays are displayed in the form of geometrical surfaces with dimensions of time, frequency, and amplitude. Alternatively, curves representing the data for individual spectrum channels can be displayed.

SPECSYSTEM leads the user through menus that guide creation of storage areas (buffers) for the incoming spectral data, set up the parameters of the plots, create reverberation displays, control transfers of data from screen to computer memory and to disk storage, and allow convenient use of the computer's other display functions. All this can be managed by users who have no knowledge of programming.

TEMPERATURE PLOTTER: FOR STUDENTS

This package monitors up to four temperatures, storing and plotting the results.

TEMPERATURE PLOTTER runs on the Apple II+, IIe and IIc. The package sells for $39.95. Temperature probes for use with the package sell two for $35 or four for $50. The vendor is Vernier Software, 2920 S.W. 89th St., Portland, OR 97225 [(503) 297-5317].

This package was designed for use with classroom experiments but may prove useful in some engineering instrumentation environments. Operation is simple and straightforward. From a main menu, the user selects the desired function, then responds to a series of screen-displayed questions and requests to implement that function.

For example, to monitor temperatures and save the results in memory, the user selects the Monitor Temperatures menu item, then types Y (yes) to a storage-wanted question, an finally types the desired length of time between recorded readings and the total number of readings desired.

The main limitations to the package are that each reading takes a minimum of one second, only four probes can be monitored, and a total of only 512 readings can be stored. There are also limitations to the accuracy of the temperature transducers and the calibration procedures.

The Analog Devices AD590 temperature transducer, in the probes for which this package is designed, can be used over the range of -55 to $+150$ degrees C. The devices are available with maximum error of 0.2 degrees C in the range of 25 to 50 degrees C. But units supplied by Vernier Software will typically have maximum errors twice as large as this. So users who have higher accuracy needs will have to purchase their own transducers.

Calibration is done by fitting the endpoints of a straight line to data from the transducer. This becomes more accurate as the temperature difference from one end of the line to the other is decreased.

Results can be displayed in Celsius, Kelvin, or Fahrenheit units. The package starts with the assumption that Celsius units are wanted. The user selects the desired units, and the package makes the necessary conversions automatically. However, the package always displays the currently selected units, so data retrieved from storage may be incorrectly labeled unless the user checks the units in which those data were originally stored and makes the appropriate adjustment.

The graphs produced by the package are simple point plots, with a different character used for the points of each of the four possible temperature plots.

Index